Doing Research in Emergency and Acute Care

Making Order Out of Chaos

Doing Research in Emergency and Acute Care

Making Order Out of Chaos

EDITED BY

Michael P. Wilson

UC San Diego Health Systems
Department of Emergency Medicine
Director of the Department of Emergency Medicine Behavioral Emergencies Research Lab, CA, USA

Kama Z. Guluma

Clinical Professor of Emergency Medicine and Research
Education Coordinator, UC San Diego Health Systems
Department of Emergency Medicine, CA, USA

Stephen R. Hayden

Professor in the UC San Diego Health Systems
Department of Emergency Medicine, CA, USA

WILEY Blackwell

This edition first published 2016 © 2016 by John Wiley & Sons, Ltd.

Registered Office
John Wiley & Sons, Ltd, The Atrium, Southern Gate, Chichester, West Sussex, PO19 8SQ, UK

Editorial Offices
9600 Garsington Road, Oxford, OX4 2DQ, UK
The Atrium, Southern Gate, Chichester, West Sussex, PO19 8SQ, UK
111 River Street, Hoboken, NJ 07030-5774, USA

For details of our global editorial offices, for customer services and for information about how to apply for permission to reuse the copyright material in this book please see our website at www.wiley.com/wiley-blackwell

Library of Congress Cataloging-in-Publication Data

Doing research in emergency and acute care : making order out of chaos / editors, Michael P. Wilson, Kama Z. Guluma, Stephen R. Hayden.
    p. ; cm.
  Includes bibliographical references and index.
  ISBN 978-1-118-64348-8 (pbk.)
I. Wilson, Michael P., 1969–, editor. II. Guluma, Kama, editor. III. Hayden, Stephen, 1961–, editor.
[DNLM: 1. Biomedical Research–methods. 2. Emergency Medicine. 3. Critical Care. 4. Research Design. WB 105]
  R850
  610.72′4–dc23

                              2015015487

A catalogue record for this book is available from the British Library.

Wiley also publishes its books in a variety of electronic formats. Some content that appears in print may not be available in electronic books.

Set in 8.5/10.5pt Meridien by SPi Global, Pondicherry, India
Printed in Singapore by C.O.S. Printers Pte Ltd

1 2016

Contents

Part 3: Getting it out there: Analyzing and publishing your study

List of contributors

Deirdre Anglin, MD, MPH
Professor of Emergency Medicine
Department of Emergency Medicine, Keck School of Medicine
of University of Southern California, Los Angeles, CA, USA

Jonathan Auten, DO
Assistant Professor of Military and Emergency Medicine
F Hebert School of Medicine, Uniformed Services University
of Health Sciences, Bethesda, MD;
Attending Physician,
Department of Emergency Medicine, Naval Medicine Center,
San Diego, CA, USA

Zubair Bayat
Cumming School of Medicine, University of Calgary, Calgary,
AB, Canada

Jesse J. Brennan, MA
Senior Research Scientist
Department of Emergency Medicine, University of California
San Diego, San Diego, CA, USA

Ashleigh Campillo, BS
UCSD Department of Emergency Medicine Behavioral
Emergencies Research (DEMBER) laboratory, University
of California, San Diego, CA, USA

Christopher R. Carpenter, MD, MSc
Associate Professor
Department of Emergency Medicine,
School of Medicine;
Director of Evidence Based Medicine
Washington University in St Louis, St. Louis, MO, USA

Daniel del Portal, MD, FAAEM
Assistant Professor of Clinical Emergency Medicine
Temple University School of Medicine
Philadelphia, PA, USA

Edward M. Castillo, PhD, MPH
Associate Adjunct Professor
Department of Emergency Medicine, University of California
San Diego, San Diego, CA, USA

Richard F. Clark, MD, FACEP
Professor of Emergency Medicine
Director, Division of Medical Toxicology
UCSD Medical Center, San Diego, CA, USA

Christopher J. Coyne, MD
Clinical Research Fellow
UCSD Department of Emergency Medicine, UC San Diego
Health System, San Diego, CA, USA

Zachary D.W. Dezman, MD, MS
Clinical Instructor
Department of Emergency Medicine, University of Maryland
School of Medicine, Baltimore, MD, USA

Louise Falzon, BA, PGDipInf
Information Specialist
Center for Behavioral Cardiovascular Health,
Columbia University Medical Center, NY, USA

Gary Gaddis, MD, PhD
St. Luke's/Missouri Endowed Chair in Emergency Medicine
St. Luke's Hospital of Kansas City;
Professor of Emergency Medicine
University of Missouri-Kansas City School of Medicine,
MO, USA

Manish Garg, MD
Professor, Emergency Medicine
Senior Associate Residency Program Director
Assistant Dean for Global Medicine
Temple University Hospital and School of Medicine,
Philadelphia, PA, USA

Kama Z. Guluma, MD
Clinical Professor of Emergency Medicine and Research
Education Coordinator, UC San Diego Health Systems
Department of Emergency Medicine, CA, USA

Prasanthi Govindarajan, MD, MAS
Associate Professor of Emergency Medicine-Medical Center Line
Stanford University Medical Center
Stanford, CA, USA

Robert Grover, MD, MPH
PGY-2
Department of Internal Medicine, The Brooklyn Hospital
Center, Brooklyn, NY, USA

Richard Harrigan, MD
Professor of Emergency Medicine
Temple University Hospital and School of Medicine,
Philadelphia, PA, USA

Stephen R. Hayden, MD
Professor in the UC San Diego Health Systems
Department of Emergency Medicine, CA, USA

Jon Mark Hirshon, MD, MPH, PhD
Professor
Department of Emergency Medicine and Department of
Epidemiology and Public Health, University of Maryland
School of Medicine, Baltimore, MD, USA

Judd E. Hollander, MD
Associate Dean for Strategic Health Initiatives
Sidney Kimmel Medical College;
Vice Chair, Finance and Healthcare Enterprises
Department of Emergency Medicine, Thomas Jefferson
University, Philadelphia, PA, USA

Austin Hopper, BS
Department of Emergency Medicine Behavioral Emergencies
Research laboratory (DEMBER), UC San Diego Health System,
San Diego, CA, USA.

Benton R. Hunter, MD, MSc
Assistant Professor of Clinical Emergency Medicine
Department of Emergency Medicine, Indiana University
School of Medicine, Indianapolis, IN, USA

Paul Ishimine, MD
Director, Pediatric Emergency Medicine Fellowship
Training Program
USCD/Rady Children's Hospital, San Diego;
Director, Pediatric Emergency Medicine
UC San Diego Health System;
Clinical Professor of Emergency Medicine and Pediatrics
University of California, San Diego School of Medicine
UC San Diego Health System, Department of Emergency
Medicine, San Diego, CA, USA

Christopher Kahn, MD, MPH
Associate Professor of Clinical Emergency Medicine
Division of Emergency Medical Services and Disaster
Medicine, Department of Emergency Medicine, University
of California, San Diego, CA, USA

David J. Karras, MD
Professor of Emergency Medicine
Assistant Dean for Clinical Education Integration
Associate Chair for Academic Affairs
Department of Emergency Medicine, Temple University School
of Medicine, Philadelphia, PA, USA

Eddy Lang, MDCU
Acting Zone Clinical Department Head and Interim Faculty
Department Head
Department of Emergency Medicine, University of Calgary,
Calgary, AB, Canada

Jennifer Lanning, MD, PhD
Resident
Department of Emergency Medicine, University of California
San Francisco, San Francisco General Hospital, CA, USA

Juan A. Luna, MA, BA
California State University San Marcos, CA, USA

Michael Menchine, MD, MPH
Associate Professor of Emergency Medicine
Department of Emergency Medicine, Keck School of Medicine
of University of Southern California, Los Angeles, CA, USA

Mary Mercer, MD, MPH
Assistant Clinical Professor of Emergency Medicine
University of California San Francisco;
Director of Performance Improvement and EMS Base Hospital
Medical Director
Department of Emergency Medicine, San Francisco General
Hospital, San Francisco, CA, USA

Alicia B. Minns, MD
Assistant Clinical Professor of Emergency Medicine
Fellowship Director, Division of Medical Toxicology
UCSD Medical Center, San Diego, CA, USA

Jarrod M. Mosier, MD
Director EM/Critical Care;
Assistant Professor Emergency Medicine,
Department of Emergency Medicine;
Assistant Professor Internal Medicine, Department of Medicine,
Section of Pulmonary Critical Care, Allergy and Sleep
University of Arizona, Tucson, AZ, USA

Sean-Xavier Neath, MD, PhD
Assistant Clinical Professor of Medicine
Department of Emergency Medicine, University of California,
San Diego, CA, USA

Kimberly Nordstrom, MD, JD
Medical Director, Psychiatric Emergency Services, Denver
Health Medical Center;
Assistant Professor of Psychiatry, University of Colorado
School of Medicine Denver, CO, USA;
President, American Association for Emergency Psychiatry
Bloomfield, CT, USA

Nas Rafi, MD
Biomedical Ethics Fellow
Assistant Clinical Professor of Emergency Medicine
UCSD Emergency Department, San Diego, CA, USA

Robert Rodriguez, MD, FAAEM
Professor of Emergency Medicine
Department of Emergency Medicine, University of California
San Francisco, San Francisco General Hospital, CA, USA

Peter Rosen, MD
Senior Lecturer, Emergency Medicine,
Harvard University Medical School
Attending Physician, Beth Israel Deaconess
Medical Center
Boston, MA, USA;
Visiting Professor Emergency Medicine,
University of Arizona School of Medicine;
Professor Emeritus Emergency Medicine, University
of California San Diego School of Medicine

Brian H. Rowe, MD, MSc, CCFP(EM), FCCP
Scientific Director, Emergency Strategic Clinical
Network, AHS;
Tier I Canada Research Chair in Evidence-based
Emergency Medicine;
Professor, Department of Emergency Medicine
University of Alberta, Edmonton, AB, Canada

George J. Shaw, MD, PhD
Associate Professor
Department of Emergency Medicine, University
of Cincinnati, Cincinnati, OH, USA

Brian Snyder, MD
Biomedical Ethics Fellowship Director
Clinical Professor of Emergency Medicine,
UCSD Emergency Department, San Diego, CA, USA

Katie L. Tataris, MD, MPH
Assistant Professor of Medicine
Section of Emergency Medicine
University of Chicago
EMS Medical Director, Chicago South EMS System Chicago,
IL, USA

Aleksandr Tichter, MD, MS
Assistant Professor of Medicine
Columbia University Medical Center, NY, USA

Vaishal Tolia, MD, MPH, FACEP
Associate Clinical Professor
Associate Medical Director
Director of ED Observation
Attending in Emergency Medicine & Hospital Medicine
Department of Emergency Medicine, University of California,
San Diego Health System, San Diego, CA, USA

**Christian Tomaszewski, MD, MS, MBA, FACEP,
FACMT, FIFEM**
Professor of Clinical Emergency Medicine;
Medical Director, Department of Emergency Medicine;
Attending in Medical Toxicology and Hyperbarics
University of California San Diego Health System,
San Diego, CA, USA

Vicken Y. Totten, MD, MS
Institutional Director for Research
Kaweah Delta Health Care District, Department of Emergency
Medicine, Visalia, CA, USA

Jacob W. Ufberg, MD
Professor and Residency Director
Department of Emergency Medicine, Temple University School
of Medicine, Philadelphia, PA, USA

Gary M. Vilke, MD, FACEP, FAAEM
Professor of Clinical Emergency Medicine
Medical Director, Risk Management, UC San Diego
Health System
Director, Clinical Research for Emergency Medicine
Department of Emergency Medicine, University
of California San Diego, San Diego, CA, USA

Julian Villar, MD, MPH
Chief Resident
Department of Emergency Medicine, University
of California San Francisco, San Francisco
General Hospital, CA, USA

Michael P. Wilson, MD, PhD, FAAEM
UC San Diego Health Systems
Department of Emergency Medicine
Director of the Department of Emergency Medicine Behavioral
Emergencies Research Lab, CA, USA

Michael Witting, MD, MS
Associate Professor
Department of Emergency Medicine, University
of Maryland School of Medicine, Baltimore, MD, USA

Peter Wyer, MD
Associate Professor of Medicine
Columbia University Medical Center, NY, USA

PART 1

Getting ready: Preparing for your research study

CHAPTER 1

Aspects of research specific to acute care

Jarrod M. Mosier[1] and Peter Rosen[2]

[1] Department of Emergency Medicine, University of Arizona, USA
[2] Emergency Medicine, Harvard University Medical School, USA

Responsibility of the academic physician

The power to save lives, and the knowledge which forms that power, is a sacred art entrusted to every physician. One can debate about whether knowledge is discovered or invented (we think it may be both), but regardless of the means of acquisition, new knowledge falls into the realm of research and, thus, of the book that you are holding. It is the responsibility of the academic physician to uncover and disseminate this knowledge. Enthusiastic young physicians commonly enter academic medicine after inspiration in seeing their accomplished mentors' body of work, only to find it frustrating that it is not easy and that it may not be possible to hit the ground running smoothly.

Indeed, many young physicians are both puzzled and dissuaded by the responsibilities faced in academic medicine. They are often willing to participate in the dissemination of knowledge, especially when this involves synthesizing others' research, giving a lecture or supervising residents and students in the clinical setting. When it comes to research and storage (i.e., the preservation of that knowledge through articles, books, etc.) many find these areas too difficult or discouraging. Both research and storage are activities that can be learned and become easier with experience. However, neither is a customary part of the student or resident curriculum and both are, therefore, very intimidating to the young physician. This chapter reflects on research as an academic responsibility for acute care and Emergency Medicine (EM) physicians and, hopefully, will give some clues on how to make it less painful and intimidating for the inspired academic physician.

Asking the right questions

The first research effort of one of the second author in medical school was an effort to produce an animal model of emphysema in rats. This was studied by building the rat a helmet with a one-way valve that it had to breathe against. The theory was that the increased pulmonary pressures would produce emphysema, but the experiment was a dismal failure. The only thing derived from the experience was an unswerving hatred of rats, which bit frequently and painfully as they were put into their helmets. The net result was that it was twenty years before the author tried any more animal research, and never again with rats.

One of the areas of intimidation is the thought that the best research (i.e., the research most likely to be funded, recognized, rewarded, and acknowledged with promotion) involves basic science. While this is partially true, it is also true that basic science is not the only form of research that is useful, funded, or desirable. Clinical and translational science is concerned with the improved quality of the practice of medicine based on evidence, and the acquisition of that evidence is of critical importance. It has become increasingly evident that the best practice of clinical medicine is based on posing the right questions (see, for example, Chapter 3). The answers to those questions are dependent both upon the quality of data that create the evidence as well as how long the evidence can be relied upon. For example, in the presence of abdominal pain, last year's pregnancy test result, no matter how well performed, is not going to help

Doing Research in Emergency and Acute Care: Making Order Out of Chaos, First Edition. Edited by Michael P. Wilson, Kama Z. Guluma, and Stephen R. Hayden.

with sorting out the etiology of this year's pain. Similarly, in the presence of chest pain, how long is last year's negative stress test result helpful and, moreover, does it matter which stress test was performed?

Yet we are taught that we must obtain certain tests to be complete, thorough, or prudent, but no one gives any information on how long information lasts to be useful, nor what to do if the test is negative when only a positive test has any useful meaning. Thus, while the basic science questions regarding the best assay for determining pregnancy or detecting at-risk myocardium while stressed are of interest, a clinical scientist is most interested in the clinical questions that guide the practice of emergency medicine. (See, for example, Chapter 4, "Evidence-based medicine: Finding the knowledge gap.")

Challenges with acute care research

How then should one commence a research project in acute care? There are many challenges to carrying out research in acute care settings, whether it is prehospital research, the emergency department (ED), or the intensive care unit (ICU). Some considerations include major hurdles such as:

- Consent: How are you going to obtain informed consent on the subjects of your study? If you want to carry out a study on resuscitation related measures, how are you expected to truly obtain informed consent when they are in respiratory distress, cardiac arrest, or are altered? Are you going to be there night and day to enroll and obtain consent from these participants?
- Where are you going to do this study? It may seem like an easy question to answer, but let us say you want to carry out a study on prehospital intubations with a new device. Are you going to put the device on every ambulance? If you want to carry out a study in the emergency department regarding a new device for an emergent procedure, where are you going to keep it? Are all the patients requiring that procedure going to go to the same place, or are they going to be spread out all over your 60 bed emergency department?
- Specialists: If you want to carry out a study with a new therapy in acute coronary syndrome, you are going to have to get buy-in from the cardiologists. Our time with these patients in the emergency department is limited, so obtaining agreements to participate from admitting services and specialists is very important and can be incredibly challenging based on your relationships with those services.
- Outcomes: What are the outcomes of your study going to be and how are you going to show that your limited time with this patient population made a difference in those outcomes?
- Blinding: How will you keep the participants and raters in your experiment blinded to their true treatment condition?
- Funding: The answer to many of the questions above is to have resources in place, but resources require funding. How and where will you obtain funding, which is increasingly harder to obtain?

Where do I start?

The initial responsibility is to define a question that needs examination. This can come from any source of inspiration, but the most useful way to begin is to think about a question from your clinical practice for which you do not know the answer. In fact, the less you know about the answer the better. If you do not know anything about the question, then any data you derive in the examination of the question will be interesting. If any data are interesting, you will be less likely to bias the results in trying to find a particular answer (see, for example, Chapter 10).

Think about cases you have seen in the emergency department. Your question may come from an observation of a dogmatic clinical practice that you do not understand the need to perform. For illustrative purposes, we will use the example of cricoid pressure during intubation. No matter how many people tell you it makes intubation safer, do we really know that to be true? If it is well studied, if the available evidence is valid, and if that evidence suggests that cricoid pressure does, in fact, increase the safety of intubation, then move on to another question. If the quest is not studied adequately, then you are on the right path. While computerized databases have made it much easier to carry out a literature search, they have a finite origin for the database, and your failure to find any literature in the computerized database does not mean that there might not have been some successful studies carried out prior to computerization. You may have to do an old-fashioned hand search. Suppose that all you have been able to find are papers on how cricoid pressure helps or hinders intubation but that there is no valid evidence that it increases safety. This suggests that the practice applying cricoid pressure to increase the safety of intubation is based on theory, which no matter how logical does not constitute evidence. You have found your propositus: the reason for doing your study. (Chapter 3, "How do I formulate a research question," gives more information.)

Roadblocks, errors, and things to avoid

The next step is to consider how to acquire the evidence. This is where most research momentum fizzles out before it even starts. In this example, the hypothesis you wish to test is whether cricoid pressure actually improves intubation safety. It would seem easy to simply set up a prospective study of intubation, where you randomize the use of cricoid pressure. If you do so, however, you will quickly encounter many of the traps of clinical research that can destroy a project.

Firstly, it is likely that very few of your faculty or colleagues will be comfortable in challenging dogma by attempting intubation without cricoid pressure. That is how they learned the technique of intubation and they are sure that it is safer than not using it. Secondly, even if they were willing to change their practice, you are dependent upon other people to acquire your data; this is fraught with error because you all are very busy clinically, such as when you work in an emergency department. Unless others share your enthusiasm for the clinical question, no one is going to be motivated to perform the additional work. Hiring research assistants to help with your study will cost a significant amount of funding that you are unlikely to get in today's economic climate. Thirdly, you will have to get Institutional Review Board approval, and even if you stimulate the curiosity of the members of that committee as to the outcome of your proposed study, they will most likely demand you have informed consent prior to each intubation. Challenges of obtaining consent for emergency procedures aside, this is an instantaneous oxymoron since, if there is no evidence whether the procedure is safe, what constitutes informed consent? Asking the subject to agree to either arm of the study, both of which might be unsafe, is not likely to get an informed consent so much as a transfer to another institution where the physicians know better what they are doing, as they do not scare their subjects before mandatory procedures.

Welcome to the world of acute care research. You found a question you are genuinely interested in, and would truly like to know the answer, but the project simply cannot be done. You might try to compromise the ideal study of a randomized prospective trial of intubation with and without cricoid pressure by doing a retrospective analysis of a group of patients who had cricoid pressure versus a control group that did not (assuming of course that you could find a group of intubations before cricoid pressure became popularized, and that there exists sufficient data to compare the two). Then you have the nightmare of analyzing records that were not completed with your study question in mind, trying to decide if your intubators represent a similar group of physicians whose intubation skills are constant, whether your subjects are a similar group of patients, and whether new equipment or technology has modified your techniques enough so that the question is no longer relevant (e.g., your colleagues now intubate with a video laryngoscope). (More information is given in Chapter 2 and Chapter 14.)

You therefore give up altogether and decide to pick a different propositus, hopefully one that will avoid similar kinds of procedural problems. It quickly becomes clear, however, that your first project needs to be very simple, easy to carry out with a small number of researchers, not dependent upon the cooperation of colleagues or another specialty, and modest in its labor and financial demands. For example, when California passed a mandatory seat belt law, one emergency medicine (EM) resident was surprised at the sudden public health claims for reduced automotive crash mortality. She picked her research team (herself), went to the nearest bridge over the freeway during some spare hours, and counted the number of cars with belted drivers. With only about 5% of the drivers wearing their seatbelts, she did not have to worry about a control group. However, she could conclude that, at that point in time, the new law had not had much impact upon the compliance of most drivers, and that the reduced mortality was merely wish-fulfillment fantasy.

Some other common errors in clinical research: It is often difficult to derive the propositus for the study. It should be clear what the original observation was that gave rise to the study other than that the authors did not have enough publications to get promoted. A clear propositus gives much greater understanding to what hypothesis is being tested.

Science, as demonstrated helpfully by Karl Popper, is based on the falsification of a hypothesis. It is not, as many lay people believe, the finding of examples of the proof of your hypothesis. The falsification is based on a study of the question in which the variance in the answer is greater than chance alone. This is not the accuracy that most people associate with science, but it is the best we can do since the observations of any differences obscure the results.

For example, suppose you are trying to determine the boiling point of water. You take a calorimeter of some kind, heat it in some way, and measure the temperature at which you spot bubbles in the water. Yet, the very act of measuring the temperature of the water during the bubbling changes the temperature of the water. Depending upon the rigor with which you wish to perform the experiment, your thermometer may be more or less sensitive to slight changes in water temperature. Since it adds little utility to the answer you are seeking, a thermometer that measures temperatures to a thousandth of a temperature degree is probably wasteful precision. Yet if you use a thermometer that only measures to a tenth of a degree, you may find a different boiling point every time you try the experiment. That is why we believe the boiling point to be 212°F, but when we actually try to prove it, we get 211, 213, 212.5, and so on and realize that the boiling point can only be the average of all the measurements.

The reason we choose a hypothesis to falsify is that it is virtually impossible to prove any hypothesis by simply finding examples of its positive presence. Thus, if the question being studied is whether cooling improves survival from cardiac arrest, you cannot just take patients in arrest, cool them, and say that your survival is better. You have to have a control group that is tested by the hypothesis that cooling is not useful, and falsify that hypothesis by showing that the cooled group did much better than the uncooled group by more than chance alone. Finding adequately matched controls can be a very difficult part of research. Case–control studies are appealing, as they solve a lot of ethical and work problems, but the evidence produced is much less compelling because causation cannot be proven. Rather, only an association can be inferred (Chapter 11).

Another very common error in acute care research is studying too small a population. This is often done because the time required to get a sufficiently large population is too great, the disease of interest is too rare, there are ethical difficulties in varying the study population, or because funding is insufficient to continue the study. It takes time to perform good research and almost nothing in our present system of doing and funding science is patient with long-term results.

We have observed an ever-increasing reliance on statistical significance, but it must also be accompanied by clinical relevance. For example, one study examined the complications of central line insertion by comparing subclavian to femoral sites. The total number of complications was not statistically different between the two locations. Does this mean the two procedures are equally safe? There was one death following a complication of the femoral line insertion. This was not statistically significant, but it is certainly clinically relevant and needs to be part of your decision making when choosing one site over another.

The converse error is reporting "trends." This comes from the difficulties presented in trying to publish negative results or in trying to obtain continued funding for a project. If the difference between the two groups is not significant, it does not matter that the difference would have been significant with only one or two more positive results. That is not a trend towards significance as much as it is a wish-fulfillment fantasy. Statistically, there is a greater probability that if the study were carried out longer, the difference would be less, not greater, because what was shown is that the difference occurred by chance alone.

We will not talk about how to get funding for projects other than to state that for initial small projects funding is probably not necessary. It is the success of pilot projects that will help one to obtain funding. Most universities have seed grants for young investigators and those sources should be looked into whenever possible. Additionally, there are also seed grants available from the specialty societies for small pilot projects (Chapter 36).

KEY POINTS

- Have a propositus that is driven by a clinical question to which you do not know the answer but are curious.
- Derive a study hypothesis that can be falsified.
- Do not depend upon colleagues, other departments or specialties, or non-academicians for data collection.
- Start small, be patient, and do not think that your first project will win a National Institute of Health grant and be published in the *New England Journal of Medicine*.
- Rather than hitting the ground running smoothly, it is like learning how to walk; we all have to start by crawling. Do not be afraid to have fun!

CHAPTER 2
Aspects of feasibility in research

Kama Z. Guluma

Department of Emergency Medicine, UC San Diego Health Systems, CA, USA

> *"I remember, when I was a resident in Emergency Medicine, I had this great idea to study cortical spreading depression (depolariza-tion) and its effect on traumatic brain injury in an animal model. After all, the department already had a prominent brain injury laboratory set up, and all I had to do was add a technique to measure cortical spreading depression to what was already being done, and I'd be set. Right? Wrong! I had no idea how to measure cortical spreading depression and couldn't find anybody at my university to show me how. Therefore, I had to take it upon myself to figure out how to do it. I'm no electrical engineer and I think ended up inadvertently measuring the effects of solar flares, instead of measuring cortical spreading depression."*
>
> Anonymous hapless resident researcher

As with many things, there are no guarantees in research. Robert Burns wrote in his 1785 poem, "The best laid schemes of mice and men go often awry, and leave us nothing but grief and pain, for promised joy!" When it comes to basic science research, the mice involved would no doubt be enthralled at this possibility (see Chapter 6, What do I need to know to get started with animal and basic science research?), but things not going as planned has costly impli-cations for researchers (and is frankly disappointing). All the preparation, diligence, intelligence, and gumption in the world will not save your research endeavor if it is not fundamentally feasible in the first place. For an endeavor, espe-cially a prospective trial, to be feasible, the following conditions must be optimized:

- Safety
- Expertise
- Compliance with study procedures
- "Recruitability"
- Sustainability.

Safety considerations

There is such a thing as a "safety study". It's a small, feasibility study in which a new intervention is tried out for the first time, carefully monitored, in a limited patient population, just to be sure that it will not harm patients. The truth of the matter, however, is that any prospective interventional clinical trial is in some way a safety study, because – while an intervention and its safety profile may be very familiar – the study inherently implies an examination of that intervention applied in a new way or using new parameters. Some things are a little more risky than others, and the higher the risk associated with an intervention (or the trial protocol), the more issues of feasibility with arise. The potential benefit of any intervention being evaluated must be weighed against the potential risk that intervention (and specifically an evaluation of that intervention) would entail.

The broad concept of "safety" impacts feasibility on multiple fronts, perceived and real:

1 **It has to look safe to get through your IRB**. A project evaluating a relatively unsafe intervention may not even get past the Institutional Review Board (IRB) at your institution. It will be "dead-on-arrival" if perceived too unsafe.
2 **It has to look safe to be accepted by your study population**. If your study does get approved, you may have a very difficult time convincing patients to consent to a study utilizing such an intervention if there is a perceived safety issue.

Doing Research in Emergency and Acute Care: Making Order Out of Chaos, First Edition. Edited by Michael P. Wilson, Kama Z. Guluma, and Stephen R. Hayden.

3 It has to look safe, period. If your intervention does not look safe, it may not be safe. If you do manage to recruit patients into the study, a truly dangerous procedure may result in an acceptably high number of **serious adverse events, or** SAEs (see Chapters 9 and 23 on safety), resulting in a very appropriate shut-down of your trial.

Do not underestimate item number 2 above. Perception is everything.

Don't take my word for it; take a real-life clinical trial, for example: Hemorrhagic shock from penetrating and blunt trauma is associated with significant mortality and is a major public health concern. Unfortunately, the logistics of storing and transporting blood make it very difficult for medics to carry it around with them in the field, ready for emergent transfusion. In the mid 2000s a multicenter clinical trial was carried out investigating the use of a blood substitute. It was a cutting-edge idea, but since the trial (starting an emergent transfusion with a blood substitute in the field) had to be performed on patients essentially dying of hemorrhage, it had to be carried out with a waiver of consent, by getting community-wide consent ahead of time. The study eventually got done and published [1], but implementation stalled (didn't happen) in one major American city because of public concerns over safety involving not only of the intervention itself but perceptions about the way patients were selected.

(**San Diego Reader** [2])

Even as you get past the considerations above and contemplate a randomized control trial of a particular intervention, you should carefully weigh the potential adverse effects of the intervention with its potential benefit, otherwise you may encounter an unpleasant safety surprise when all is said and done.

Take another real-life clinical trial, for example: Hypervolemic hemodilution (giving very large volumes of intravenous fluids) was a promising intervention studied as a therapy for acute ischemic stroke until about the 1990s. Great idea, right? Why not dilute the patient's blood so that it has more favorable rheological properties and flows more easily past a cerebrovascular occlusion? … or through tenuous brain collaterals?

When put to the test, however, hypervolemic hemodilution did not work out quite as planned. In one trial, 5.5% of patients given this treatment died within the first five days, compared with only 1.6% of control patients [3], and the further investigation – no matter use – of this type of therapy was disparaged by prominent experts in the field [4]. It turns out that hypervolemic hemodilution may dilute the oxygen carrying capacity of the blood (no surprise) and worsen cerebral edema (no surprise), neither of which are good for a patient with a stroke.

The reality is that because the disease processes inherent in the acute care environment or emergency department involve high morbidity and high mortality, the seminal interventions and research trials involved in addressing them may be inherently riskier than in other healthcare environments. The management of safety is an integral part of assuring feasibility.

Expertise and infrastructure

The importance of having the expertise to design study procedures, carry out study procedures, and analyze and interpret study results cannot be overstated. It is never a good idea to engage in a study project with the anticipation that you will garner the expertise needed or will develop the needed infrastructure as you go along (as did the hapless investigator in the introductory vignette). If this is unavoidably going to be the case, this development should be part of the research plan (i.e., be part of the study itself), with end points and milestones clearly articulated.

This should by no means be interpreted, however, as an advisement to avoid studies in which you or your co-investigators do not have certain areas of expertise. In fact, the opposite is encouraged, with the proviso that you seek out individuals with the necessary expertise as collaborators. This not only allows you to implement the study you desire, but enables you and your collaborators to learn from each other and grow experientially from the collaboration.

Here's an example of a collaboration that merged expertise: In a study by Chan and colleagues, a collaboration between emergency physicians and law enforcement officers (of whom at least one was a co-author) enabled a study of the effects of "pepper" spray on respiratory function [5]. In the study, 35 subjects were exposed to oleoresin capsicum (OC) or placebo spray, followed by 10 minutes of sitting or being put in a "prone maximal restraint position", while spirometry, oximetry, and end-tidal CO_2 levels were collected. Physicians typically have little expertise in the proper application of law enforcement restraint techniques, and the involvement of law enforcement officers as co-investigators was an important asset in this study.

Compliance with study procedures

"We had a great idea. We were going to do a prospective emergency department study to see if draining, irrigating, and then suturing abscesses closed would lead to better outcomes than the simple incising, draining, and packing we were doing … But, despite a ton of patients with abscesses coming through our emergency department every week, we hardly got any study patients; while many of our colleagues liked the idea, when it came right down to it they were not willing to enroll patients for us."

Alicia Minns, MD

The procedures in your research study must be doable, on many fronts. It is unlikely that you yourself will be enrolling every patient and personally carrying out all study procedures on them (unless you have procured full-time funding to put yourself at the research site 24/7). You will, therefore, inevitably need the (likely unpaid) help of your colleagues or others, or subinvestigators. Given this, the following definitely have to be taken into account:

1 The procedures imposed on your subinvestigators should not significantly impact work flow (unless you are rewarding them with lavish gift cards and free buffet meals; but – please – before considering this, see Chapter 8, "Ethics in Research").
2 The procedures imposed on your subinvestigators must not be too technically unfamiliar to them.
3 The procedures imposed on your subinvestigators must not be unacceptable to a majority of them (for example, *"I'm not going to enroll any of my patients in that study comparing pain medications to hypnosis for abdominal pain – I don't believe in hypnosis, and I just can't deprive my patients of pain medications"*).
4 In animal studies (and human studies), time windows for procedures and assessments should be ergonomic.

The first of these considerations can be attended to with good, a priori, study planning, which may entail visualizing yourself as an uninvested subinvestigator and empathically exploring what may or may not be palatable to you. It may require a trial run of study procedures (for example, in preparation for a stroke study he was a principal investigator on, this author – much to the amusement of nursing staff – once rolled an empty stretcher from the emergency department, up some elevators and into a treatment area, with himself as a simulated patient, just to assess if procedures and the time-frames they needed to be implemented in were feasible).

The second and third considerations can be attended to with careful and thorough investigator training and orientation prior to trial initiation. It is always best to survey potential subinvestigators, collaborators, and helpers *prior* to finalization of study design, as critical design flaws or issues may be exposed and addressed ahead of time.

The final consideration, with regards to animal studies, also applies to follow-up periods in human studies. For example, carelessly setting up a 36-hour time window for a re-evaluation in an animal study just because it "seems right" or because a prior published report used that time window, when 24 hours or 48 hours would be just as scientifically valid, may have you coming into to your laboratory at three in the morning so that you do not end up violating your own protocol (more about preclinical research logistics is covered in Chapter 6). The more you can take into consideration before you finalize (or even start writing up) a study protocol, the better.

Talking about ergonomic time-windows: In a controlled study by Gennis and colleagues designed to assess the efficacy of soft cervical collars in the early management of whiplash-injury-related pain, the initial plan was to call patients every week for up to six weeks or until they were pain free [6]. However, by two months into the study, per the authors, it became evident that this was too impractical, so the protocol had to be changed to a much more palatable follow-up scheme: a single phone call at six weeks post-injury.

If an example of poor investigator compliance is required, how about a trial which couldn't even be done? In 1995, Brooker and colleagues had hoped to implement a large, publicly-funded a study to train nurses in emergency departments in the United Kingdom to screen all their patients for alcohol problems, with a view to identifying a sample of problem drinkers to participate in a randomized controlled trial of health education plus brief counselling versus health education alone.

However, despite 16 654 patients showing up to the emergency departments during the recruitment phase of the study, only 20% of them were screened by the nurses, of whom only 19% were identified as problem drinkers, eventually leaving only 264 patients eligible for entry to the trial, of whom a majority refused to enter. The trial had to be abandoned. The authors tried to figure out what happened and on surveying the nurses learned they were facing a number of problems, including stress and poor morale amongst the nursing teams, differences in perception concerning the value of research between nurse managers and the nurses actually doing the work at the bedside, and the inadequacy of training in study procedures [7].

"Recruitability"

"Recruitability" refers to three core concepts:

1 The incidence of your study condition-of-interest has to be high enough that you can complete the study in a reasonable time-frame (if at all).

"I put together this trial to evaluate a treatment for patients with middle cerebral artery (MCA) strokes at my hospital, but – lo and behold – I could hardly get any patients ... It turns out my hospital had a relatively low rate of patients presenting with strokes to begin with, and I did myself in by further narrowing the field down to MCA strokes only."

Anonymous

---

2 Those patients with the target condition have to be consentable.

"We wanted to put together a prospective trial evaluating the utility of head CT for minor head injury in patients with acute alcohol intoxication. It turned out to be very difficult to gain consent from an acutely intoxicated patient – as in, impossible."

Michael Wilson, MD

Patients who are generally not consentable (or difficult to consent) include the acutely intoxicated, the psychotic, and the delirious (really anyone with an altered perception) presenting emergently and with no family who can give surrogate consent. Unless you are able to get a waiver of consent from your IRB, you will face almost insurmountable challenges with these subsets of patients.

3 Those patients with the target condition have to want to consent to your study, at least most of the time.

"I had a great randomized, prospective clinical trial evaluating the use of an intraosseus (IO) line versus getting a central line in intravenous drug abusers without any veins, because an IO line is so much quicker, and probably safer. For some reason, however, whenever I mentioned that getting a 'needle put into your bone' was an option, some patients would not consent to the study."

Alfred Joshua, MD

The signing of a consent to your study represents an alignment between a potential study subject's personality, fears, prior experience and understanding, and his/her informed assessment and expectations of the details, risks and benefits of enrolling in your study. Even if there are no data to support it, if a patient perceives an issue with a trial procedure, or has a visceral aversion to it, his or her decision to consent will be unduly influenced. Appropriate study patient selection (via inclusion and exclusion criteria) and appropriate choice (or delivery) of intervention are ways to minimize this issue. Simply doing a simulation in your head of what it would be like to be a patient contemplating consent to be enrolled in your trial might reveal issues you had not thought of.

> **It doesn't even have to be the thought of being poked in the bone with a sharp object that might scare patients away from your trial. It can be an easily-overlooked financial detail. Take a real-life clinical trial as an example**: Shen and colleagues carried out a study with an hypothesis that a designated outpatient syncope unit in the emergency department would improve diagnostic yield and reduce hospital admission for patients presenting with syncope [8]. Their inclusion criterion was syncope of undetermined cause, in a patient with intermediate risk for an adverse cardiovascular outcome, meeting the general guidelines for consideration of hospital admission.
>
> When the trial had been completed, 795 patients had met the inclusion criteria, but only 262 of them consented to the study. What happened here? We're talking about a stay in an observation unit, aren't we? The authors indicated they were not sure exactly why so few of the eligible patients consented to be in the study, but suggested that it may have had to do with insurance deductibles. This makes sense; patients typically have to pay a higher insurance deductible for care in an emergency department if they are not admitted to the hospital, and this fact may have dissuaded them from consenting to be in a trial in which they might be randomized to a stay in an outpatient unit.

Sustainability considerations

Lastly, but not least, one has to anticipate sustainability issues. This pertains specifically to prospective interventional studies and incorporates questions about financing, industry partner support, changes in the legislative or market landscape in which you are working, emerging trials being done elsewhere that might influence the interpretation or validity of your results, and time.

Ask yourself the following questions:

- Is there a concurrent trial or research endeavor being (or about to be) done elsewhere that might pre-empt your study plan or make your results obsolete? Are you using an intervention – telemedicine via hand-held smartphone devices, for example – that utilizes rapidly evolving technology that might be obsolete (making your methodology or outcome measures irrelevant to clinical care) by the time you finish your study?
- If your trial is a drug or device trial, will the industry sponsor providing the drug or device for the trial remain engaged and continue to provide support? Or are there emerging financial constraints, Food and Drug Administration (FDA) determinations, or market developments (e.g., a competitor with a much more marketable drug or device) that would make use of that particular drug or device unsupportable in the long term?
- If your study is going to be funded from a specified funding source for a specified amount, what type of unexpected diversions of funding need to be anticipated?
- Will you (or your research team) have time to carry the endeavor through from beginning to the end – that is, time to do background literature searches, write up protocols and other trial-related documents, obtain IRB and administrative approvals, recruit enough patients to carry out the study, do a quality check on data, and then analyze the results? Even if you do have the time, is your trial going to take too long for its own good? Time makes wine and cheese better, but it can make a clinical trial start to pull apart at the seams and require "patches".

> **Having to change key trial parameters mid-course due to evolving regulatory environment is a real possibility, even for large multicenter trials. Take the ATLANTIS study as an example:** The ATLANTIS study, finally published in 1999, first began in August 1991 and was initially designed to assess the efficacy and safety of intravenous recombinant tissue-plasminogen activator (rt-PA) administered to patients within 0–6 hours of onset of an acute ischemic stroke. However, it had to be temporarily stopped due to a safety issue with hemorrhages in patients treated between 5 to 6 hours. Upon a planned re-initiation of the trial (now called ATLANTIS "Part B") with a 0–5 hour window, it turned out rt-PA had, in the interim, been approved by the FDA for treatment of stroke in patients presenting within 0–3 hours of onset. The trial was, therefore, restarted using a 3–5 hour treatment window [9].

KEY POINTS

- Pick the safest approach to investigating an intervention.
- Study procedures should be easy to follow and understand, and should fit into investigator work-flow.
- The incidence of your study condition-of-interest has to be high enough to complete a trial in a feasible time frame.
- Your potential study patients have to be consentable.
- Your study procedures have to be palatable to your potential study patients.
- Consider your potential research endeavor a "ship" that has to navigated through roiling waters of (i) changes in funding, (ii) changes in industry support, (iii)) evolving legislative and market conditions, and (iv) evolving knowledge from work being done contemporaneously elsewhere.

References

1 Moore, E.E., Moore, F.A., Fabian, T.C. *et al.* (2009) Human polymerized hemoglobin for the treatment of hemorrhagic shock when blood is unavailable: the USA multicenter trial. *J Am Coll Surg*, **208**(1):1–13.

2 San Diego Reader (2005) Bad Blood? Experimentation south of I-8. http://www.sandiegoreader.com/news/2005/jul/28/bad-blood/ (last accessed 22 April 2015)

3 Scandinavian Stroke Study Group (1987) Multicenter trial of hemodilution in acute ischemic stroke. I. Results in the total patient population. *Stroke*, **18**(4):691–699.

4 von Kummer, R., Back, T., Scharf, J. and Hacke, W. (1989) Stroke, hemodilution, and mortality. *Stroke*, **20**(9):1286–1287.

5 Chan, T.C., Vilke, G.M., Clausen, J. *et al.* (2002) The effect of oleoresin capsicum "pepper" spray inhalation on respiratory function. *J Forensic Sci*, **47**(2):299–304.

6 Gennis, P., Miller, L., Gallagher, E.J. *et al.* (1996) The effect of soft cervical collars on persistent neck pain in patients with whiplash injury. *Acad Emerg Med*, **3**(6):568–573.

7 Brooker, C., Peters, J., McCabe, C. and Short, N. (1999) The views of nurses to the conduct of a randomised controlled trial of problem drinkers in an accident and emergency department. *Int J Nurs Stud*, **36**(1):33–39.

8 Shen, W.K., Decker, W.W., Smars, P.A. *et al.* (2004) Syncope Evaluation in the Emergency Department Study (SEEDS): a multidisciplinary approach to syncope management. *Circulation*, **110**(24):3636–3645.

9 Clark, W.M., Wissman, S., Albers, G.W. *et al.* (1999) Recombinant tissue-type plasminogen activator (Alteplase) for ischemic stroke 3 to 5 hours after symptom onset. The ATLANTIS Study: a randomized controlled trial. Alteplase Thrombolysis for Acute Noninterventional Therapy in Ischemic Stroke. *JAMA*, **282**(21):2019–2026.

CHAPTER 3

How do I formulate a research question?

Michael P. Wilson

Department of Emergency Medicine, UC San Diego Health Systems,
Department of Emergency Medicine Behavioral Emergencies Research Lab, CA, USA

> *"I really wanted to do research, but I couldn't think of a research question. When I did think of one, it was already a chapter in someone's textbook."*
>
> A resident researcher

Formulating the right question is not only the first step in doing research but the most important part. Ask a question that is too basic, and your research will either be completely uninteresting or already answered. Ask a question that is too complex, and, well, your research will be undoable.

In order to succeed, a research question must be the right question. In other words, it must have the following characteristics:

- A question that is interesting (to you).
- A question that is interesting (to readers).
- A question that can be answered within the time you have available (see also Chapter 2, "Aspects of feasibility in research").
- A question that can be translated into a hypothesis.
- A question that can be answered ethically (see also Chapter 8, "Ethics in research").

Characteristics of an interesting question

One of the first questions that is usually asked by novice researchers is "How do I come up with a question?" Well, congratulations! If you have gotten that far, you have already have! In other words, you have proven that you can ask questions ("How do I ask a question?" is really just another question!).

Curiosity cannot be taught, but it certainly can be refined. If you are curious enough to ask questions, then this chapter is for you. Hopefully, after reading this chapter you will be able to ask the right question. This sounds easier than it actually is, but once you have accomplished this, the rest of this book will help you test your new question in a meaningful way.

Although you have obviously just proven that you can ask questions, the trick is asking questions that are relevant to your medical practice. Sources of these questions are everywhere, but usually come out of your ordinary every day decision making. If you have ever scratched your head and wondered why your attending or fellow resident just did THAT, you have got the makings of a good research question. Other great sources include questions that are contained in journal articles or review books, especially the sections entitled "Questions for future research." If that does not give you any ideas, try asking your colleagues. What kinds of things have they always wanted to know about their practice? Do different doctors practice different ways? If so, this is another great place to start asking questions.

If you are reading this book, then you are likely interested in researching acute care. This means that you should focus your questions on conditions that arise suddenly (think heart attack, strokes, or trauma), are life threatening (think pulmonary embolus), or are seen often in acute care settings like the emergency department (think psychiatric emergencies). Within these broad areas, there are many different possible questions. Some researchers study the basic

Doing Research in Emergency and Acute Care: Making Order Out of Chaos, First Edition. Edited by Michael P. Wilson, Kama Z. Guluma, and Stephen R. Hayden.
© 2016 John Wiley & Sons, Ltd. Published 2016 by John Wiley & Sons, Ltd.

science or physiology of these conditions; others focus on the emergency department burden of these diseases; while others focus instead on their clinical treatment.

Regardless of which area you choose, the best questions are fairly similar in some important way. Thanks to some of the pioneers in acute care research, we have a mnemonic that helps us remember how to define the best questions. The best questions really are the FINER ones. That is, they are feasible, interesting, novel, ethical, and relevant [1].

Making a question interesting

> *"The more I thought about it, I just couldn't see myself sticking electrodes in rats' heads for even a month."*   Kama Guluma, MD

The first step in making a research question interesting is making it interesting to you. What have you always wanted to know more about? What wouldn't you mind reading a few dozen articles about? You and you alone must find the subject sufficiently fascinating to spend hours collecting and analyzing data. On the other hand, you must balance what you are interested in with the interests of your readers. In other words, you will have to answer a question that other people find interesting too.

How do you figure out what your colleagues find interesting? Ask them [2,3]. You can also search internet databases like PubMed (see Chapter 5, "How to do an efficient literature search"). There, you can figure out what other people have already found interesting by reading what they have written on the subject. If a topic has attracted other researchers, even if your question specifically has not been answered, chances are good that your research project will be interesting to others as well. Reading prior literature is not only a good way to find out what other researchers think is interesting, but is also a great way to find out what investigations have already been published. Nothing could be worse than completing a research project that you thought was novel only to find out that someone else already did the same study – but with better design and more participants than you!

Having said all that, you must also answer a question that is relevant to your practice. If you ask a question about whether patients that come to the emergency department are pleasant and satisfied, this will hardly change clinical practice or sway the opinions of your colleagues. If, on the other hand, you ask whether giving information to patients about the current wait time in the emergency department has the effect of making them both more pleasant and more satisfied, you are well on your way to a good question.

Time and resources to answer a question

Your question also must be answerable in the time that you have. Be realistic. If you are currently a resident working more than 60 hours a week, answering any research question, let alone a complicated one, is a daunting task. You simply will not be able to conduct a multicenter prospective trial on the latest drugs for cardiac arrest (see Chapter 2, "Aspects of feasibility in research"). In fact, you should not even try. No one likes seeing a project start with enthusiasm … only to die a few months later because the investigator "didn't have time." On the other hand, if you can set aside a few hours a week for your research project, you are much more likely to finish it … but it may take several months or even longer depending on the complexity of your question.

Translating a question into a hypothesis

Once you have asked a question that is relevant, that has not been answered before in a convincing way, and that you have time to answer, you must refine your question by turning it into a testable statement. For most researchers, this is the hardest part.

Turning your question into a testable hypothesis means that you need to translate your question into an outcome. Instead of asking, for example, whether patients that receive information about the emergency department are more satisfied with their visit, ask instead which patients, which information, and satisfaction about what. Here are some more examples:

- *Question: Which drug is better?*
- Hypothesis: Drug A is best for treating a particular (well-defined) condition as measured by mortality.
- *Question: Is high blood pressure at emergency department triage bad?*

- Hypothesis: Initial high blood pressure at emergency department triage (as defined by blood pressure >140/90) most often resolves during the emergency department stay, and there are no long-term adverse consequences.
- *Question: Can CT scanning be used to detect deep venous thrombosis?*
- Hypothesis: CT scanning is as accurate as ultrasound at detecting deep venous thrombosis in the lower extremities, but is more accurate at identifying deep venous thrombosis in the pelvis.

As you can see by these examples, a testable hypothesis is a question that can be answered in a concrete way.

By the way, refining a hypothesis to this level can sometimes take a lot of work. Here is an example from our patient satisfaction question above which we might rephrase in the following manner: "Will patients in the emergency department for the next six months who receive information at triage about how the emergency department works rate the satisfaction with their visit more highly than patients who do not receive this information?" [4] This moves beyond a question and gets us most of the way to a good hypothesis. Now, we just have to answer a few more details about how the patients who receive the information and how the patients who do not receive the information are selected, who will give this information and how, and which survey we will use to measure their satisfaction, and we have an excellent research hypothesis! (Incidentally, you will find information in other parts of this book about submitting your new hypothesis to the Institutional Review Board, basic statistics for analyzing your data, and writing up your research project for publication, so keep reading.)

Ethical concerns

Almost any study conducted raises the possibility of ethical concerns. Although it might seem unlikely that a question-naire about patient satisfaction could provoke ethical concerns of any kind, look at it from the patient's perspective. Can the patients truly answer the survey however they wish? What if their answers are unflattering to the department? Will their treatment be changed if patients name staff who they think were rude or will they be charged more after the visit? There are quite a number of such concerns in any project, and collecting data in a responsible and ethical manner is of paramount importance. (See other chapters in this book, such as, Chapter 16 "How to design a study that everyone will believe: Ethical concepts for special populations in emergency research," Chapter 8 "Ethics in research: How to collect data ethically," and Chapter 9 "Safety in research: How to ensure patient safety," for more information.)

KEY POINTS

- Research should be FINER: feasible, interesting, novel, ethical, and relevant.
- Research questions should be interesting both to you and to potential readers.
- Research questions should be answered within the time you have available.
- You can turn a research question into a testable hypothesis by stating it in terms of a discrete measurable outcome.
- Your research project should be one that can be answered ethically.

References

1 Kwiatkowski, T. and Silverman, R. (1998) Research fundamentals: II. Choosing and defining a research question. *Acad Emerg Med*, **5**:1114–1117.
2 Cairns, C.B., Bebarta, V.S. and Panacek, E.A. (2012) How to pick an emergency medicine research topic. In: V.S. Bebarta and C.B. Cairns (eds) *Emergency Care Research – A Primer*. American College of Emergency Physicians, pp. 7–10.
3 Krishel, S. and Baraff, L.J. (1993) Effect of emergency department information on patient satisfaction. *Ann Emerg Med*, **22**:568–572.
4 Lewis, L.M., Lewis, R.J., Younger, J.G. and Callaham, M. (1998) Research fundamentals: I. Getting from hypothesis to manuscript: An overview of the skills required for success in research. *Acad Emerg Med*, **5**:924–929.

CHAPTER 4

Evidence-based medicine: Finding the knowledge gap

Eddy Lang[1] and Zubair Bayat[2]

[1] Department of Emergency Medicine, University of Calgary, AB, Canada
[2] Cumming School of Medicine, University of Calgary, AB, Canada

The ultimate goal of the research endeavor is to create new and useful knowledge that can improve clinical care. That can be a daunting task at first glance because many of the most relevant research questions appear to have been answered already and often with studies that have taken years to design and execute at considerable expense. Do not get discouraged – the good news is that this chapter will provide you with unique perspectives that will allow you to identify gaps in clinical knowledge that might not be all that obvious. The objective of this chapter is to use the frameworks of evidence-based medicine and implementation science to identify gaps in existing knowledge and practice for most of the clinical questions that acute care providers face on a daily basis. In fact, once you have a closer look at the tools and concepts that this chapter describes, I think you will agree that there is a great deal more that we do not know about how to improve patient care than we do know about. Furthermore, enlightening these unknowns can be achieved with manageable research projects.

Evidence synthesis/systematic reviews

Increasingly, major funding agencies are demanding that researchers provide a detailed analysis of all of the existing evidence around a health topic before releasing funds. This makes good sense, since it would be unwise to bankroll an effort that does not complement or add to the current state of knowledge. This was not lost on the Institute of Medicine in 2012 when it released its report entitled "Finding What Works in Healthcare – Standards for Systematic Reviews" [1].
    Systematic reviews are defined as:

> "…a review of a clearly formulated question that uses systematic and explicit methods to identify, select, and critically appraise relevant research, and to collect and analyze data from the studies that are included in the review. Statistical methods (meta-analysis) may or may not be used to analyze and summarize the results of the included studies. Meta-analysis refers to the use of statistical techniques in a systematic review to integrate the results of included studies." [2]

Importantly, systematic reviews are in and of themselves scientific works and a form of clinical research. They require a well developed methodology laid out in a scientific protocol and should be registered with an international registry of reviews like PROSPERO (http://www.crd.york.ac.uk/NIHR_PROSPERO/), just as you might register a prospective randomized study with the National Institutes of Health (https://clinicaltrials.gov) The largest database of high quality and continuously updated systematic reviews can be found in the Cochrane Library and is termed the Cochrane Database of Systematic Reviews (http://www.thecochranelibrary.com/). This database contains several thousand systematic reviews and protocols for reviews that are in development, but admittedly only covers a fraction of the totality of biomedical knowledge that can be gleaned from clinical research.
    Systematic reviews have their critics who would note that, if the nature of an existing evidence base is replete with methodologically-flawed research, then you are not doing anyone any favors by pooling data from this work and attempting to draw meaningful conclusions. There is also debate whether the strongest evidence comes from a meta-analysis or an adequately sized randomized controlled trial. This perspective, while commonly espoused is likely short-sighted for a number of reasons (Box 4.1).

Doing Research in Emergency and Acute Care: Making Order Out of Chaos, First Edition. Edited by Michael P. Wilson, Kama Z. Guluma, and Stephen R. Hayden.
© 2016 John Wiley & Sons, Ltd. Published 2016 by John Wiley & Sons, Ltd.

Box 4.1 Reasons for performing and basing decision making and policies on systematic reviews.

1 Pooling studies may provide increased certainty around estimates of effect, increasing the ability to see effects that would not be apparent from single trials.

2 Noting that the estimates of effect, whether they apply to diagnostic or therapeutic interventions, are similar or the same across studies performed in different settings and with different populations adds to the robustness and generalizability of the systematic review findings.

3 It is important to know if study findings agree with each other. Systematic reviews that employ meta-analyses (pool analyses of existing data) can provide measures of heterogeneity that informs our understanding of effects across studies and whether studies should be pooled in the first place.

4 Heterogeneity, when observed, is not necessarily problematic as long as it can be explained. In fact, one of the reasons that systematic reviews can be valuable and useful is that they can undertake a prespecified subgroup analysis that enlightens our understanding of the effect of an intervention; for example, medication X works to prevent admissions in severely ill patients but not in the moderately ill.

5 Publication bias, be that the result of suppressed data, or demotivated investigators who choose not to develop their projects into manuscripts for peer review is an important concern in the biomedical literature. Fortunately, systematic reviews can evaluate for the presence of publication bias in some instances through statistical and visual methods. Funnel plots and Eggner's test for publication bias are particularly useful in this regard.

As you explore a clinical subject that is of interest to you from a research perspective, a high quality systematic review that aligns with your topic will be very informative when it comes to determining the state of knowledge on a typical topic. What may transpire as you seek out a systematic review on a given topic is that you will learn that one does not exist, is not in development, or that the most recently published version is out of date, with new relevant evidence that could help refine the conclusions. This could represent a unique and important opportunity to fill an existing gap in knowledge. Even if several studies already exist on a given topic, without a systematic review it would be very difficult for frontline clinicians to make sense of the totality of evidence related to a clinical problem they face in either the realm of diagnostics or therapeutics.

In performing a systematic review, it is necessary to search the literature for relevant publications, to screen the identified publications and assess them for suitability, to perform a qualitative analysis of the suitable publications, and, finally, to perform a quantitative synthesis (meta-analysis) of the analyses identified (http://www.prisma-statement. org/). Essential team members include a health information specialist who can assure a comprehensive search of multiple biomedical databases, other co-investigators who can critically appraise the component studies that will be identified, as well as a clinical content expert who can provide guidance and perspective. A number of resources exist on how to conduct a systematic review but many systematic reviewers find it useful to work backward from quality criteria for the conduct of reviews, such as the AMSTAR criteria (http://amstar.ca/index.php), or tools for reporting systematic reviews, for example, PRISMA (http://www.prisma-statement.org/).

Structured critical appraisal

The need for a clinical trial is often born from an analysis of existing best evidence on a clinical topic. Any medical trainee who has ever attended a critical appraisal or journal club session can attest that by appearances and the nature of the discussion, there is no paucity of study flaws, perceived or real, that plague many if not most of the research that addresses acute care. But how important are the study flaws that can be discovered in reviewing primary research and are these limitations a threat to the validity of the reported results? Or would they be expected to have more impact on the application of the findings to bedside care? These questions may be difficult for someone with epidemiologic training to answer with certainty, let alone a healthcare trainee charged with presenting a critical analysis of an article. Fortunately, there are a myriad of tools that can help young academics evaluate the risk of bias in nearly every category of biomedical research and publications (Table 4.1).

Engaging in structured critical appraisal is not only of value in determining if a specific piece of primary literature can inform clinical practice but it can also point to opportunities to repeat studies with the problematic component corrected. For example, researchers in France noted that the literature on the impact of family presence was based entirely on observational studies at high risk of bias and chose to conduct a landmark randomized controlled trial suggesting that the practice was beneficial. [5] Occasionally, after encountering a challenge in practice, formulating it as a research question, performing a systematic review and a critical appraisal, a researcher finds that reliable evidence exists, but that

Table 4.1 Research and biomedical publication evaluation tools.

Category	Instrument	Functionality
Randomized controlled trials	CONSORT	Checklist and flow diagram facilitating complete and transparent reporting of trial findings and aiding in critical appraisal and interpretation. (http://www.consort-statement.org/)
Diagnostic accuracy studies	QUADAS 2 [3]	Analyzes four key domains to rate bias and applicability of primary diagnostic accuracy studies. (http://www.bris.ac.uk/quadas/resources/quadas2.pdf)
Prognosis studies	QUIPs [4]	Six sources of bias assessed to provide valid assessments of answers to prognostic questions.
Systematic reviews	PRISMA	27-item checklist facilitating the transparent and complete reporting of systematic reviews and meta analyses. (http://www.prisma-statement.org/)
Clinical practice guidelines	AGREE II	23-item tool assessing the methodological rigor and transparency with which clinical practice guidelines are developed. (http://www.agreetrust.org/)

common practice stands in contradiction to it. For instance, the Ottawa Ankle Rules have been validated repeatedly as a sensitive bedside gauge of which patients are in need of radiography, but the usage of these rules in clinical practice is inconsistent. [6] In cases like this, a structured critical appraisal can signal the researcher that knowledge translation, rather than further data collection and synthesis, is required to address the gap in common practice.

Knowledge translation

The Institute of Medicine has also pointed out between the health care we currently live and work in, and the one which we could potentially enjoy, there exists not just a gap but a chasm. [7] This vast deficiency in the delivery of quality health care is characterized by disparities and the failure of the fruits of biomedical science to become integrated into routine practice. Arguably, we could do more to improve the outcomes of our acute care patients and restore rational decision making to our healthcare environment by implementing what we know to be effective and eliminating what we know is ineffective and harmful or driven by perverse incentives. [8]

With this in mind as a backdrop, it should become evident that researchable gaps are not only represented by gaps in knowledge in the literature, but can be explored as gaps or variations in acute care medicine as delivered by a representative sample of providers. While identifying gaps, disparities and variations in care in a rigorous and reliable manner is an important avenue of inquiry and often readily accomplished, as it relies on retrospective designs using chart reviews and administrative data, it does not tell the whole story. Reasons for not adhering to evidence-based practice can be complex and unexpected and an analysis of the barriers to evidence-based care can also constitute an important contribution to the literature.

Ultimately, however, you can know all there is to know about the exact nature, severity and causes of practice gaps in acute care and you will be no further ahead when it comes to proving, through research, how to improve it. This realization has spawned the field of Knowledge Translation (KT), known synonymously with implementation science in some circles. [9] While traditional biomedical science has asked questions that are of a nature whereby interventions or tests are compared against a given standard of care, that is, is treatment A better than treatment B for the care of disease C, KT research takes a different slant. It accepts that a given treatment or management strategy is better than another, assuming a systematic review supports that contention, and instead asks if implementation strategy A, informed by an understanding of relevant barriers, is more effective and yields superior outcomes to implementation strategy B. As such, KT research and interventions are necessary to bridge the gap between the modification of best practices, and those practices being adopted as new standards of patient care. Essentially, the field of KT is suggesting that we cannot hope to achieve truly evidence-based care without engaging in evidence-based implementation (Table 4.2).

Conclusion

Healthcare providers in acute care and other medical fields and settings are surrounded by gaps of a myriad nature, including bodies of evidence in need of synthesis, key studies that need to be repeated with improved methodology,

Table 4.2 Knowledge translation interventions matched to barriers of evidence uptake.

Barriers to evidence uptake	Knowledge translation interventions
Lack of knowledge regarding effective interventions	Educational interventions
Complexity of therapies and lack of availability of guidance at the bedside	Order sets/computerized physician order entry
Limited self-awareness, i.e., providers (mistakenly) believe they are following evidence	Audit and feedback
Skepticism about efficacy of an intervention	Opinion leader methodology, i.e., respected colleague espouses the benefits
Practice isolation, i.e., physicians located in a remote location and not exposed to evidence	Academic detailing
Busy work-flow with no time to offer evidence-based therapies	Reminders (electronic or otherwise)

and real-life gaps in practice that are urgently in need of closure. The discrepancies often provoke questions that merit a review of the literature, and a critical appraisal of the existing data and analyses. In performing this analysis, the healthcare provider can determine whether further research or synthesis is necessary to eliminate the gap, or whether there is a deficit in knowledge translation, and can take appropriate action to remedy the situation. These gaps are the fuel and substrate for igniting fires of creative research endeavor that can improve care and outcomes for the acutely ill patients we care for every day.

KEY POINTS

1 **Evidence Synthesis:** Clinical questions are rarely answered by single studies – nor should they be – since all good science should be reproduced to assure validity and applicability. As such, bodies of evidence need to be considered in their totality to understand the true current state of affairs around a clinical problem or potential innovations in care.

2 **Structured Critical Appraisal:** There is no such thing as the perfect clinical study and no scientific investigation is infallible. The challenge is to identify when research is so greatly at risk of getting it wrong that it needs to be repeated in a manner that corrects for those gaps in study integrity.

3 **Knowledge Translation:** More often than not, the problem we face in acute care medicine is not that we do not know what works well, but rather that we are not acting on best evidence or, potentially worse, we are doing things that are harmful or wasteful. Knowledge Translation or Implementation Science looks at measuring, understanding and overcoming these real-life clinical gaps in care.

References

1 Institute of Medicine (2011) Finding What Works in Health Care: Standards for Systematic Reviews, http://www.iom.edu/Reports/2011/Finding-What-Works-in-Health-Care-Standards-for-systematic-Reviews.aspx (last accessed 25 April 2015).

2 Higgins, J.P.T. and Green, S. (2011) *Cochrane Handbook for Systematic Reviews of Interventions*, Version 5.1.0 [updated March 2011]. http://handbook.cochrane.org/ (last accessed 25 April 2015).

3 Whiting, P.F., Rutjes, A.W., Westwood, M.E., *et al.* (2011) QUADAS-2: a revised tool for the quality assessment of diagnostic accuracy studies. *Ann Intern Med*, **155**(8):529–536. doi: 10.7326/0003-4819-155-8-201110180-00009.

4 Hayden, J.A., Côté, P., and Bombardier, C. (2006) Evaluation of the quality of prognosis studies in systematic reviews. *Ann Intern Med*, **144**(6):427–437.

5 Jabre, P., Belpomme, V., Azoulay, E., *et al.* (2013) Family presence during cardiopulmonary resuscitation. *N Engl J Med*, **368**(11):1008–1018. doi: 10.1056/NEJMoa1203366.

6 Holroyd, B.R., Wilson, D., Row, B.H., *et al.* (2004) Uptake of validated clinical practice guidelines: experience with implementing the Ottawa Ankle Rules. *Am J Emerg Med*, **22**, 149–155.

7 Institute of Medicine (2001) Crossing the Quality Chasm: A New Health System for the 21st Century, http://www.iom.edu/Reports/2001/Crossing-the-Quality-Chasm-A-New-Health-System-for-the-21st-Century.aspx (last accessed 25 April 2015).

8 Venkatesh, A.K. and Schuur, J.D. (2013) A "Top Five" list for emergency medicine: a policy and research agenda for stewardship to improve the value of emergency care. *Am J Emerg Med*, **31**(10):1520–1524. doi: 10.1016/j.ajem.2013.07.019.

9 Lang, E.S., Wyer, P.C., and Haynes, R.B. (2007) Knowledge translation: closing the evidence-to-practice gap. *Ann Emerg Med*, **49**(3):355–363.

CHAPTER 5

How to carry out an efficient literature search

Aleksandr Tichter[1], Louise Falzon[2], and Peter Wyer[1]

[1] *Columbia University Medical Center, NY, USA*
[2] *Center for Behavioral Cardiovascular Health, Columbia University Medical Center, NY, USA*

> *"I'm interested in doing a project on CHF. Now what?"*
>
> A junior faculty member

Once you have decided on a general research topic, the next step is to gauge the volume of literature that has been published in the area, so as to determine how you can make the most meaningful contribution. Your two best friends during this part of the research process are a sound familiarity with efficient, goal-oriented literature searching and your local librarian. The librarian will help with the proverbial "deep dive", but first you have to wade into the shallow end on your own.

Part I: Surveying the research landscape

Like most things in life, the goal of any literature search is to maximize efficiency, without sacrificing quality. The best initial approach, therefore, begins with resources that provide information in a dependable, albeit succinct format in order to gain an overview of best evidence and expert opinion relevant to your topic of interest. These so-called "summaries" consist primarily of electronic, peer-reviewed texts and evidence-based practice guidelines.

Electronic textbooks, like **UpToDate**© (http://www.uptodate.com/home) are a favorite among residents and physicians in private practice for a reason (Figure 5.1). Their summary of research and background information can be quickly and easily adapted to bedside clinical practice. The same virtues make these types of resources similarly efficient in providing an overview of your research topic, with a description of current knowledge gaps, controversies, ongoing studies, and areas for further investigation. Several different vendors provide this type of content, and include **Dynamed**© (https://dynamed.ebscohost.com) (Figure 5.2), American College of Physicians **(ACP) Pier**© (http://pier.acponline.org), and *British Medical Journal* (BMJ) **Clinical Evidence**© (http://clinicalevidence.bmj.com) (Figure 5.3), which are all worth investigating, depending on your institution's subscriptions. Each of these resources offer natural language queries and are useful not only due to their content but also their references.

Most practice guidelines can be found by searching a single resource, the **National Guideline Clearinghouse (NGC)**© (www.guideline.gov), which, in addition to links to the guidelines themselves, provides expert commentary, systematic comparisons of guidelines that address similar topics, and the ability to perform a side-by-side comparison of the guidelines of your choosing. The purpose of reviewing guidelines related to your research topic is not to answer a specific question *per se*, but, rather, to identify recommendations that are based on low-level evidence and, therefore, inviting of further investigation.

Another type of resource that, if available, can provide a sense for the research landscape is a "synthesis". Syntheses consist of original systematic reviews and meta-analyses, which, as the term "systematic" implies, use an organized and

Doing Research in Emergency and Acute Care: Making Order Out of Chaos, First Edition. Edited by Michael P. Wilson, Kama Z. Guluma, and Stephen R. Hayden.
© 2016 John Wiley & Sons, Ltd. Published 2016 by John Wiley & Sons, Ltd.

Predictive models — A variety of predictors of survival have been identified in patients with HF, such as peak VO2, New York Heart Association (NYHA) functional class, left ventricular ejection fraction, and markers of the adequacy of tissue perfusion. (See "Predictors of survival in heart failure due to systolic dysfunction".)

Although these risk factors correlate with survival on a statistical basis in a large population, their ability to predict survival in individual patients is limited. As a result, a number of retrospective analyses have been used to develop predictive models that utilize multiple indicators to generate a more accurate estimate of prognosis [26-29].

Potential benefits of using prognostic models for HF include the following [30]:

- Enables patients and families to have a realistic expectation of the prognosis
- Enables appropriate allocation of resources, including transplantation, mechanical circulatory assist devices, and implantable defibrillators
- Enables selection of therapies most likely to positively affect the quality and quantity of life
- Promotes open, honest communication between clinicians, patients, and their families to define the goals of therapy.

Potential hazards of using prognostic models for HF include the following [30]:

- The model was derived from a different population of patients
- Patient compliance, preference, or attitudes are not incorporated
- New therapies become available, making the models obsolete
- The patient is not in compensated HF or is not on evidence-based therapies
- Uncertainty in applying the model to an individual patient cannot be quantified and this uncertainty may be difficult for clinicians to effectively explain to patients and their families
- Scores from the models replace informed, compassionate, clinician-patient conversations

Given the limitations of prognostic models, use of a prognostic model should supplement rather than replace the judgment of the clinical team [30]. A study of the predictive accuracy of physicians and HF nurses for estimating risk of hospitalization and death among patients with advanced HF found that nurse estimations of mortality added significantly to the derived prognostic model but physician estimations did not [31]. It was hypothesized that the nurses were better versed in patient psychosocial characteristics that impact HF outcomes.

EFFECT model — The EFFECT model was derived, tested, and intended to be used in patients hospitalized for HF [26]. The derivation cohort included 2624 patients in the EFFECT study, who presented with HF at 34 hospitals in Ontario, Canada between 1999 and 2001. The model was then validated in 1407 patients presenting between 1997 and 1999.

Multiple clinical characteristics, including both HF-related factors (respiratory rate, systolic pressure, blood urea nitrogen, and serum sodium concentration) and comorbidities (eg, chronic obstructive pulmonary disease [COPD], anemia, malignancy) were correlated with 30-day and one-year mortality. Points were assigned to each significant predictor; the sum of the points results in a risk score ranging from ≤60 (very low; 30-day mortality <1 percent and one year mortality <10 percent) to >150 (very high; 30-day mortality >50 percent and one year mortality >70 percent).

An on-line calculator for this risk model is available at www.ccort.ca/CHFriskmodel.aspx.

Figure 5.1 UpToDate© search: "heart failure prognosis".

methodical approach to compile the wealth of existing evidence on a particular topic. While the question addressed by a typical synthesis may be overly narrow for the purposes of your exploratory search, it will, nevertheless, be valuable in providing background information relevant to the topic, commentary on the included studies, as well as references worthy of further perusal. Perhaps the most well-known source of syntheses is the Cochrane Database of Systematic Reviews (CDSR)© (http://www.thecochranelibrary.com), whose publications are authored by internal Cochrane review groups, organized by either organ system or disease process, and focus exclusively on questions related to therapeutic interventions and diagnostic test accuracy. Although reflecting a high standard of quality, the CDSR is only one source of systematic reviews. Such reviews can be done on any research question and are published throughout the medical literature. They can easily be found via a **PubMed**© (www.ncbi.nlm.nih.gov/pubmed) search, by applying the *"Article types"* filter, or by utilizing *"Clinical Queries"*, which is discussed in more detail later. A source of independently appraised synopses of systematic reviews on a broad range of topics is the Database of Abstracts of Reviews of Effect (DARE)© (http://www.crd.york.ac.uk/CRDWeb), which is included in the Cochrane Library and can also be accessed without a subscription.

Although not typically considered to be of rigorous methodologic quality, narrative review articles addressing your topic of interest are another reasonable place to begin scanning the research milieu. These can be found by conducting a simple **PubMed** search and, under the *"Article types"* filter in the upper left hand corner, clicking on the *"Review"* link (Figure 5.4).

One useful feature of **PubMed** is the *"Titles with your search terms"* box in the right-hand column of the search results (Figure 5.5), which, if selected by clicking *"See more"*, will display only those results that contain your search term in the title.

Prediction rules:

- multivariable risk scores[2]
  - validated multivariable risk scores can be useful to estimate subsequent risk of mortality in ambulatory or hospitalized patients with heartfailure (ACCF/AHA Class IIa, Level B)
  - risk scores for patients with acutely decompensated heartfailure include
    - ADHERE Classification and Regression Tree (CART) Model (JAMA 2005 Feb 2;293(5):572), commentary can be found in JAMA 2005 May 25;293(20):2467, ACP J Club 2005 Jul-Aug;143(1):25 📖 EBSCOhost Full Text
    - American Heart Association Get With The Guidelines Score (Circ Cardiovasc Qual Outcomes 2010 Jan;3(1):25 full-text poster PDF)
    - EFFECT Risk Score (JAMA 2003 Nov 19;290(19):2581), commentary can be found in ACP J Club 2004 May-Jun;140(3):80 📖 EBSCOhost Full Text online calculator can be found at Canadian Cardiovascular Outcomes Research Team
    - ESCAPE Risk Model and Discharge Score (J Am Coll Cardiol 2010 Mar 2;55(9):872)
    - OPTIMIZE HF Risk-Prediction Nomogram (Circ Heart Fail 2011 Sep;4(5):628 full-text)
- **ADHERE risk tree validated for predicting in-hospital mortality**
  - based on cohort of 65,275 hospital records of adults presenting to United States hospitals with acutely decompensated heartfailure, retrospective derivation cohort of 33,046 hospitalization episodes from 2001 to 2003, and prospective validation cohort of 32,229 hospitalization episodes from March to July 2003
  - if blood urea nitrogen (BUN) < 43 mg/dL (30.7 mmol/L)
    - if systolic blood pressure 115 mm Hg or higher, in-hospital mortality 2.14% in derivation cohort, and 2.31% in validation cohort
    - if systolic blood pressure < 115 mm Hg, in-hospital mortality 5.49% in derivation cohort, and 5.67% in validation cohort
  - if BUN 43 mg/dL (30.7 mmol/L) or higher
    - if systolic blood pressure 115 mm Hg or higher, in-hospital mortality 6.41% in derivation cohort, and 5.63% in validation cohort
    - if systolic blood pressure < 115 mm Hg
      - if serum creatinine < 2.75 mg/dL (243.1 mcmol/L), in-hospital mortality 12.42% in derivation cohort, and 13.23% in validation cohort
      - if serum creatinine 2.75 mg/dL (243.1 mcmol/L) or higher, in-hospital mortality 21.94% in derivation cohort, and 19.76% in validation cohort
  - Reference - JAMA 2005 Feb 2;293(5):572, commentary can be found in JAMA 2005 May 25;293(20):2467, ACP J Club 2005 Jul-Aug;143(1):25 📖 EBSCOhost Full Text, summary can be found in Am Fam Physician 2007 Apr 15;75(8):1231 full-text
- **alternative validated predictive index (EFFECT rule) for mortality after hospital admission for heartfailure**
  - online calculator can be found at Canadian Cardiovascular Outcomes Research Team
  - derived from Enhanced Feedback For Effective Cardiology Treatment (EFFECT) study
  - details of predictive index
    Click for Details
    - based on retrospective cohort of 4,031 community-dwelling patients presenting to Canadian hospitals with heartfailure, derivation cohort of 2,624 patients from 1999 to 2001, and validation cohort of 1,407 patients from 1997 to 1999
    - score derived from factors easily determined within hours of hospital admission
    - score derivation varies slightly for 30-day prediction and 1-year prediction
      - 1 point for each year of age
      - systolic blood pressure (in mm Hg) for 30-day score is -60 points if 180 or higher, -55 points if 160-179, -50 points if 140-159, -45 points if 120-139, -40 points if 100-119, -35 points if 90-99, - 30 points if < 90; subtract 10 more points for 1-year score
      - add 1 point for each mg/dL (0.714 mmol/L) units of BUN up to maximum 60
      - add 10 points if sodium < 136 mEq/L
      - add 10 points if cerebrovascular disease
      - dementia adds 20 points for 30-day score, 15 points for 1-year score
      - add 10 points if chronic obstructive pulmonary disease (COPD)
      - hepatic cirrhosis adds 25 points for 30-day score, 35 points for 1-year score
      - add 15 points if cancer
      - hemoglobin < 10 g/dL adds 10 points to 1-year score (not used in 30-day score)
    - mortality rates predicted by scores
      - score 60 or less predicts 0.4%-0.6% mortality at 30 days and 2.7%-7.8% mortality at 1 year
      - score 61-90 predicts 3.4%-4.2% mortality at 30 days and 12.9%-14.4% mortality at 1 year
      - score 91-120 predicts 12.2%-13.7% mortality at 30 days and 30.2%-32.5% mortality at 1 year
      - score 121-150 predicts 26%-32.7% mortality at 30 days and 55.5%-59.3% mortality at 1 year
      - score > 150 predicts 50%-59% mortality at 30 days and 74.7%-78.8% mortality at 1 year
    - Reference - JAMA 2003 Nov 19;290(19):2581, commentary can be found in ACP J Club 2004 May-Jun;140(3):80 📖 EBSCOhost Full Text, summary can be found in Am Fam Physician 2007 Apr 15;75(8):1231 full-text

Figure 5.2 Dynamed© search: "heart failure prognosis".

Prognosis

Top

The prognosis of heart failure is poor, with 5-year mortality ranging from 26% to 75%.[9] Up to 16% of people are re-admitted with heart failure within 6 months of first admission. In the US, heart failure is the leading cause of hospital admission among people over 65 years of age.[9] In people with heart failure, a new MI increases the risk of death (RR 7.8, 95% CI 6.9 to 8.8). About one third of all deaths in people with heart failure are preceded by a major ischaemic event.[10] Sudden death, mainly caused by ventricular arrhythmia, is responsible for 25% to 50% of all deaths, and is the most common cause of death in people with heart failure. Women with heart failure have a 15% to 20% lower risk of total and cardiovascular mortality compared with men with heart failure (risk after adjustment for demographic and social economic characteristics, comorbidities, cardiovascular treatments, and LVEF).[11] The presence of asymptomatic LVSD increases an individual's risk of having a cardiovascular event. One large prevention trial found that the risk of heart failure, admission for heart failure, and death increased linearly as ejection fraction fell (for each 5% reduction in ejection fraction: RR for mortality 1.20, 95% CI 1.13 to 1.29; RR for hospital admission 1.28, 95% CI 1.18 to 1.38; RR for heart failure 1.20, 95% CI 1.13 to 1.26).[12] The annual mortality for people with diastolic heart failure varies in observational studies (1–18%).[7] Reasons for this variation include age, presence of coronary artery disease, and variation in the partition value used to define abnormal ventricular systolic function. The annual mortality for left ventricular diastolic dysfunction is lower than that found in people with systolic dysfunction.[12]

Figure 5.3 (BMJ) Clinical Evidence© search: "heart failure prognosis".

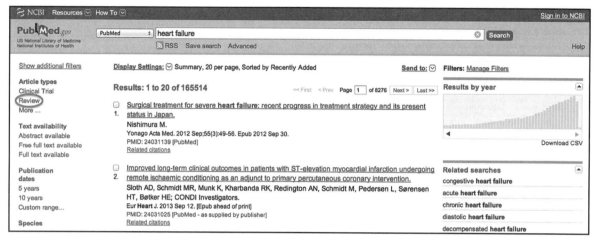

Figure 5.4 PubMed *"Article Type (Review)"* search [Source: Reproduced with permission of National Library of Medicine (NLM)].

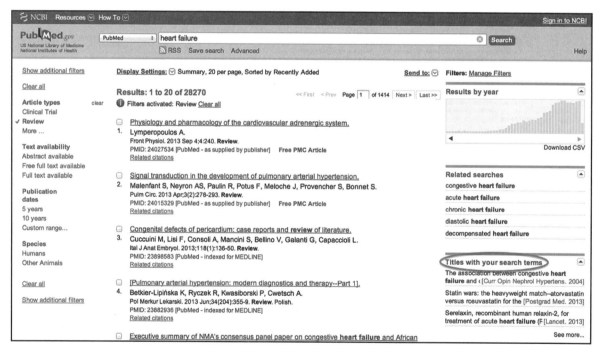

Figure 5.5 PubMed *"Titles with your search terms"* search [Source: Reproduced with permission of National Library of Medicine (NLM)].

If a particular citation piques your interest, you can click on it to find if the overall content of the abstract seems consistent with what you were looking for. If so, there is another box on the right-hand side within the abstract display entitled, *"Related citations in PubMed"* (Figure 5.6). Here, you can select to either *"See reviews"* or *"See all,"* in which case PubMed will follow an internal algorithm to display a list of citations related to that which you originally selected.

There have recently been developed search engines that facilitate the process by simultaneously searching multiple resources in response to specified search terms and providing results organized according to resource-type.

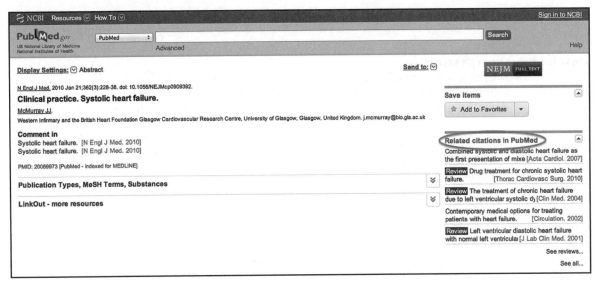

Figure 5.6 PubMed "*Related citations in PubMed*" search [Source: Reproduced with permission of National Library of Medicine (NLM)].

One example is the **Trip Database**© (http://www.tripdatabase.com), which displays filters on the right-hand side of the screen and organizes its output based on the classification of its publisher. For example, Cochrane reviews are classified under "Systematic Reviews", whereas articles published in the *New England Journal of Medicine*, are found under "Key Primary Research". Trip Database will give you a snapshot of the major research based papers and publications for your topic. Select one or two key words or phrases (not sentences), enter them into the search box and voila!

Finally, no search would be complete without at least some attempt at "Googling". The same virtues that have made Google© (http://www.google.com) the world's most popular search engine contribute to its utility in surveying the research landscape. Its simplicity, ease of use, and speedy retrieval of relevant results are invaluable in performing an efficient background search targeting not only journal articles but also websites, blogs, and podcasts through which experts in the field provide commentary regarding standards of care, the current state of knowledge, and ongoing controversies surrounding your topic of interest.

Overall, the use of this general approach, scanning the resulting titles and abstracts, and finding a few references from a systematic review that are close to your question will provide a great departure point in orienting you to the topic, and in helping you to become familiar with the vocabulary the authors use to describe it. Asking colleagues and consultants with particular knowledge of an area for suggestions is also a great idea.

> *"I read through the literature, and think I want to focus on something related to identifying which CHF patients can be safely discharged from the ED. Where do I go from here?"*
>
> A junior faculty member

Part II: The deep dive

Now that you have identified your general research topic, the next step of the process will be to perform an exhaustive search similar to that which would be undertaken in the process of conducting a systematic review. You will need your local librarian's help with this part of the literature search, as it involves structuring your terms in a systematic way and using advanced techniques to get to the most relevant references. However, it will be a big help if you have taken the time to become an informed consumer. By familiarizing yourself with the important search concepts, and identifying a few key articles to help guide the discussion, you will save time and effort that can be invested elsewhere.

Developing a search strategy

Your preliminary search should have covered the spectrum of summary and synthesis-type resources, and served to familiarize you with both the relevant knowledge gaps, as well as the key concepts and breadth of terminology used in the study of your research question. It is the same concepts and terminology that you will now use to develop your search strategy.

The first step is to create a list of the most relevant words or phrases you encountered during your preliminary search. If you are unsure as to which ones best represent the concept of interest, an easy tactic is to borrow the PubMed medical subject heading (MeSH) terms common to the articles you reviewed in Part I. These can be found at the bottom of the abstract display (Figure 5.7).

For the heart failure example used above, the key words might include:

- Congestive heart failure
- Emergency medical services
- Mortality

The above method applies to all types of research questions (e.g., basic science, epidemiological, etc.). However, if your question happens to be a clinical one, another approach to keyword identification involves defining the question in terms of the kind of clinical action or reasoning that is at issue (therapy, diagnosis, prognosis or harm), and organizing it into component words or phrases, using the commonly employed "Patients-Interventions-Comparisons-Outcomes" (PICO) framework, each element of which corresponds to an individual search term.

Table 5.1 is a tabulated summary of common PICO constructs for the four categories of clinical questions. While providing a broad overview, it should be noted that, depending on the context, there are many possible variations on

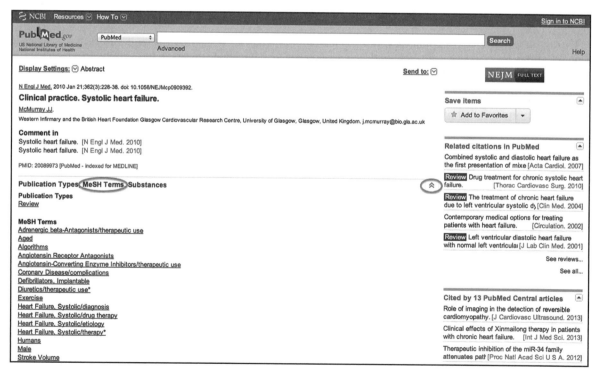

Figure 5.7 PubMed *"medical subject heading (MeSH)"* search [Source: Reproduced with permission of National Library of Medicine (NLM)].

PICO phrasing, and several different potential study designs that correspond to each of the four categories of clinical questions. To obtain a more in-depth understanding of and facility with PICO formulation and linking study design to clinical question type will require further reading of dedicated evidence-based medicine articles or texts, the content of which lie beyond the scope of this chapter [1, 2].

> *"I've identified mine as a "Prognosis" question and rephrased it as follows:*
> P: adult patients presenting to the emergency department with CHF exacerbations
> I: what are the risk factors
> C: N/A
> O: for 30-day mortality
> *How can I find the best articles to bring to my librarian?"*
>
> A junior faculty member

Performing the search

The types of articles that are likely to be of most interest to you at this stage of planning your research project will be primary studies, papers which inform you of how similar projects have been designed and run. Your librarian will be able to advise on the most appropriate databases to search, but they will probably include two principal types (Table 5.2).

PubMed

Although an all-out **PubMed** search may seem like a daunting task, which produces thousands of results that you will need to screen one-by-one for relevancy, there are a few tricks that can make the process much more manageable. We emphasize that you will need the help of a librarian to do this effectively. If you aim to increase knowledge in an area, your ship will sink before leaving port if you have mis-identified existing relevant knowledge.

The *"MeSH Database"* feature allows you to not only search for MeSH headings based on the keywords you identified during search strategy development, but also to simultaneously "build" your PubMed search, one MeSH heading at a time (Figure 5.8). The result is a much more manageable output of articles, which can be efficiently scanned for relevant titles in significantly less time than a traditional keyword search.

For searching terms related to clinical questions, *"Clinical Queries"* is a **PubMed** feature that limits results to specific "Clinical Study Categories", which should now be familiar to you: Therapy, Diagnosis, Prognosis and Harm (**PubMed**

Table 5.1 PICO constructs for the four categories of clinical questions.

Question type	(P)opulation	(I)ntervention	(C)omparison	(O)utcome
Therapy	Patient with a particular disease	Therapeutic intervention	Control	Likelihood of clinical outcome
Diagnosis	Patient with a symptom	Diagnostic test	Gold standard	Accuracy in identifying disease
Prognosis	Patient with a symptom	Performance of a predictor or rule on clinical outcome	N/A	Accuracy in predicting likelihood of outcome
Harm	Patient with a particular disease	Therapeutic, diagnostic or prognostic intervention	Control	Likelihood of adverse outcome

Table 5.2 Principal types of database.

Database type	Study type	Source
Primary databases	RCT, Cohort, cross-sectional, case–control	• PubMed • Clinical queries • Emergency medical abstracts
Ongoing research studies	RCT, cohort, cross-sectional, case–control	• Clinicaltrials.gov

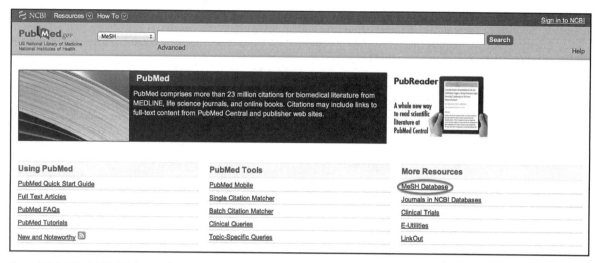

Figure 5.8 PubMed *"(MeSH) databas"* feature [Source: Reproduced with permission of National Library of Medicine (NLM)].

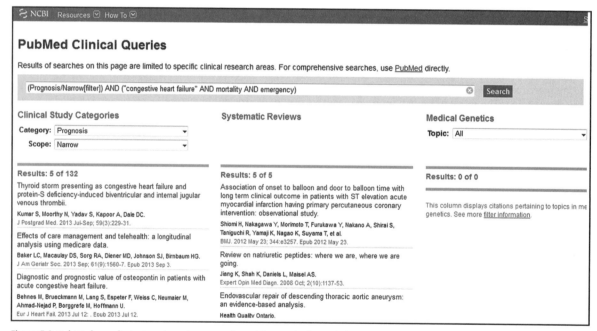

Figure 5.9 PubMed search strategy for primary studies – "Congestive heart failure" AND "mortality" AND emergency [Source: Reproduced with permission of National Library of Medicine (NLM)].

calls this one "Etiology"). In addition to the four primary question types, **PubMed** further breaks down Prognosis, by providing a fifth option specifically for "Clinical Prediction Guides". *Clinical Queries* also allows you to move from a "broad" to a "narrow" search strategy, which serves to improve the "specificity" of the results at the expense of "sensitivity".

Apart from "Clinical Study Categories", *Clinical Queries* also allows for limiting the search results to systematic reviews, which can be helpful once you have reached the "synthesis" stage of your search process as outlined in Part I.

An example of a search strategy for primary studies in PubMed Clinical Queries might look as shown in Figure 5.9.

A more exhaustive search would employ advanced techniques such as:

- Searching using subject heading terms and text words (words found in the title or abstract).
- Using synonyms for text word terms.
- Using "OR" to combine terms representing the same concept
- Using "AND" to find articles in which all of your concepts are present
- Using the truncation symbol (*) to find all variable word endings (e.g., death* would find death OR deaths).
- Using search limits to narrow down to your specific age group, gender, or study design.

The example in Figure 5.10 illustrates these techniques in PubMed.

Clinicaltrials.gov

Clinicaltrials.gov is a web site that was launched in 2000 and is maintained by the National Library of Medicine (NLM). The database was created in response to the Food and Drug Administration Modernization Act of 1997 (FDA MA) and subsequent amendments made in 2007, which, in an effort to reduce publication and selective outcome reporting bias (among other things), mandated that all controlled clinical investigations of FDA-regulated drugs or devices be registered. Its purpose is to maintain a publicly available catalog of both ongoing and completed clinical trials for the benefit of clinicians, researchers and laypeople alike (https://clinicaltrials.gov).

Clinicaltrials.gov is an invaluable resource for your "deep dive", in that it allows you to determine not only the extent to which your question has already been investigated, but also whether any related trials are ongoing, and at what stage of completion they are in. Its basic search should be approached in the same way as a typical PubMed key word search. However, it has supplemental user-friendly features, such as the ability to search by disease, intervention, sponsor or location, which help to make the searching experience more efficient.

Google

While Google© is unquestionably useful during Part I of the search process, its value when performing a "deep dive" remains unclear. Google Scholar©, in particular, has been praised by some as offering "one stop shopping" for literature retrieval needs, and has been shown to index the same articles included in systematic reviews performed using more

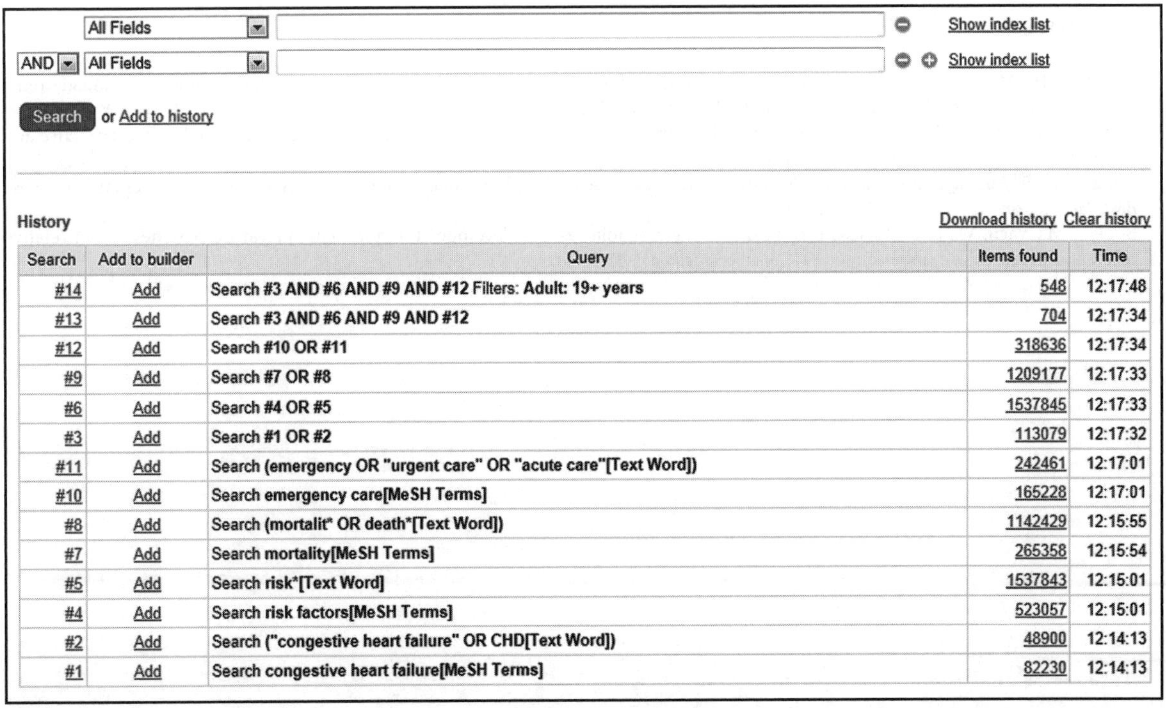

Search	Add to builder	Query	Items found	Time
#14	Add	Search #3 AND #6 AND #9 AND #12 Filters: Adult: 19+ years	548	12:17:48
#13	Add	Search #3 AND #6 AND #9 AND #12	704	12:17:34
#12	Add	Search #10 OR #11	318636	12:17:34
#9	Add	Search #7 OR #8	1209177	12:17:33
#6	Add	Search #4 OR #5	1537845	12:17:33
#3	Add	Search #1 OR #2	113079	12:17:32
#11	Add	Search (emergency OR "urgent care" OR "acute care"[Text Word])	242461	12:17:01
#10	Add	Search emergency care[MeSH Terms]	165228	12:17:01
#8	Add	Search (mortalit* OR death*[Text Word])	1142429	12:15:55
#7	Add	Search mortality[MeSH Terms]	265358	12:15:54
#5	Add	Search risk*[Text Word]	1537843	12:15:01
#4	Add	Search risk factors[MeSH Terms]	523057	12:15:01
#2	Add	Search ("congestive heart failure" OR CHD[Text Word])	48900	12:14:13
#1	Add	Search congestive heart failure[MeSH Terms]	82230	12:14:13

Figure 5.10 Exhaustive PubMed search using advanced techniques [Source: Reproduced with permission of National Library of Medicine (NLM)].

traditional searches across a variety of databases [3]. However, despite its high sensitivity, indexing that includes the breadth of both primary and gray literature, and ability to use Boolean operators, subsequent analyses have called into question the ability of Google Scholar© to yield precise, reproducible search results [4]. These limitations are largely due its changing content and relatively opaque "PageRank" algorithms. In general, Google Scholar© is an important tool in the armamentarium of the research scientist but cannot yet be relied upon exclusively, and at the expense of due diligence to prospectively identify the most relevant citations during this stage of the process.

Summary

Once you have completed your search and identified a handful of the most relevant articles, the final step is to schedule a meeting with your institutional research librarian, who will provide further guidance and help you to strategize regarding the next steps.

KEY POINTS

- Begin with a broad search using "summary" and "synthesis" type resources to get a sense for the research landscape in your area of interest, and narrow down your question based on the results.
- Once you have a specific question in mind, make a list of the words or phrases most representative of the concept of interest.
- Perform a more comprehensive search with a focus on original, primary studies, while utilizing database specific tricks to ensure a manageable number of results
- Always consult with a research librarian

References

1 Guyatt, G.H., Meade, M.O., Richardson, S., *et al.* (2008) What is the question? In: G.H. Guyatt, D. Rennie, and M.O. Meade (eds) *User's Guide to the Medical Literature: A Manual for Evidence-Based Clinical Practice*, 2nd edn, pp. 17–28, McGraw-Hill, New York, NY.
2 Silva, S.A. and Wyer, P.C. (2013) The roadmap: a blueprint for evidence literacy within a scientifically informed medical practice and learning model. *Eur J Pers Cent Healthc*, **1**(1):53.
3 Gehanno, J.F., Rollin, L., and Darmoni, S. (2013) Is the coverage of Google Scholar enough to be used alone for systematic reviews? *BMC Med Inform Decis Mak*, **13**(7):1–5.
4 Boeker, M., Vach, W., and Motschall, E. (2013) Google Scholar as a replacement for systematic literature searches: Good relative recall and precision are not enough. *BMC Med Res Methodol*, **13**:1–24.

CHAPTER 6

What do I need to know to get started with animal and basic science research?

George J. Shaw

Department of Emergency Medicine, University of Cincinnati, Cincinnati, OH, USA

> *"…I wish my experiment would work for more than 2 days in row!!!"*
>
> Fellow Graduate Student

This chapter is written with a broad audience in mind. Firstly it is that of the newly-qualified Emergency Medicine faculty member who either has a PhD in a basic science or who has a undertaken a research fellowship to obtain bench skills in basic science. This type of individual has started on the road to becoming a Principal Investigator (PI) and having a laboratory with their name on it; this is much easier if you already have a good working knowledge of the experimental skills and techniques needed to conduct the research you have in mind [1]. So if you want to be a basic science PI, step 1 is to get some experience in it, either through formal coursework (Master's, PhD, or similar), or working in someone else's laboratory. The second type of individual is the clinician, resident, or even medical student who is interested in carrying out a basic science project, but may not want to pursue this as a career. Both of these audiences are addressed in this chapter.

Developing a basic science research career in Emergency Medicine (EM) is a viable career option for the appropriately trained newly-qualified EM faculty member. Both clinical and basic science research projects are, typically, hypothesis driven, strive to obtain useful data, and then attempt to make some sense (sometimes or even usually failing) of the data. As a result, most EM residents have some idea of what these terms mean, and likely some idea of how to carry out a clinical trial. The skills needed to perform a clinical trial carry over quite well to basic science and vice versa.

Conducting basic science or animal research requires the following:

- Laboratory space.
- Equipment and supplies.
- Choosing the right model.
- Laboratory workers (graduate students, residents, laboratory technicians, postdoctoral fellows…).
- Mentors and collaborators.
- Funding.

Laboratory space

In the beginning of your career, your laboratory needs to be a designated space with appropriate utilities. You will likely need to negotiate for this up front with your Chair, as it can be difficult to get. There is not a lot of unused laboratory space in a typical academic medical center. This sounds obvious, but you need to have enough room for your equipment, your supplies, and for your people. Put up a name plate for it; pretty typical is to use your last name and call it, for example, "The Smith Lab." This promotes a sense of identity and ownership for your laboratory and the people in it.

Make sure it has the appropriate utilities; if you are doing polymerase chain reactions, you need access to distilled water. If you are working with ultrasound, you need lots of power strips. You will absolutely need Internet access;

Doing Research in Emergency and Acute Care: Making Order Out of Chaos, First Edition. Edited by Michael P. Wilson, Kama Z. Guluma, and Stephen R. Hayden.

this is how people (including you) get and read scientific papers. It should also have a few desks and some bookcases for your laboratory personnel; this gives them a place to work and to keep their stuff. Also, there is no such thing as too many electrical outlets. In addition, if you are performing animal experiments or cell culture work, you need: (i) a fume hood (critical for cell culture, and animal studies, re: perfusions, tissue post-processing, preps, inhalational anesthesia, etc.); (ii) access to a vacuum line; (iii) access to an oxygen source is convenient if in a medical center environment (otherwise have to change out O_2 tanks); (iv) an indoor walk from a vivarium (it is always awkward – and dangerous – to walk between buildings with experimental animals). If possible, and it may not be, the laboratory should be fairly close to your designated office. That way, your people can find you, and vice versa.

Equipment and supplies

Obtaining equipment can be easier than you think. A major source of equipment can be a mentor or collaborator who is discontinuing an experiment. The equipment used in that experiment can be "lent" to you, typically in return for an agreement that their students can use it to get data in the future if needed. Also, medical researchers are migratory and people move their laboratories from one institution to another all the time. That 800 lb. vibration-isolation table is probably something they really do not want to ship, and they wouldd rather see it used productively than not. I have found very useful equipment just roaming the halls after someone either moves or downsizes their laboratory. This is called 'dumpster diving,' and is an accepted procurement technique in basic science. It also works for laboratory office furniture.

From an administrative standpoint, major laboratory equipment belongs to the department that the investigator was affiliated with. Therefore, it is good practice (and good manners) to let that department know that you would like to "borrow" that piece of equipment. After obtaining agreement and permission to borrow it, I usually draft a letter to the Chair of said department indicating (i) what I am borrowing, (ii) what it will be used for, and (iii) where it will be located. When that Department is audited by the University bean counters, they can then easily find and point to where their old equipment is.

Used equipment can also be found on the internet, but you have to be careful. Firstly, you may have no way of knowing whether it is in working order or not, and getting it fixed can cost as much as buying it new. Secondly, many university procurement offices have problems ordering equipment from an internet-based vendor, so be sure to check the procedure accounting for this with whoever places orders at your institution. Finally, laboratory equipment can suffer the same aging phenomenon that computers and software do; after some period of time, the manufacturer will no longer support it. This makes it riskier to get really old equipment that you may not be able to get serviced or repaired.

Supplies are usually one of the smallest parts of your budget, but without them you cannot get any data. The only exception is medications; certain medications – especially if in a drug class that is under patent – can be quite costly and it is best to secure a supply agreement from a drug manufacture if testing a drug. It is a good idea to delegate keeping track of supplies and laboratory ordering to someone in your laboratory to avoid running out at inauspicious times, like the day after your block of four night shifts. Many institutions mandate inventory control, especially of hazardous materials, so you will need to know the location and amount of every hazardous reagent in your laboratory and have a centralized location for the Material Safety Data Sheet (MSDS) pertaining to each. In addition, proper disposal containers will have to be on hand and proper disposal procedures will have to be adhered to. The use of radioactive materials will almost assuredly require special training (and even more special disposal procedures), so if you have a choice as to whether or not to use them, choose wisely (hint, hint). Also, do not forget the more trivial supplies, such as gloves and reagents; it is hard for your personnel to run experiments without them. And although I said that you should delegate supply ordering to someone in your laboratory, it is a good idea to know how much is going out the door. I set limits on purchases for my laboratory; over a certain threshold I need to at least know about it. For example, if the order is less than $200, it can just be purchased, if its $200–1000, I should know in advance. If it is greater than $1000, I need to be involved in the decision to purchase. In addition, the PI must be involved in major capital purchases; most universities set this as a piece of equipment costing more than $5000. Involve your Department's business personnel early in such large purchases; they often must be "bid out," particularly in state institutions.

Choosing the right model

Choosing the right model, either *in vitro* (test tube) or *in vivo* (animal model), is a difficult but important decision. Federal funding agencies, particularly the National Institutes of Health (NIH), have recently placed more of an emphasis on the "translational" or "bench-to-bedside" aspects of medical research. As a result, grant review committees typically want an animal model in your grants, or at least an approach that can lead to verification of your approach in an animal model. However, the use of an animal model results in a whole new level of scientific and regulatory effort for the nascent PI. In most universities, the IACUC (Institutional Animal Care and Use Committee) reviews and approves or disapproves grant protocols that use animal models. In addition, the expense of such models is not trivial.

Overall, there are fairly well-defined animal models for various disease processes. For example, research questions about cardiovascular physiology can be addressed quite well in porcine, sheep, and canine models. Questions about toxicology, pharmacology and sepsis have been addressed in the literature in small animal models, such as rats, mice, and rabbits. Finally, various genetically altered rat models are readily available for drug and genetic disease studies. It is likely not a good idea to try and develop a brand new animal model for your research question. In my experience, such an approach leads to a third of the grant reviewers accepting your model, a third hating it, and a third feeling lukewarm about it. A better idea is to collaborate with someone who already has an animal model in place, and collaborate with them.

Laboratory workers

These are the personnel who perform the day-to-day work of your laboratory. It is a common mistake, especially early in one's career, to think that you, yourself, can get the data you need. After all, your Chair has you working only 24 clinical hours per week – that is 4–5 days that can be used to get data. WRONG!! This will not work on a long-term basis, and it has to do with the fact that your job as an up-and-coming Principal Investigator (PI) is a very different one from what you have been used to as a resident, graduate student, or even postdoctoral fellow (postdoc). Your new job is to: (i) devise and accomplish the overall scientific goals of the laboratory, (ii) ensure that things are running smoothly, and (iii) keep things funded. You will need people in your laboratory on a full-time basis to enable you to do all of this.

The next question is "who should I hire and where do I find them?" In the beginning of establishing your laboratory, undergraduate student workers may be your best bet. Many universities have cooperative education programs whereby undergraduate students can get work or research experience. Many of these individuals want to go to medical school and working in your laboratory can help them build their resume for this. It will not hurt their chances to have an abstract or a publication to show the Admissions Committee either, so be generous with the credit. In my experience, these students can be very dedicated, hard working, and a major asset to the laboratory. The downside is that it is unusual to find an undergraduate that will have experience in running your particular experiments, so training for them on your part might be needed.

After a few years of doing basic science at your institution, you will start getting asked to join other Departments as "secondary faculty." Joining these other departments is helpful for you and your laboratory for a multitude of reasons, but, very importantly, can provide access to graduate students. These are individuals who are working on obtaining a Master's or PhD, and need supervised research experience (and data) to do this. This can work out very well for both parties, the student gets a laboratory to work in and a dissertation supervisor, you as the PI get a dedicated individual working in your laboratory and getting data.

Keep in mind that there is more of a commitment on your part to a graduate student than to a student worker; after all, the graduate student is working to get an advanced degree. It is your responsibility as their advisor to make sure they are on track in their research and getting what they need from you and your laboratory. In addition, you are making a commitment to keep the student funded for potentially three years or more. Be sure to take these responsibilities into account prior to hiring a graduate student; this is only fair to them and to your secondary department.

A postdoctoral fellow is an individual who has completed their PhD but wants additional experience in order to transition to the role of a tenure-track faculty member. The completion of such a fellowship, typically 2–3 years or so, is very common in the basic sciences prior to becoming a tenure-track Assistant Professor. A fellow acts more as an independent investigator than a graduate student. In larger laboratories, they may be responsible for the day-to-day supervision of the graduate students in addition to their project. If you have the funding, they can be an invaluable asset to your laboratory as they can accomplish more than a graduate student or student worker. Postdocs are less interested in working in their exact particular field than in finding an interesting project in someone's laboratory. If you are contemplating a new research endeavor, a postdoctoral fellow can really help get it "up and running."

As with a graduate student, there are academic responsibilities on your part towards a postdoc. They wish to advance their career and to be able to demonstrate to future academic employers that they can perform the functions of a tenure-track faculty member. Therefore, they want (and need) publications and presentation opportunities.

They also need experience in grant writing. It is incumbent upon you as their advisor to provide such opportunities, and to make sure they stay on track in their research.

Mentors and collaborators

A mentor is an invaluable asset to your development as a basic scientist. A mentor is a senior, well-established investigator, who takes a personal interest in you and your career, and is willing to provide guidance along the way. Although there are an increasing number of senior PIs in emergency medicine, there are still very few basic scientists in our field. It is, therefore, likely that you will have to go outside the specialty to find a mentor. You should try and find someone willing to take on this role for you as early as possible in your career.

Your basic science mentor can provide guidance and advice, and early on may be willing to provide initial projects and laboratory space. I got started with my mentor by working on a specific project in her laboratory during my elective time as a fourth year resident. This resulted in several joint abstracts and publications, and ultimately several grants. This was an invaluable experience, and really got my basic science career going. We still collaborate (going on about 14 years) on projects of mutual interest.

The mentor–mentee relationship is a two-way street. Both parties must benefit, or the relationship is not helpful for anyone's career. Your mentor can help you get your basic science career off the ground by aiding you with laboratory space early on, collaboration with their ongoing projects, and helping you get your first grant funding. In return, you can assist your mentor by providing access to clinical data and samples, engaging in advising and clinical shadowing experiences for your mentor's students and postdocs, and being willing to give basic science lectures and presentations for their undergraduate and graduate courses. Such a relationship will also accelerate the progress of your joint research projects, and the ongoing development of both labs.

Although the term seems obvious, collaborators are other scientists with whom you conduct research. In basic science, such individuals may have useful measurement techniques or models that can help your joint projects. For example, in my laboratory we make liposomes as a method to package and deliver thrombolytic medications. An important parameter to know for these preparations is the diameter of the liposomes [2]; they have to be small enough to flow through the smallest capillaries (approximately 8–10 microns), but large enough to contain a reasonably useful amount of thrombolytic medication. We do not have the ability to determine the size of these liposomes, but my collaborator has a "zetasizer." Without going into too much detail, a zetasizer is a device that measures the diameter of small particles suspended in a fluid by determining their "electrophoretic mobility," or how they move in the fluid when an electric field is applied. Rather than use precious grant dollars to obtain this very expensive device, and then have to learn how to use it (not trivial), we ask our collaborators to measure the diameter of these liposomes for us. This yields a joint publication and they get to use our IX-71 Olympus inverting microscope in return. In summary, finding and developing collaborations is a very useful way to augment your laboratory's science and to come up with new projects that may help the both of you.

Funding

This topic is covered in detail in Chapter 36, but some aspects as they apply to the basic science researcher are discussed here. Firstly, especially early in your career, there is no such thing as a "too small" grant. Look around your institution for grants for early investigators. Getting one of these funded is a great way to buy some equipment, hire a laboratory technician, and get things off the ground. Also, "success breeds success" for grants. If you establish a track record of writing and obtaining some small grants, reviewers will be better inclined to help you get bigger ones.

Secondly, plan for the long term. Your project just may have started, and you might be getting some data, but it is not too early to start writing the next grant. The NIH grant process takes at least a year, and usually two (or more), so you should be writing the next proposal now. In addition, you will need letters from collaborators and colleagues for that NIH proposal, and these can take some time to get. Earlier is better.

Thirdly, do not feel you must stay rigidly within your particular research area. In the current funding environment, it helps to be flexible about what you are studying. This is something of a balancing act; you do not want to go too far from your area of expertise as this would not be credible with reviewers, but you do need to keep the laboratory going. Also, consider applying to other sources of funding in addition to NIH [3], such as private foundations and industry.

"So you want to do a single preclinical study?" An approach for the ad hoc investigator

I am a firm believer that doing or being involved in a basic science project can be a lot of fun. In my career, I have had great ideas for projects come from fellow faculty, residents, medical student, nurses, respiratory therapists, and undergraduates. So, if you do not do basic science for a living, but want to do a project in it, go for it!

The quickest way to get started is similar to the advice I have for the new PI; find out who works in your subject area (or close to it), and go talk to them. On average, this is a fairly congenial and democratic bunch and they are more than willing to discuss their research, their field, and your idea. Such discussion will also help in turning your proposed project or idea into a testable hypothesis. This is a crucial step in the formulation of any project. Once you have a hypothesis, you can figure out what kind of data you need to answer the research question. Is it mortality data? Is it physiologic information? This information will also help in figuring out who to collaborate with and the type of preclinical model that would be useful. I strongly encourage collaboration for the ad hoc investigator; it is easier to get the work done and most PI's welcome collaboration. Usually, they have lots of ideas and not enough people to help.

KEY POINTS

- Get formal or informal basic science training in the experimental techniques you will use.
- Do not forget to negotiate for laboratory space.
- Hire someone to work in the laboratory full-time as soon as possible in your career.
- Find a basic science mentor, and remember it is a two-way street.
- Building collaborations is a GREAT way to extend your laboratory's capabilities.
- NO grant is too small … small ones can buy things, too, and help your CV.

References

1 Ley, T.J. and Rosenberg, L.E. (2005) *The physician-scientist career pipeline in 2005: build it, and they will come. JAMA*, **294**(11):1343–5131.

2 Shaw, G.J., Meunier, J.M., Huang, S.L., *et al.* (2012) *Ultrasound-enhanced thrombolysis with tPA-loaded echogenic liposomes. Thromb Res*, 2009. **124**(3): 306–310.

3 Yang, O.O. (2012) *Guide to Effective Grant Writing*, 2nd edn. Springer, New York.

CHAPTER 7

The IRB process: How to write up a human studies protocol

Christian Tomaszewski

Department of Emergency Medicine, University of California San Diego Health Sciences, San Diego, CA, USA

Introduction

If you are going to carry out clinical research, then you will have to deal with an Institutional Review Board (IRB). Your local IRB reviews all research involving human subjects while acting as an advocate for subjects' rights and welfare. Approaching the committee can be quite daunting and even intimidating. You will have to convince a group of five or more physician scientists, along with a lay community member, that they should let you subject a group of volunteers or patients to a research intervention. You will have to show them that risks are minimal compared to the potential benefit to be garnered answering your worthwhile research question.

Because of unethical practices from the past, including heinous "research" from Nazi Germany, we now have a systematized way to approve ethical human research. The tipping point in the United States was the Tuskegee Study conducted in Georgia from 1932 to 1972 by the US Public Health Service ([1]; Chapter 8). Hundreds of African American males with syphilis were not given access to penicillin, even when it was accepted treatment in 1947 and wives and children contracted the disease. Public outcry focused on the lack of informed consent and undue influence of the subjects. In response, the US government established regulations for IRBs in 1974 to protect human subjects in research studies [2].

In 1981, Federal policies for protection of human subjects were codified as the common rule within the Health and Human Service regulation known as 45 CFR (Code of Federal Regulation) part 46 [3]. This rule of ethics applies to government funded research in the United States, but almost all academic institutions hold their researchers to the same standard regardless of funding. Thus, as an investigator you will be expected to comply with your local IRB in determining appropriate consent. The IRB in turn is responsible for review of your research as well as record keeping. Failure in compliance can result in the federal Office for Protection from Research Risks coming and suspending all federally funded research at your home institution [4].

Key issues

So you have an idea for a clinical study and you want IRB approval. In addition to writing up your research plan, you will have to approach your local IRB for permission to do the study. As you fill out their forms, you will need to be cognizant of the following to have a successfully approved ethical study:

- What goes to the IRB?
- What studies are exempt from IRB Review?
- What are the elements of informed consent?
- Are you avoiding undue influence or coercion of subjects?
- Do you have vulnerable subjects in your study?
- Can you compensate subjects for participating in your research project?
- Do you need a Health Insurance Portability Accountability Act (HIPAA) authorization to do research?
- Can you do actual research without a HIPAA authorization?
- Are you going to have a placebo and, if so, how do you justify one group not getting standard of care?

Doing Research in Emergency and Acute Care: Making Order Out of Chaos, First Edition. Edited by Michael P. Wilson, Kama Z. Guluma, and Stephen R. Hayden.

- What about true emergency research where you need an exception to informed consent?
- How should investigators address the possibility of incidental findings with potential clinical significance in their study subjects?
- Do IRBs feel I need any special training to do research?
- Can I start my study after the IRB receives all my paperwork?

What goes to the IRB?

IRBs are entrusted with protecting the rights of human research subjects. You must submit any research or investigation that involves humans. This is particularly true if your intent is to contribute to generalizable knowledge through presentation at scientific meetings or publication. If you are not clear on whether what you are doing is human research or not, it never hurts to contact your local IRB and review your project with them.

What studies are exempt from IRB review?

Case reports, case series, and quality improvement (QI) or quality assurance (QA) projects are not generally submitted to IRBs. For case reports and reviews, you are really doing a minimal risk review of medical records after the fact. For QI/QA, the purpose is to improve hospital performance without increasing risk to patients, except perhaps loss of confidentiality, which is a minimal risk. It is not designed for publication, although certainly later you may want to publish your results and most medical journals will require proof of IRB exemption. In that case you should submit the study to the IRB.

IRBs also recognize certain categories of research that are so low risk that they can be expedited and done without informed consent. According to the "Common Rule" 45 CFR 46.101(b), potential exempt categories include [3]:

- Prospective educational research.
- Noninvasive routine procedures.
- Surveys.
- Research involving the collection or study of existing data, documents, records, pathological specimens, or diagnostic specimens.

However, there are several caveats with regard to these exemptions. First of all, you need to make sure that you do not include vulnerable subjects, for example, pregnant women, prisoners, children, or decisionally-impaired subjects. The study, by design, must be minimal risk. To be exempt, you cannot collect personal health identifiers (PHIs). A PHI is defined as individually identifiable health information created or received by healthcare providers regarding the physical or mental condition of an individual. Demographics such as name, address, medical record number, birth date, and full face photos are obvious PHIs. Things like zip code (<20 000 population) and older age extremes (>89 years) are included if the population subset is so small that the patient could be identified. To comply with the Health Insurance Portability and Accountability Act, Privacy Rule, the confidentiality of all PHI must be maintained throughout the research and thereafter as well. Figure 7.1 shows an algorithm for deciding if IRB approval is needed.

What are the elements of informed consent?

For almost all studies, especially prospective, you will need to obtain informed consent from each of your subjects. As per the Office of Human Research Protections, your informed consent form, at the minimum, should include the following [3]:

- Statement that the study involves research.
- Purpose of the research.
- Expected duration of participation.
- Identification of procedures that are experimental.
- Risks to subject.
- Benefits to subject, if any.
- Alternative course of treatment, if any.
- Description of how confidentiality of records will be maintained.
- Compensation or treatment available if injury occurs.
- Whom to contact for questions.
- Statement that participation is voluntary and no penalty for nonparticipation or withdrawal.
- Number of subjects in study .

The informed consent form should be written in lay language, at the eighth grade level or below. You should definitely avoid medical jargon as you detail what the subject should expect in what is clearly an investigational study.

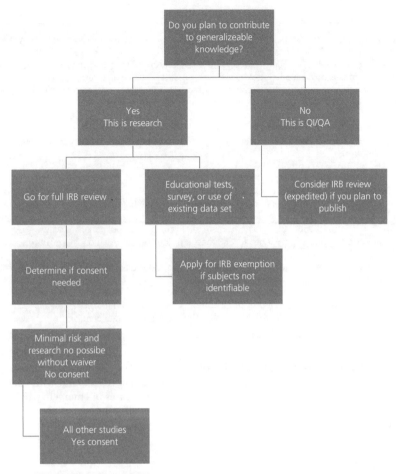

Figure 7.1 Algorithm for seeking IRB approval for human subject research.

Are you avoiding undue influence or coercion of subjects?

It is common to get medical students and fellow healthcare employees to enroll in your study. They are convenient and you might think that they know what they are getting into. One such case involved a 24-year old healthy laboratory technician named Ellen Roche who died after participating as a healthy volunteer in an asthma study (Box 7.1). One issue raised if using a volunteer from the same division, especially a subordinate, could have led Ellen to be unduly influenced to participate and take risks she normally would not have taken on her own [4].

In the case of Ms. Roche, she was offered $365 for completion of an asthma study at her home institution that killed her. Does that represent an undue inducement? Namely, was she offered goods, in this case money, that were excessively attractive and resulted in her doing things she would normally have objected to, based on risk or fundamental values? Remember, this was basic science research on a healthy subject with risks, but no potential for benefit. This is very different from a therapeutic trial where ill patients might have some hope of benefit. Some ethicists noted that because Roche was an employee at the university she may have felt coerced or unduly induced to volunteer.

Along with undue influence, you will also need to avoid coercing subjects into your study. Coercion is the presence of threat or harm if a subject refuses to participate. Educators deal with this issue all the time when they try to enroll their own students in research. If class credit is offered, most offer an alternative non-research participatory path for the same credit. To avoid coercion, just make sure that you are not enrolling direct reports, that is, people who work for you or depend on you for an evaluation or grades.

Box 7.1 The Ellen Roche story.

Ellen Roche was a 24-year old technician at the John Hopkins University asthma and allergy center [5]. She was asked to participate in a study looking at airway reactivity. One of the drugs used in the study, hexamethonium, had been withdrawn years earlier by the US Food and Drug Administration (FDA) due to efficacy and safety concerns. In the study it was being used to suppress bronchial protective effects of deep inspiration in healthy subjects. On 4 May 2001, she received hexamethonium 1 gm by inhalation. The next day she developed cough and dyspnea, which over the first week was accompanied by pulmonary infiltrate and reduction in FEV1. By 12 May 2001 she was in the ICU, intubated, and suffered from both ARDS and bilateral pneumothoraces. She died on 2 June 2001 with refractory hypotension and multiorgan failure. Ellen Roche was a healthy volunteer that had nothing to gain from this study.

The Office for Human Research Protection investigated and accused the Hopkins IRB for failing to take proper precautions. Highlights of their findings were:

- The investigator did not inform the IRB that the first subject (Ellen was the third) developed a cough and dyspnea for one week after the hexamethonium exposure. IRBs expect that all significant adverse effects will be reported in a timely manner.
- The consent form did not mention that the drug was not a routine medication but rather an experimental, FDA unapproved drug.
- Under potential risks in the consent form there was no mention of potential pulmonary toxicity. In fact, there were older studies in the literature which were missed, suggesting that hexamethonium could cause pulmonary toxicity.
- The study was not reviewed at a properly convened full IRB meeting. Hopkins had relied on an executive subcommittee to approve the study.
- Although Ellen worked at the same laboratory as the researchers, there was the perception that she may have been coerced into the study, although the university concluded she had not.

The final result of the Roche case was that John Hopkins University was not allowed to resume research activities until 22 July. And, at that time, studies with greater than minimal risk to subjects were still suspended pending further review [6].

Do you have vulnerable subjects in your study?

Ellen Roche, as a research subject, may have been vulnerable. As a direct report, and with coercion, she may have exhibited decreased capacity to make the right decision. There are many cases in emergency research where you may come in contact with vulnerable subjects. The most notable are pregnant women, children and prisoners. All of the following can also be vulnerable, depending on the study:

- Embryos and fetuses.
- Mentally disabled individuals.
- Subjects in emergency situations.
- Educationally disadvantaged subjects.
- Economically disadvantaged subjects.
- Marginalized social groups.
- Individuals with incurable or fatal diseases.

If you include such subjects, you will be required to take extra safeguards and paperwork. You must make sure that they truly can make an *informed* decision in consenting to your study. If the study includes individuals with reduced capacity or decision-making impairments, some form of cognitive prescreening may be useful. Alternatively, if the patient is completely incapacitated, you may use a legally authorized representative as in surrogate consent (Box 7.2). It is good to keep in mind that consent capacity is a spectrum and, depending on the complexity and risks involved, you may have to increase your safeguards depending on the patient and the risks involved.

Can you compensate subjects for participating in your research project?

If you decide to compensate subjects, whether they be healthy subjects or patients, the IRB will look closely at your compensation scheme. Compensation can be money or gifts given in remuneration for time and inconvenience for participation. Although not necessary, if you have money, especially in a grant, it is nice to share that with subjects. Reasonable inducements are especially useful if you are worried about patients and/or subjects returning for follow up. Compensation for their travel is certainly fair. But make sure you do not make such compensation excessive because the IRB may consider it undue influence, which could cloud a subject's decision to participate. Also, make sure it is fair. If the subject completes half of the visits, they should at least be entitled to half of their promised travel money.

Box 7.2 The pediatric seizure study.

One of the most vulnerable subjects in research is a patient suffering from an emergency life-threatening condition. Toss in the fact that they are unconscious, and children, and you have a potential nightmare in attempting to get informed consent. This is exactly what researchers faced when they sought to test the efficacy of lorazepam compared to diazepam for status epilepticus in children [7].

To address the consent issue, the investigators decided to invoke the Exception from Informed Consent for Emergency Research regulation, 21 CFR 50.24. However, this did not absolve the researchers from ultimately getting consent. Instead, they did their homework. The researchers approached patients with known epilepsy and their parents a priori in the clinic in order to get consent. If a child showed up in status epilepticus that was not already consent, they would attempt to get consent from parents or surrogates at the emergency visit. For the few cases where the unconsented child presented alone, they would instead get consent from the parents as soon as they arrived. This meant that some patients were entered without consent. This was obviated by their community outreach and education plan along with oversight from the FDA, an independent ethics panel, safety monitors, and, ultimately, the individual IRBs.

In the end, the study took four years of hard work at 11 centers to enter 273 patients. The result was a manuscript in the *JAMA* that showed equipoise between both treatments. In this age of intermittent drug shortages, it is nice to know that either drug works well.

Do you need a HIPAA authorization for research?

If the research involves review of person-identifiable medical records, or the study results in new information that is added to medical records (such a test of a new diagnostic or therapeutic agent or device), then it is using or creating PHIs. This makes it subject to the Health Insurance Portability Accountability Act (HIPAA) Privacy Rule provisions. A signed HIPAA authorization is required in consenting study participants. Although federal regulations allow the HIPAA language to be included in the consent, some states, such as California, require a separate "stand-alone" HIPAA authorization form.

Can you do actual research without a HIPAA authorization?

If you are not doing prospective research on actual patients, but just want to review medical records, then you will need a waiver of HIPAA authorization, also known as a waiver of consent. This HIPAA waiver may be also useful if you trying to screen medical records looking for prospective patients. Per the Common Rule, in order to use PHIs in either of these instances, you have to me*et al.*l of the following criteria:

- The use or disclosure of PHIs involves no more than minimal risk.
- Granting of waiver will not adversely affect privacy rights and welfare of the individuals.
- The project could not practicably be conducted without a waiver and the use of PHIs.
- The privacy risks are reasonable relative to the anticipated benefits of research.
- A plan to protect identifiers from improper use and disclosure.
- A plan to destroy the identifiers at the earliest opportunity.
- Written assurances that PHIs will not be re-used or disclosed for other purposes.
- Whenever appropriate, subjects will be provided with additional pertinent information after participation.

If all of these conditions apply, then most IRBs will grant you the waiver to complete your chart review without consenting patients.

Are you going to have a placebo and, if so, how do you justify one group not getting standard of care?

If you decide to have a placebo arm in your study, you are to be commended for adding a valid comparison. However, be careful because there are additional risks in using placebos. Your study may be invalid clinically because you did not compare your treatment to standard of care. Also, you may place your subjects at risk if they have to avoid routine medication to be in the placebo arm. For example, many asthma studies with a placebo arm will include close monitoring and rescue therapy especially for the control group. In psychiatric studies, there is the very real danger of self-harm to those subjects randomized to placebo arms. My advice is to avoid placebo-controlled trials when using patients, unless there really is no viable current standard of care. For volunteer studies, you are certainly encouraged to use a placebo arm to insure more robust science.

What about true emergency research where you need an exception to informed consent?

Foreign countries are currently taking the lead in emergency research. For example in 2009, the French actually randomized 655 patients who needed emergent intubation to ketamine versus etomidate [8]. If the patient was incapacitated and no surrogate was available, they enrolled patients without prior consent. Technically, we cannot do that in the United States except through community assent (Box 7.2 details a successful example). The FDA Final Rule 21 CFR 50.24 [9] allows for enrollment of patients without prior consent for emergency research, but strict criteria must be met:

- There must be a life-threatening condition requiring immediate intervention.
- Available treatments are not satisfactory.
- Obtaining informed consent from the subjects or surrogates is not feasible.
- You cannot pre-identify subjects.

Although using this rule allows you to proceed without immediate informed consent, you still have homework in terms of additional protections for your subjects:

- Consult with representatives of and ensure public disclosure to the community in which the study will be conducted regarding risks, benefits, and need for waiver.
- Public disclosure after completion of the study to let the community know the results.
- Independent data monitoring committee for oversight.

This is a very costly and time consuming process, usually involving advertisements and public hearings. And even then, there have been untoward outcomes (Box 7.3).

How should investigators address the possibility of incidental findings with potential clinical significance in their study subjects?

In the course of your research, you may find something incidental in your subjects. For instance, an MRI in a cognitive study may reveal a mass. Such apparent medical abnormalities may have clinical implications that are unrelated to the topic under study. Examples include:

- Blood study showing an potential untreated infection or even anemia.
- Mental status screening indicates a serious psychiatric condition.
- Brain imaging reveals a structural abnormality.

Although there are no policies on how to handle incidental findings, one should be prepared to deal with these contingencies. Preemptively, a plan to address such findings can be included your research plan and even in the consent form.

Do IRBs feel I need any special training to do research?

Most IRBs now require completion of the appropriate training in human research protection. One of the most popular is the Collaborative Institutional Training Initiative (CITI) training module provided on-line by the University of Miami (www.citiprogram.org). The CITI Program's Human Subjects Research content includes two tracks, one with a biomedical focus and the other designed for the social, behavioral, and educational disciplines, each of which covers the historical development of human subjects' protections as well as current information on regulatory and ethical issues. In addition, most IRBs require training regarding the research aspects of HIPAA, particularly if you are working with patients.

Box 7.3 The artificial hemoglobin story.

In the 1990s, the United States had issues with guaranteeing the safety of the nation's blood supply. So researchers turned to substitutes that were based on hemoglobin but produced aseptically. The first trial with a product known as Polyheme resulted in increased mortality in the experimental group versus the control real blood group [10]. It appears that the problem with these products is that free hemoglobin can accumulate and cause hypertension along with direct renal damage. However, the resulting public outcry had nothing to do with science. The bigger issue was that subjects were assigned to the artificial hemoglobin group without their consent. Public Citizen, a consumer rights advocacy group, sued the FDA questioning the safety of these studies [11]. As a direct result of such trials, both IRBs and the FDA have increased scrutiny of these types of studies, ensuring that all criteria for exception to informed consent in emergency research are followed in future studies.

Can I start my study after the IRB receives all my paperwork?

Obviously you cannot start your study until the IRB approves it. You may be lucky on your first pass and get approval pending a few changes or clarifications. Alternatively, if there are issues, they may defer or even reject it. Do not despair. Read your letter and call to clarify the issues. You can still resubmit, provided you address these issues. You may either make the required changes in your informed consent or research protocol, or give a reasonable explanation as to why you disagree with their conclusions.

Once you start your study, remember that you are not done with the IRB. They can audit you at any time. Additionally, if you decided later to make a changes in your study, you must supply an amendment for their approval. Also, if you plan to go beyond a year in terms of data collection or analysis, you will need to go back to the IRB for continuing approval.

Conclusion

Yes, research can be fun and rewarding, especially if it advances improvements in emergency care, but you as a researcher will need to keep your patient's rights in mind. As you fill out the IRB paperwork, keep in mind the Common Rule that encompasses the following requirements:

- Respect for persons – ensure a complete and concise consent form.
- Beneficence – make sure the benefits of your research outweigh any risks.
- Justice – protect your research subjects, especially vulnerable ones, from coercion.

The goal of the IRB is to protect your subjects. With their help, you will have an ethical worthwhile project, helping to insure sound publishable research.

KEY POINTS

- Quality improvement projects do not need to go the IRB if your intent is not to contribute to generalizable knowledge, but if you ultimately publish the journal may require it.

- For consent forms, make sure you clarify risks and alternatives, including the option of receiving treatment outside the study, in lay language.

- Make sure, if applicable, you address protection of vulnerable subjects, including those that could be decisionally impaired or feel coerced into participating in your study.

- You will need a waiver of HIPAA authorization if you want to data "snoop" in medical charts for enrolling subjects or collecting data.

- In emergency research always try to get informed consent from the subject or use a surrogate, otherwise you will have to consider pre-identifying subjects or more costly community assent.

References

1 Jones, J.H. (1993) *Bad Blood: The Tuskegee Syphilis Experiment*. Free Press, New York.
2 US Department of Health, Education and Welfare (1979) *The Belmont Report: Ethical Principles and Guidelines for the Protection of Human Subjects of Research*. www.hhs.gov/ohrp/policy/belmont.html (last accessed 29 April 2015).
3 United States Department of Health & Human Services (2009) *Code of Federal Regulations: Title 45 Public Welfare, Part 46 Protection of Human Subjects*. http://www.hhs.gov/ohrp/humansubjects/guidance/45cfr46.html (last accessed 29 April 2015).
4 Steinbrook, R. (2002) Protecting research subjects – The crisis at Johns Hopkins. *N Engl J Med*, **346**:716–720.
5 Becker, L.C., Bower, R.G., Faden, R., *et al.* (2001) Report of internal investigation in to the death of a volunteer research subject. http://www.hopkinsmedicine.org/press/2001/JULY/report_of_internal_investigation.htm (last accessed 29 April 2015).
6 Savulescu, J. and Spriggs, M. (2002) Current controversy: The hexamethonium asthma study and the death of anormal volunteer in research. *J Med Ethics*, **28**:3–4.

7 Chamberlain, J.M., Okada, P., Holsti, M., *et al.* (2014) Lorazepam vs diazepam for pediatric status epilepticus: a randomized clinical trial. *JAMA*, **311**(16):1652–1660.

8 Jabre, P., Combes, X., Lapostolle, F., *et al.* (2009). Etomidate versus ketamine for rapid sequence intubation in acutely ill patients: a multicentre randomised controlled trial. *Lancet*, **374**(9686), 293–300.

9 United States Department of Health & Human Services (2013) *Guidance for Institutional Review Boards, Clinical Investigators, and Sponsors: Exemptions from Informed Consent Requirements for Emergency Research: March 2011 (updated April 2013)*. http://www.fda.gov/downloads/RegulatoryInformation/Guidances/UCM249673.pdf (last accessed 29 April 2015).

10 Moore, E.E., Moore, F.A., Fabian, T.C., *et al.* (2009) Human polymerized hemoglobin for the treatment of hemorrhagic shock when blood is unavailable: The USA multicenter trial. *J Am Coll Surg*, **208** (1):1–13.

11 Natanson, C., Kern, S.J., Lurie, P., *et al.* (2008). Cell-free hemoglobin-based blood substitutes and risk of myocardial infarction and death. *JAMA*, **299**(19), 2304–2312.

CHAPTER 8

Ethics in research: How to collect data ethically

Nas Rafi and Brian Snyder

UCSD Emergency Department, San Diego, CA, USA

So you have formulated a good research question, done the background literature search to arrive at its relevance and ability to be answered, but did you think about whether or not your research project was ethical? Nowadays that is a normal question to ask, but, as you will see, it was not always the case.

What does it mean to conduct ethical research and why is it important?

> *"I came up with a great research idea that's never been done before and is a very relevant question: What percentage of patients with an acute MI will survive without any medical intervention?"*
>
> An enthusiastic resident researcher who has yet to consider the importance of ethics in research

Ethical considerations are necessary when conducting research on human beings. To understand why, we are going to review:

- The philosophical foundation of experimental research.
- Historical case studies that have shaped how human research is conducted.
- The establishment of the Belmont Principles.
- The ethical standards to which we are held today as regulated by the Institutional Review Board (IRB).

The philosophical foundation of experimental research

A physician's moral obligation to his or her patient is almost as age-old as the medical profession. Take the Hippocratic Oath, for instance, which was established in ancient Greece during a time when Zeus decided the fate of his minions – and clearly he adhered to no such oath. You were making a commitment to medical ethics before you even knew it, when you took the same or similar oath in medical school. Inherent in that oath is the promise to do no harm [1]. And where could that be more applicable than in the setting of experimental research, where you're not necessarily treating someone's disease but investigating means of potential treatments? This is particularly true (and you will see this be addressed later in the Belmont Principles) if the treatment does not pertain to those who are serving as research participants. As it is a physician's duty to protect his/her patients, all the more as researchers, it is our duty to protect human participants.

Historical case studies that have shaped how human research is conducted

The first documented research experiments were the vaccination trials in the 1700s where physicians used themselves (the principle of informed consent was definitely met here) or family members as research participants. Once these trials started being conducted on family members or others, the participants were not necessarily informed of

Doing Research in Emergency and Acute Care: Making Order Out of Chaos, First Edition. Edited by Michael P. Wilson, Kama Z. Guluma, and Stephen R. Hayden.

the dangers associated with such experiments. The testing of the smallpox vaccine by Edward Jenner on his son and neighborhood children is a good example of this. On the other hand, Louis Pasteur conducted all his vaccination trials on animals until he felt like the death of his first human test subject, a nine year old boy suffering from rabies, was inevitable. Only then did he use him as a human subject. (And that young boy, Joseph Meister, became the first person to be successfully treated for rabies [2].)

Later came days when medical professionals were not held in such high regard when it came to their research endeavors. At the end of World War II, for instance, approximately two dozen German physicians and researchers were put on trial for the murder of concentration camp prisoners who were used as research participants. The trial became known as the Nuremberg Trials, in which fifteen of the researchers were found guilty. (Seven of these researchers were subsequently sentenced to death by hanging; eight were sentenced to time in prison.) Out of this trial came the Nuremberg Code, which was the first international document outlining requirements for conducting research on human participants. First and foremost among this code was the principle that "the voluntary consent of the human subject is absolutely essential [2]".

Unfortunately, physically injurious research on vulnerable, un-informed populations was not only taking place outside of the United States. The Red Wing Studies of 1941, for instance, were conducted on schizophrenic patients and inmates (between the youthful ages of 17–32) for the purpose of investigating the arrest of cerebral blood flow in humans. This was done by using a rapidly inflating cuff placed around the neck of the subject until cessation of blood flow for up to 100 seconds, leading to a sequence of responses including unconsciousness, dilated pupils, tonic/clonic movements, loss of bladder and, eventually, bowel control, and appearance of pathological reflexes.

Despite the declaration of the Nuremberg Code, shady and sometimes outright criminal research continued. The Willowbrook Hepatitis Study took place in 1955 at an institution for mentally disabled children in Staten Island, New York. The purpose of this study was to determine the natural history of viral hepatitis and the effectiveness of gamma globulin as an inoculating agent against the disease. Over 15 years, more than 700 children at Willowbrook were involved in the studies, which fell into two categories. The first used children who were already at Willowbrook. Researchers injected some of these children with gamma globulin (the experimental group) and did not inject others (the control group). The degree of immunity to hepatitis was observed over time. In another series, researchers gave newly-admitted children gamma globulin. A subset of these children was then deliberately infected with hepatitis A virus obtained from other sick children. Those who had received protective antibodies but were not deliberately infected served as controls. Hard to believe that this took place 60 years ago, right?

The researchers' defense of the study was that most new children would become infected with hepatitis within the first year at the institution (recent estimates put the risk of contraction between 30 and 50%). Although consent was obtained from parents, they were not fully informed of the potential dangers of involvement. Furthermore, the children of parents who gave consent got priority enrollment into the facility, potentially a form of coercion [3].

However, research participants may not only be physically harmed as in the Willowbrook studies, but also mentally harmed. Perhaps one of the most interesting examples of this is the Obedience to Authority Study, also known as the Milgram experiment. This study was meant to determine the willingness of study participants to obey an authority figure who instructed them to perform acts that conflicted with their conscience. The participants, who were recruited volunteers, were told the experiment would study the effects of punishment on learning ability. Although participants were lead to believe they had an equal chance of playing the role of a student or of a teacher, the experiment was set up so that all participants played the role of teacher. The learner was an actor working as a cohort of the investigator. The subject was instructed to punish the learners' errors by administering increasing levels of electric shocks, even to the point of unconsciousness and potential death (although no real shocks were actually administered). The participants who asked to withdraw from the study were told they had to continue to administer shocks. Sixty-three percent of participants administered "lethal shocks" despite the learners' painful screams. At the conclusion of the experiment, participants were debriefed and showed great relief upon finding that they had not harmed the learners but many were deeply disturbed by the extent of their willingness to inflict harm just so as not to resist authority [3].

How about something that would seem fitting for a horror movie? ... Morales and colleagues published details of a trial in 1957 in which they took 11 patients in a psychiatric ward and endotracheally intubated them, anesthetized them with intravenous thiopental, gave some of them a high (C4–T1) spinal block with procaine to prevent shivering, and then cooled them to a rectal target temperature around 30°C using a rubber cooling blanket and alcohol, all to evaluate the effects of hypothermia on renal function. By the way, the hypothermia itself was being studied as an experimental treatment for psychiatric disease [4] ....Ouch! No mention was made about informed consent and one has to wonder if these hospitalized psychiatric patients in 1950s USA truly consented to the seemingly quite uncomfortable procedures described. It is more likely than not that they had no choice in the matter...

Another famous study that shaped research ethics is known as the Tuskegee Study of Untreated Syphilis in the Negro Male. In 1932, the Public Health Service initiated a study to document the natural history of syphilis in African American men. When the study began, there was no proven treatment for the disease. Investigators enrolled 600 black men in Alabama, 399 of whom had syphilis and 201 without the disease who served as controls. The study was not only conducted without informed consent, but the men were deliberately misinformed about the purpose of the study. The men were told they were going to be treated for "bad blood," a nonspecific local term used to describe several ailments including syphilis, anemia, and fatigue. In exchange for taking part in the study, the men received free medical examinations, free meals, and burial insurance. The study was initially planned to last six months but ended up lasting for forty years after the decision was made to follow the men until death.

In addition to invasive procedures like spinal taps which ,were falsely presented as a necessary and free treatment, this experiment was continued years after a safe and effective treatment for syphilis (penicillin, of course) was developed in the 1940s. In fact, the men enrolled in the study were followed until 1972 without being offered penicillin or the option to quit the study. The study resulted in 28 deaths, 100 cases of disability, and 19 cases of congenital syphilis. The public outcry that ensued ultimately resulted in a 10 million dollar settlement that included lifetime medical benefits and burial benefits to the survivors, their wives, widows, and offspring. The study also prompted a Presidential apology in 1997. Federal regulations were developed and implemented with the aim of protecting future human research participants [2].

The establishment of the Belmont Principles

In 1974, as media coverage of the Public Health Service syphilis study waned, Congress authorized the formation of the National Commission for the Protection of Human Subjects in Biomedical and Behavioral Research. This represented a codification of the principles of the Nuremberg Code into American law. It was the task of this commission to identify basic ethical principles necessary to conduct human research as well as develop guidelines to ensure that all human research would be conducted in accordance with these principles. The National Commission published the so-called Belmont Report in 1978 [3]. The Belmont Report continues to be a required reading for everyone involved in human subject research (that includes you) and established three basic ethical principles important for human research: autonomy (respect for persons), beneficence, and justice.

The Belmont Principles: Respect for persons
Based on the writing of philosopher Immanuel Kant, this principle necessitates the treatment of human participants as autonomous individuals who are not used as a means to an end. As such, we must allow people to make decisions for themselves and provide even further protection to those with limited autonomy, much like we strive to do in our clinical endeavors.

An autonomous individual is one who has:

- Mental capacity for self-determination, also known as decisional capacity.
  - Decisional capacity is the ability to make a decision regarding medical treatment. This is made up by the ability to:
    (i) receive information; (ii) process and understand information; (iii) deliberate; and (iv) make and articulate a choice.
- Willfulness, the ability to act independently of others' dominance.

As such, participants can be considered fully autonomous when they have the capacity to understand and process information and the free will to volunteer without pressure [5].

The practical application of this principle means we need to:

- Obtain (and document) informed consent.
  - For a subject to provide informed consent, he/she must have decisional-making capacity. Additionally, the patient should, to the extent possible, have an understanding of the proposed intervention and its risks and benefits. This principle applies outside the realm of research as the American College of Emergency Physicians (ACEP) summarizes in its code of ethics: "Emergency physicians shall communicate truthfully with patients and secure their informed consent for treatment, unless the urgency of the patient's condition demands an immediate response."
- Protect those who have diminished autonomy (vulnerable populations).
  - Diminished autonomy could be due to a medical condition, as sometimes seen in emergency department patients with life threatening conditions unable to consent to treatment. But remember, there are numerous types of vulnerability: cognitive vulnerability (whether due to cognitive impairment or language barriers); institutional vulnerability (prisoners); economic vulnerability (participants in need of money/shelter/goods); and social vulnerability (people belonging to undervalued groups such as those addicted to drugs or alcohol).
- Protect the privacy of research participants.
  - Protecting the privacy of individually identifiable health information that can be linked to a particular person, just as we do when practicing clinically (HIPPA, anyone?).

The Belmont Principles: Beneficence

Similar to the concept of non-maleficence (not doing harm) that is sworn by medical students when taking the Hippocratic Oath, the principle of beneficence emphasizes the need to maximize benefits when conducting human research [5].

The practical application of this principle means we need to:

- Abstain from research that does not have a positive risk/benefit ratio.
  - As physicians, beneficence is inherent to our practice. Even so, sometimes our work requires us to cause patients relative harm in in pursuit of treatment (chemotherapy in cancer treatment, for instance). As researchers, we must take this a step further to ensure that research conducted on human participants is more beneficial than harmful, particularly because we are not providing a validated therapy as we do in our clinical practice.
- Utilize procedures with the least amount of risk.
- Ensure the ability to perform said procedures and handle any potential risks.

The Belmont Principles: Justice

This principle necessitates the fair treatment of participants as well as the need to design research so that its benefits and burdens are equally distributed [5].

The practical application of this principle means we need to:

- Select participants equitably.
- Utilize the least vulnerable research populations possible.
- Ensure there is no potential conflict of interest between the investigators and the participants.

The intention of the National Commission with the creation of this report was that each of these three principles would carry an equal amount of weight [5], although it is quite conceivable that these three principles may not be congruent with each other. For example, the principle of respect for persons may suggest that we should restrict the use of developmentally disabled persons in research because they may have relatively limited autonomy. However, the principle of justice suggests that participants should be equitably chosen so that everyone has an equal opportunity to benefit from research. In light of such potential conflicts, it is important to remember that no one principle outweighs another but that each should be considered independently on a case-by-case basis.

The ethical standards to which we are held today

So now we know the basic ethical principles that guide how research is conducted, as well as the controversial and historic cases that led to their establishment. But how are these principles enforced and what does that mean to research in the acute setting or emergency department? [6]

All human research in the United States is subject to federal regulations. The purpose of these regulations is to protect the human participants involved by:

- Institutional assurances, a mechanism by which all institutions are subject to federal regulations when it comes to human subject research, regardless of the source of funding.
- Informed consent, which includes providing the subject with information, answering any questions that may improve the subject's comprehension, and finally, obtaining voluntary agreement of the subject to participate in the study.
- Review by an IRB, a regulatory board guided by the ethical principles delineated by the Belmont Report [7].

The Institutional Review Board

The IRB is a review committee established to protect the rights and welfare of human research participants. IRB review and approval is required for research involving human participants that is regulated by the federal government. The IRB is composed of at least five members from both genders that come from varied professions. There must be at least one member who has a non-scientific background, at least one member with a scientific background, and at least one member who is not otherwise affiliated with the institution [8].

The IRB has the authority to:

- Approve research.
- Disapprove research.
- Modify research.
- Conduct continuing reviews.
- Observe/verify changes.
- Suspend or terminate approval.
- Observe the consent process and the research procedures.
  IRB applications minimally contain information that allows members to assess:
- Anticipated risk/benefit analysis.
  - Identification and assessment of risks and anticipated benefits.
  - Determination that risks are minimized and are reasonable in relation to potential benefits.
- Informed consent process and documentation.
- Assent.
  - The affirmative agreement of a minor or decisionally-impaired individual to participate in research, as well as documented permission (informed consent) from legally recognized surrogates.
- Selection of participants.
  - Equitable selection in terms of gender, race, ethnicity.
  - Benefits are distributed fairly among the community's populations.
  - Additional safeguards are provided for vulnerable populations.
- Safeguards.
  - Ensure individual participants' privacy and that the confidentiality of the information collected during the research is monitored (especially data that includes "Protected Health Information" that may identify a subject).
- Research plan for collection, storage, and analysis of data.
- Research design/methods.
  - Are appropriate, scientifically valid and, therefore, justify exposing participants to research risks.
- Additional information that may be necessary if the research involves special populations (for instance, incarcerated participants, children, pregnant women, and those with diminished mental capacity).
  In addition, the IRB must review:
- The qualifications of the principal investigator (PI) and collaborators.
- A complete description of the proposed research.
- Provisions for the adequate protection of rights and welfare of participants.
- Compliance with pertinent federal and state laws/regulations and institutional policy.
- Clinical brochures/investigator protocols (for FDA-regulated research) [8].

Once this information is presented, reviewed and approved, it is then that clinical research can begin. Which means the process of obtaining and documenting informed consent from participants has already been delineated. So making sure your research population has decisional making capacity to understand the purpose, the process and the interventions of the research with which they are to be involved, as well as any possible risks (and benefits), is of utmost importance.

Almost all research requires informed consent. Exceptions to this occur rarely and only in specific circumstances [9]. Research that involves very little risk to the subject and in which consent cannot feasibly be obtained, for instance, may sometimes be allowed to proceed with a waiver of informed consent. Projects that collect and analyze data without affecting care decisions that lead to "minimal risk" to participants may be granted a waiver of informed consent. Examples of these kinds of studies are chart reviews in which consent is impossible, observational studies that do not record Protected Health Information (individually identifiable health information), studies that use de-identified data sets, or pre-existing specimens [7]. Intervention trials that involve participants that cannot provide consent (such as resuscitation trials) require much more preparation, including community disclosure and outreach. To conduct this kind of research, you will need much more than this book as a guide (Chapter 16 provides some more information about this).

So, as you can see, getting a research project approved by the IRB is no small feat, and each IRB may be different in its requirements. However, that approval is the first leap into the deep sea of clinical research. Now that you have a better understanding of what constitutes ethical research, you can begin to get your feet wet. Yet, as you embark on your journey, you may come across unexpected ethical challenges. Federal regulations are in place to set up basic guidelines, but unexpected ethical dilemmas may arise at any point. There are not always clear answers, particularly in the acute setting of the Emergency Department, where most decisions, including the decision for participants to consent, are very much time-limited. The areas where the most can still yet be learned are often the same areas that are most difficult to research, from the Alzheimer's patient who lacks the decisional making capacity to give consent to the patient in status asthmaticus who may say yes to anything in a moment of distress. Such challenges are unique to the field of Emergency Medicine, so it is imperative that any potential ethical dilemma that may arise be considered well beforehand [10]. Sound and professional judgment is the foundation of bioethics and the same holds true for ethics in research. The Society for Academic Emergency Medicine (SAEM) Code of Conduct endorses members engaging in research to "strive to safeguard the public and protect the vulnerable. As a researcher, one vows competence, compassion, respect, impartiality, integrity and responsibility" [11].

Summary

The lessons of time have brought about principles and regulations to help aid the process of experimental research on human participants, but there is no substitute for well thought-out design, sound judgment, and good intentions. Our eager resident in the beginning of the chapter has good intentions but lacks a design that thoroughly considers the ethical implications of the research. The proposal not only includes patients who likely would not be able to give consent due to medical vulnerability, but the study itself will likely cause harm to patients for whom we already have a proven treatment. This violates the principles of autonomy, beneficence, and justice, which means that getting IRB approval for such a study would be a nearly impossible feat. So, keep these fundamental principles in mind when formulating your research question and throughout the duration of your project. If you remain mindful of these important ethical considerations, your research will have the integrity necessary to be a meaningful contribution to the field (as well as be much more likely to be approved).

Ultimately, remember that just as it is our duty to protect our patients and do our very best to treat their diseases, successful medical research aims to do the same.

KEY POINTS

- Ethical considerations are absolutely necessary when conducting research on human beings.
- Just as we swore an oath to protect our patients as physicians, all the more as researchers it is our obligation to protect human subjects.
- Notorious historical research on human subjects, such as the Nuremberg experiments and the Tuskegee Study, ultimately led to the establishment of the Belmont Principles in an effort to keep such atrocities from occurring again in the name of medical research.
- The Belmont Principles identify the three basic ethical principles that underlie all human research: respect for persons, beneficence and justice.
- The Institutional Review Board (IRB) is a federally regulated review committee established to protect the rights and welfare of all human research subjects.
- Research in the emergency setting brings with it a unique set of challenges including, but not limited to, time limitations and the difficulty of obtaining informed consent from a patient in distress. Thus, it is that much more imperative that the ethicality of the research being conducted is considered prudently in advance.

References

1 Beauchamp, T.L. and Childress, J.F. (2001) *Principles of Biomedical Ethics*. Oxford University Press, New York.
2 US Department of Health & Human Services, National Institute of Health (nd) *Bioethics Resources on the Web*. http://bioethics.od.nih.gov/index.html (last accessed 29 April 2015).
3 Levine, R.J. (1986) *Ethics and Regulation of Clinical Research*, 2nd edn. Urban and Schwarzenberg, Baltimore, MD.
4 Morales, P., Carbery, Y., Morello, A., and Morales, G. (1957) Alterations in renal function during hypothermia in man. *Ann Surg*, **145**(4):488–499.
5 US Department of Health, Education and Welfare (1979) *The Belmont Report: Ethical Principles and Guidelines for the Protection of Human Subjects of Research*. www.hhs.gov/ohrp/policy/belmont.html (last accessed 29 April 2015).
6 Iserson,K.V. (1986) *Ethics in Emergency Medicine*. Williams & Wilkins, Baltimore, MD.
7 US Department of Health & Human Services, Office for Human Research Protections (OHRP) (nd) *OHRP Policy and Guidance library*. http://www.hhs.gov/ohrp/policy/index.html (last accessed 29 April 2015).
8 Office for Human Research Protections (OHRP) (1993) *Institutional Review Board Guidebook*. http://www.hhs.gov/ohrp/archive/irb/irb_guidebook.htm (last accessed 29 April 2015).
9 US Department of Health & Human Services (2011) *Guidance for Institutional Review Boards, Clinical Investigators, and Sponsors; Exception from Informed Consent Requirements for Emergency Research: March 2011 (updated April 2013)*. http://www.fda.gov/downloads/RegulatoryInformation/Guidances/UCM249673.pdf (last accessed 29 April 2015).
10 Jesus, J., Grossman, S.A., Derse, A.R., *et al.* (2012) *Ethical Problems in Emergency Medicine: A Discussion Based Review*. John Wiley & Sons, Ltd, Chichester, UK.
11 Larkin, G.L. (1999) A code of conduct for academic emergency medicine. *Acad Emerg Med*, **6**(1):45.

CHAPTER 9

Safety in research: How to ensure patient safety?

Robert Grover[1] and Vicken Y. Totten[2]

[1] Department of Internal Medicine, The Brooklyn Hospital Center, Brooklyn, NY, USA
[2] Department of Emergency Medicine, Kaweah Delta Health Care District, Visalia, CA, USA

> "Primum non nocere"
> "First, do no harm"
>
> Hippocratic Corpus: Epidemics

All physicians, whether in clinical practice or in research, just like in the classical era, still want to not only "do good", but also to "do no harm".

To protect our patients, and to do no harm, we consider:

- Privacy (Chapter 24; violation of confidentiality may itself cause harm).
- Protecting our patients from harm in our study. What harms could possibly happen from this study? Think hard.
  - What possible adverse events might happen and what should we do if they occur?
  - How do we (and our sponsors) monitor our trials?
  - What are the reporting requirements?

Remember that most studies in emergency medicine and acute care are not drug studies. For example, you have seen people uncomfortable on backboards. What are the harms of lying on a hard backboard? Being on a backboard can cause back pain. What could you do to minimize this harm? Padding? Limiting the time on the board? Maybe it would be hard to take a deep breath. Could they get hypoxic? Would the risks be the same for children and adults? What risks to their safety would there be? How would you know? You could ask adults or children who can talk. If no, perhaps you could use a pulse oximeter? Or, you might check a peak flow, and see how hard they breathed.

Well, OK, asking someone to lie on a board till they hurt, it is obvious there could be harm – or at least pain – to subjects. But there could not be any harm to a survey, could there? Maybe. What about, for example, asking about HIV? What possible risks to the subjects could there be from that? Perhaps they would be embarrassed about being asked to participate? Perhaps, just because you asked, will they feel offended or think you are judging them, or suspecting them of risky behaviors? What can you do in advance to minimize the potential harms? How about a fact sheet in advance? Maybe a poster or pamphlets in the lobby alerting them to the possibility to help advance medical science would allow for an indirect approach to asking them to participate? Remember, even retrospective data analysis poses some risk. This is discussed under adverse events, but remember, even the smallest breach of privacy is in itself a harm to the patient.

> Now it is your turn. Suppose you want to see if a tourniquet around the abdomen stops blood flow to a flaccid postpartum uterus. What potential harms might there be? List them. How could you avoid or minimize them?

Doing Research in Emergency and Acute Care: Making Order Out of Chaos, First Edition. Edited by Michael P. Wilson, Kama Z. Guluma, and Stephen R. Hayden.
© 2016 John Wiley & Sons, Ltd. Published 2016 by John Wiley & Sons, Ltd.

Thinking about all possible risks is something that you want to work into your protocol even before you start your study. Think about and describe the risks in your study, and include plans for how to manage these events, should and when they occur, in to your study plan.

Outline:
- It is your job to protect your subject.
- It is your job to report EVERY adverse event, and investigate if it could possibly be related to what your investigational intervention was – even if it isn't likely.
- It is your job to keep really good records. Depending on how bad the event is, you may have to:
  - Stop the study right away.
  - Notify your grantor (if you have one), notify your IRB or ethics board.
  - Investigate the event.
  - Just keep track of how many events there are.
  - Report the adverse events at your annual research report to your IRB or IRB equivalent.

  It is your job (or that of your safety monitoring committee) to decide if there are more adverse events than expected by chance and, if so, to decide if this is related to the research, and if it is to stop the study.

How do we protect patients in our studies?

By the very nature of a research study, you are trying to learn the unknown. Therefore, while we cannot eliminate all risk, we can, and should, think about what could go wrong. How will we monitor subjects for a safety issue? If things go wrong, what will we do? Is there a back-up plan? How about several?

If you are able to figure out the cause of a problem, it may open the door to refining the experimental protocol. Or a whole new question! When you learn the underlying mechanism or cause, you not only have the opportunity to prevent a condition, but the adverse effect itself may have potential as a therapy for some other malady.

Maybe you haave heard that minoxidil is now used to treat male pattern baldness. Did you know that minoxidil was developed to treat hypertension? It is still used for that indication. Doctors noticed that some hypertensives were growing their hair back! So they wondered if it would be even more effective if applied directly to the scalp. This is one, serendipitously noted, adverse effect that turned into a whole new question, followed by investigation of the effect, and finally a whole new product line. (This became a main topic in the literature as early as 1983 in "Reversal of androgenic alopecia by minoxidil, lack of effect of simultaneously administered intermediate doses of cyproterone acetate" [1].

Adverse events

An adverse event is a harmful or undesired effect. There are lots of different kinds of potential adverse events. Getting sick, hurting or dying are all commonly considered adverse events. Even embarrassment or loss of privacy can be considered an adverse event! Some adverse events are clearly the result of participating in your study: discomfort from a blood draw, inconvenience from answering a lot of questions, allergic reactions, or known and unknown treatment effects. Others, like getting hit by a car while crossing the street coming out of the supermarket, probably are not. But, you never can tell! For research purposes, ANY adverse event, for whatever reason, should be documented and investigated [2]. Even the car accident: you document it, and describe why it is highly unlikely this was related to the scalp treatment for baldness (or whatever your study was about).

Adverse event monitoring – How long is necessary?

The nature of the study will guide your monitoring period. Of course, this is subjective and should be guided by common sense. Certain interventions, such as new chemotherapy or the placement of a prosthetic, might require a lifetime of follow up. A survey with no follow up might require only privacy monitoring once the answers are handed in. Other temporary interventions, such as a new antibiotic, might require a few months of monitoring after a 10-day course. What would you monitor for? Any recurrence of the infection? Opportunistic infections? Subsequent organ dysfunction? (Think chloramphenicol and bone marrow suppression!) Monitor long enough to ensure both efficacy and safety.

Multicenter studies need to be protocolized – Why?

Multicenter studies need to have protocols for adverse event monitoring. Remember the old joke that when you have five doctors in a room, you will get at least eight opinions? The same thing happens with adverse events. Rather than relying on the opinions of investigators at many sites, a formal, or standardized adverse reporting protocol will reduce variation between sites and ensure potential adverse events are uniformly analyzed and or recorded.

Risk Levels

Minimal Risk: "The risk of participation is not greater than that encountered in daily life or by routine physiological or psychological testing" [3, Chapter 3].
   More than Minimal Risk: Any risk greater than Minimal Risk.

Adverse Event: Undesirable medical, psychological, or other signs or symptoms related to participation in a study.
   Severe Adverse Event: Adverse Event that causes hospitalization, is life threatening, disabling or is teratogenic.

Attrition: Loss of study participants to follow up, regardless of the causation: "Not Related"/"Possibly Related"/"Definitely Related"
   Not Related: There is no relationship.
   Probably or Possibly Related: There is likely or possibly a relationship between a cause and the observed outcome.
   Definitely Related: The event has a known causal relationship and no other cause is possible.

MedDRA coding

MedDRA is a proprietary organ-based classification system used for technical specifications of pharmaceuticals, vaccines, and medical devices [4]. The copyright is owned by the ICH (International Committee on Harmonization of Technical Standards) and is provided for free to regulators, and academics (outside Japan. Inside Japan there is a nominal fee.) It is licensed to for-profit entities based in part upon their annual revenues.
   MedDRA is a multilingual system designed to allow operation across language barriers by assigning all terms to an eight digit code [5].

FDA reporting requirements

In the United States, the FDA (Food and Drug Administration, which is an agency of the Department of Health and Human Services) requires manufacturers of drugs and medical devices to report any adverse events that they learn of themselves or which are reported to them. The FDA may investigate reports either before or after taking an action based on the report. While physicians and others are able to file reports of a potential adverse event anytime, there is no requirement that physicians do so. Still, "post marketing surveillance" (the voluntary reporting of adverse effects) is another way to "do good" and "do no harm."

Post marketing surveillance is important for other reasons also. Drugs are initially tested for safety in healthy people, then for efficacy in people with the condition it is designed to treat. It is not possible to test the drug together with all other medicines or comorbidities that the patient might have. Post marketing surveillance is truly the ultimate test for safety in the general population, and many rare but important adverse events may not be detected before this stage [6]. Every physician who notices and reports a potential adverse effect is helping to improve medical practice!

Post marketing surveillance is the ongoing monitoring of drug safety that occurs once a drug becomes commercially available. The FDA continues to collect Adverse Event Reports; for example, through FAERS (Federal Adverse Event Reporting System) [7] and VAERS (Vaccine Adverse Event Reporting System). These data seek rare side events (for example drug, interactions) that could alert us to previously undetected risks associated with the medication.

For example: In the 1980s, PhenFen (or Fen Phen) was hailed as a miracle drug for weight loss. Phenteramine and the fenflura-mine were both thought to be safe; fenfluramine had been in use for decades. The combination was marketed for a decade before it was discovered that fenfluramine had a significant risk for causing pulmonary hypertension and valvular defects. This effect was only discovered through post marketing surveillance.

When you are doing research, you do not have the option to NOT report an adverse event. The Principal Investigator (PI) needs to know. The sponsor (if there is one) needs to know. Your IRB needs to know. Every single thing needs to be reported so that it can be analyzed, and its relationship to the intervention ascertained. However improbable it is that your intervention caused or was related to the adverse event, if it is possible then it must be reported. (Remember the guy hit by a car leaving the supermarket? Could it be that your drug caused him to lose his peripheral vision?) While severe adverse events should make the PI take immediate action, following the Institutional Review Board's approved plan is the best course of action [8, 9].

FDA IND (investigational new drug) and IDE (investigational device exemption)

The FDA requires direct notification for these particular types of research in the event of any severe adverse event, or any unanticipated adverse event.

It is possible that an adverse event will not possibly happen to all persons. Even in persons at risk of the adverse event, the underlying mechanism that caused the adverse event may be of therapeutic benefit in other circumstances. Thalidomide was a drug discovered to have great sedative and anti-emetic effects. Unfortunately, many women who used thalidomide for nausea of pregnancy delivered babies without arms or legs, "phocomelia." (Phocomelia is a disorder where the limb buds differentiation is prematurely terminated resulting in the child having limbs like flippers.) As a result, thalidomide developed such a bad reputation that it is medicolegally almost untouchable. (In 2013, a Spanish Court found the drug's original developer, Grunenthal, responsible for the malformations suffered by the Spanish thalidomide babies. The court has ordered them to pay the legal costs and tens of thousands of Euros to each of the victims in compensation [10].)

However, thalidomide is still an effective sedative. Dr Jakob Sheskin was treating a man with erythema nodosum leprosum (ENL); the man could barely move and was having great difficulty sleeping. Dr Sheskin remembered thalidomide. Since the man couldn't possibly get pregnant, he cautiously offered it to his patient. The man was able to sleep, and in the morning was actually able to get up on his own! Since then, thalidomide has be used for ENL. Dr Sheskin's observation and report of the patient's symptoms and their resolution led to improved treatment of people around the world.

Your meticulous note taking may help to uncover an adverse event (or a beneficial side effect!). Figuring out how it happened may uncover an unexpected therapeutic property of the agent.

Data safety monitoring plans and data safety monitoring boards

Large trials with more than minimal risk often require special monitoring in the form of data safety monitoring plans or data safety monitoring boards. Small trials involving potentially high risk procedures (e.g., first-in-human treatments) may also benefit from such monitoring, albeit on a smaller scale. Data safety monitoring plans are required by the US National Institutes of Health (NIH) of all human subject studies that they fund. You can have one for any other research, too. It depends on the potential risks to subjects. If embarrassment about the subject matter is the greatest risk, the study is likely "minimal risk" and probably does not need a data safety monitoring plan. On the other side of the spectrum, if death is a potential side effect, you clearly have a more than minimal risk study, and you definitely need a formal safety board. When the risk of the study is not at either extreme, how do you know if you need a data safety monitoring plan or data safety monitoring board? This is a judgment call and your organizations' IRB will decide. How long the study lasts is also a factor. If the whole intervention and data collection takes five minutes, and you or your data collector will be present the whole time, you may not need a separate data safety monitoring plan! If the study lasts for months, and you do not see your subjects often, you might not notice subtle but potentially serous changes if you are not looking. And since you might be biased, it is better if someone who is not otherwise connected with the study, sometimes called an "Independent Safety Monitor", is looking over your shoulder to make sure that there is not an excess of adverse events. In other words, while in many cases the Principal Investigator may prepare an annual summary of the adverse events and any other safety issues that arose during the study, in more complex studies, or studies with larger medical risks, adverse events may have an independent board to review reports.

Data safety monitoring boards can stop a trial if it becomes apparent that the new treatment is futile, has safety issues, or has sufficient evidence to prove efficacy.

For example: The study of a vaginal estradiol soft gel capsule "TX 12-004-HR" was stopped early, because it was shown to achieve comparable vaginal estradiol levels to "Vagifem®", the currently FDA approved treatment for the postmenopausal changes that occur in the female reproductive tract. This study was concluded early not just due to showing comparable therapeutic efficacy, but rather due to the demonstration that it could achieve this with a reduced side effect profile [11]. The side effects of this type of treatment are believed to be due to the systemic rise in estradiol, and the new product showed a substantially decreased level of systemic estradiol absorption compared to the current treatment (Vagifem®).

Another example: The NIH Stenting versus Aggressive Medical Management for Preventing Recurrent Stroke in Intracranial Stenosis (or SAMMPRIS) was also stopped early [12]. The researchers expected that intracranial arterial stenting would decrease the risk of stroke or death by about 35%. Unfortunately, the data showed that the rate of complications was increased by nearly a factor of three! This study showed that there was a substantially increased risk of death and stroke in patients who received intracranial stenting. It would have been unethical to continue the study: it was too dangerous.

Still another example: The Strategies for Management of Antiretroviral Therapy (SMART) study was stopped on grounds of futility rather than safety [13]. The researchers had theorized that although there might be an increase of AIDS-related complications, the increase would be more than balance by a decrease in metabolic, cardiovascular and other complications. The study found AIDS progressed twice as fast, so the expected benefit was not worth it.

Clinical trial monitors, contract research organizations, and clinical research associates

The FDA has stipulated that a sponsor of medical research must monitor that research. Many academic medical centers, universities, and other institutions perform this internally with their own monitoring boards. There are also a number of specialized firms called Contract Research Organizations (CROs). While CROs may help to monitor research, there are also people who we will call Clinical Research Associates (CRAs) who can also help to do research.

The role of "research assistant", "research associate", "and clinical research coordinator," and so on is not standardized. What do you expect when you hear "Clinical Research Associate"? A doctor who is affiliated with the hospital principally as a researcher? Maybe, but the CRA might be an undergraduate student out to pad his medical school application, too. While these terms may sound analogous to academic rank, they are not. These terms have not yet been standardized. They can be used interchangeably in research job postings on web sites ranging from "www.apds.org" to "www.residentswap.com". What the Department of Surgery at Mount Sinai in New York calls a "research coordinator", is the "research assistant" at another site. Some Research Associates are team members without a doctorate; in other places only an MD without residency training would qualify. Still others are nurses, trained undergraduates, and foreign medical graduates or have other credentials.

On the other hand, "Research Fellow" is a more standardized title. This is a physician gaining special expertise in research methods and actively doing research. Typically, the Research Fellow has already completed a residency. Other Research Fellows have PhDs; more typically, these are called "Postdoctoral Fellows".

The CRO is a third party that acts on the behalf of the research sponsor to verify subject welfare, adherence to study protocol, and compliance with research regulations, as well as to confirm database entries with source documents. It even trains clinical investigators to assure that measurements are done uniformly across centers. While a sponsor may delegate monitoring to a CRO, the sponsor still remains responsible for ensuring that these functions are performed [14, p. 18].

KEY POINTS

- It is your moral, legal, and professional duty to protect your patient.
- Keep excellent records to improve patient safety and study efficacy.
- You need to keep track all adverse effects and investigate every possibility.
- The FDA requires manufactures (of drugs and medical devices) to report adverse events.
- The FDA requires sponsors of research to monitor their research.
- The NIH requires data safety monitoring plans for research it funds that involve human subjects.
- Adverse events may be caused by the research (e.g., a new treatment).
- Iatrogenic events are those that are caused by the doctor.
- Clinical trial monitors are outside groups employed by research sponsors to monitor study progression, events, and reporting.

References

1 Vermorken AJ. (1983) Reversal of androgenic alopecia by minoxidil: lack of effect of simultaneously administered intermediate doses of cyproterone acetate. *Acta Derm Venereol*, **63**(3):268–269. http://www.ncbi.nlm.nih.gov/pubmed/6192653 (last accessed 30 April 2015).
2 University of South Carolina (nd) *Adverse Event (AE) Reporting Guidelines*. orc.research.sc.edu/PDF/AEGuidelines.pdf (last accessed 5 June 2015).
3 US DHHS (1993) *Institutional Review Board Guidebook, Chapter III, Basic IRB Review*, Office for Human Research Protections (OHRP). www.hhs.gov/ohrp/archive/irb/irb_chapter3.htm (last accessed 30 April 2015).
4 ICH (2011) *Introductory Guide, MedDRA Version 14.0*, ICH (International Committee on Harmonization of Technical Standards) .http://www.who.int/medical_devices/innovation/MedDRAintroguide_version14_0_March2011.pdf (last accessed 5 June 2015).
5 ICH (nd) *How to use MedDRA*, ICH (International Committee on Harmonization of Technical Standards) http://www.meddra.org/how-to-use/support-documentation/english (last accessed 5 June 2015).
6 FDA (2013) Safety – Report a Problem. www.fda.gov/Safety?ReportaProblem/QuestionsandAnswersProblemReporting/default.htm#why (last accessed 30 April 2015).
7 FDA (2014) FDA Adverse Events Reporting System (FAERS) http://www.fda.gov/Drugs/GuidanceComplianceRegulatoryInformation/Surveillance/AdverseDrugEffects/ (last accessed 30 April 2015).
8 US DHHS (nd) *Institutional Review Boards (IRBs)*, Office for Human Research Protections (OHRP). http://www.hhs.gov/ohrp/assurances/irb/index.html (last accessed 5 June 2015).
9 US DHHS (2009) *Code of Federal Regulations, Title 45, Documentation of informed consent*, Office for Human Research Protections (OHRP) http://www.hhs.gov/ohrp/humansubjects/guidance/45cfr46.html (last accessed 5 June 2015).
10 AFP (2013) Five decades on, Spain court convicts thalidomide maker www.breitbart.com/news/954500c1-b416-440f-a27d-1a03a8f74fbf/ (last accessed 5 June 2015).
11 Market Watch (2014) TherapeuticsMD reports positive PK study results for its estradiol vaginal capsule VagiCap™ (TX 12-004-HR) for treatment of vulvar vaginal atrophy (VVA). http://www.marketwatch.com/story/therapeuticsmd-reports-positive-pk-study-results-for-its-estradiol-vaginal-capsule-vagicap-tx-12-004-hr-for-treatment-of-vulvar-vaginal-atrophy-vva-2014-01-28?reflink=MW_news_stmp (last accessed 30 April 2015).
12 SeniorJournal (2011) Brain stenting appears to increase strokes in highest risk cases; study stopped. http://seniorjournal.com/NEWS/Health/2011/20110908-BrainStenting.htm (last accessed 30 April 2015).
13 National Institutes of Health (2006) International HIV/AIDS trial finds continuous antiretroviral therapy superior to episodic therapy. http://www.nih.gov/news/pr/jan2006/niaid-18.htm (last accessed 30 April 2015).
14 US DHHS (2013) *Guidance for Industry: Oversight of Clinical Investigations – A Risk-Based Approach to Monitoring*. www.fda.gov/downloads/drugs/guidancecomplianceregulatoryinformation/guidances/ucm269919.pdf (last accessed 30 April 2015).

Further reading

COSEPUP (1995) *On Being a Scientist, Responsible Conduct in Research*, 2nd edn. Committee on Science, Engineering, and Public Policy (COSEPUP), National Academy of Sciences/National Academy of Engineering/Institute of Medicine. http://www.nap.edu/search/?term=on+being+a+scientist (last accessed 5 June 2015).
Rand Corporation (nd) Standards for High-Quality Research and Analysis. http://www.rand.org/standards.html (last accessed 30 April 2015).
University of Washington (nd) *Researcher's Guide, Proposal Development*. www.washington.edu/research/guide/dsmp.html (last accessed 30 April 2015).

PART 2

Getting it done: Doing your research study

CHAPTER 10

How to design a study that everyone will believe: Minimizing bias and confounding

Michael Witting

Department of Emergency Medicine, University of Maryland School of Medicine, Baltimore, MD, USA

> *"I'm not going to the hospital. My dad died there."*
>
> A confounded person

When I was a young investigator, a reviewer wrote that my study design allowed bias. Considering that this was just one of pages of criticisms, I thought to myself, in a high-pitched voice, "So there's a little bias." It was only later in my career that I learned that bias and confounding are major issues, perhaps the biggest threats to study validity. Make sure you have done what you can to minimize them before you start collecting your data.

Bias

There are two types of error – random and systematic. A lot of research education focuses on statistics (alpha error, beta error, power, significance, p values – some of these terms even mean the same thing!), but these concepts apply to quantifying random error. Bias, or systematic error, applies to all other types of error. As much as I like the geeky aspects of statistics, it is better to be an expert in minimizing bias. Fortunately, you can usually limit bias by thoughtful study design.

Generally, researchers are interested in seeing whether there is a relationship between an "independent" and "dependent" variable. This terminology implies that there is such a relationship, which is the hypothesis of the study. The null hypothesis is that there is no relationship. As Figure 10.1 shows, bias can be "toward the null" or "away from the null." [1, 2]

Broad categories of bias
Selection bias
Selection bias refers to selection for getting into a study or being selected for the study intervention. Convenience sampling often leads to selection bias, since those enrolled are often different from those not enrolled for some reason or another. This is especially an issue in cross-sectional studies where one is trying to obtain a prevalence estimate or characterize emergency department visitors.

Selection bias can also affect the population enrolled in a randomized trial. If patients are too ill to consent, this will tend to select for patients with less severe disease. This may bias the study toward the null, as there is less opportunity for an intervention to show a difference in mild disease.

> If one is designing a study of an early intervention to decrease admissions in asthma, one must be aware that excluding a population with severe disease will tend to decrease one's ability to detect a difference if one exists. Use of explicit eligibility criteria will limit the likelihood of selecting only those who are unlikely to benefit from the intervention.

Doing Research in Emergency and Acute Care: Making Order Out of Chaos, First Edition. Edited by Michael P. Wilson, Kama Z. Guluma, and Stephen R. Hayden.
© 2016 John Wiley & Sons, Ltd. Published 2016 by John Wiley & Sons, Ltd.

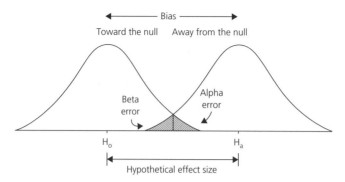

Figure 10.1 Relationship between inferential statistics and bias. In planning a study, investigators desire a sample size that will allow detection of a difference between an alternate hypothesis value (H$_a$) and a null hypothesis value (H$_o$). Larger sample sizes minimize alpha and beta error, which are types of 'random error.' Bias, also known as 'systematic error,' can shift the entire curve.

Non-response bias in surveys is another form of selection bias. When selection bias in enrollment is a concern, you can carry out additional sampling to assess its significance. For example, in a survey with a low response rate, you could recontact non-responders to get a sample of late responders. Late responders tend to be closer to non-responders than to initial responders; if the late group gives responses similar to those of the initial group, then it is likely that non-responders would also [1].

> Many inexperienced investigators planning a survey will send a questionnaire to the entire sampling frame by e-mail. This method is destined to have a low response rate and select those who have the greatest interest in the subject, thus introducing selection bias. A better method is to choose a random sample and plan to re-contact those who do not respond initially.

Selection bias can also refer to selection for an intervention. For example, an investigator might wish to study the real-world effect of thrombolytic therapy on good outcomes in stroke. However, patients might be selected for thrombolytic therapy based on their comorbidities or initial presentation. If patients are selected for therapy based on milder presentations and fewer comorbidities, this will lead to a bias away from the null. If, on the other hand, more severe stroke cases get thrombolytic therapy, this will bias toward the null, assuming thrombolytic therapy is truly better. This is also an example of confounding, which we will cover later on. Though a patient may be assigned an intervention, he may not choose to take it (*compliance bias*). Also, investigators may offer additional interventions (co-interventions) to patients they know are in the treatment group that would not be offered to a control group.

> In a randomized trial, some patients assigned an intervention may not take it, leading to a potential reduction in effect size. Though it is tempting to limit analysis to those who took the intervention, it is important to analyze patients as randomized, the "intention to treat" analysis. Non-compliant patients tend to have poor outcomes, so it is important to keep these patients assigned and analyzed equally between groups. Furthermore, non-compliance is a real-world phenomenon that is greater with less comfortable treatments, and compliance should be factored into the effect size.

Information bias

Information bias refers to biased acquisition of information obtained from patients in the study. There are many types of information bias. *Recall bias* relates to case–control studies: patients with disease are better able to remember exposures they think relate to their disease than are those without disease. Biased measurement would also fit into this category. *Unblinding* can create bias in the processing of information and also in the application of co-interventions (see Selection bias); unblinding generally tends to bias away from the null. *The Hawthorne effect* refers to the tendency of workers (or participants) to alter their behavior when they know they are being studied. *Observation bias* refers to bias in the way patients are observed in the study; if patients in one group have better follow-up, they will have more opportunity to have disease diagnosed or bad outcomes noted [1].

A common problem in studies of emergency department patients is poor follow-up, a case of **observation bias**. Often, rates of losses to follow-up are higher than differences in effect between groups, begging the question of whether those dropping out had differing rates of bad outcomes. For example, a study may find that a medication decreased return visits by 10%, but 30% were lost to follow-up. How many went to another hospital because they were unhappy with the new treatment? Losses to follow-up can be minimized by enrolling only patients with good contact information and by using proxies, relatives or friends that can be contacted in case the patient is not available. The importance of losses to follow-up can be characterized by comparing baseline variables between those lost to follow-up versus those remaining in the study.

Misclassification bias refers to putting participants in the wrong categories, either of the dependent variable or independent variable. In the thrombolytic example, this would be wrongly assessing whether a patient had thrombolytic therapy (independent variable) or a good outcome (dependent variable). *Non-differential misclassification* tends to bias toward the null, and *differential misclassification* can bias toward or away from the null, depending on how it goes. For example, in a study with patient weight as an outcome, an imprecise scale applied to both groups would cause non-differential misclassification, but a scale that reads high, applied only to the treatment arm, would cause differential misclassification [1].

Special situations involving bias
Bias in diagnostic studies
A few types of bias are applicable to studies of diagnostic tests or clinical findings related to disease. These studies generally compare a diagnostic test or finding with a criterion, or gold, standard for the presence of disease. *Spectrum bias* relates to the severity of disease; diseases are easier to diagnose when they are in their severe stages, and studies that include only severe cases will have an inflated estimate for sensitivity. *Incorporation bias* occurs when a test under scrutiny is incorporated, or included, in the criterion standard test; this frequently occurs when tests of early cardiac markers are included in making the diagnosis of myocardial infarction. *Work-up bias, or verification bias*, occurs when only patients with certain characteristics are referred for definitive testing. Selectively working up those with disease and assuming that those not worked up are without disease biases toward higher sensitivity and specificity. For example, if you are interested in the sensitivity of a difference in systolic pressure in the two arms to detect aortic dissection, work-up bias can occur when that factor leads to testing [3].

Investigators derived a score to predict necrotizing fasciitis, the LRINEC (Laboratory Risk Indicator for Necrotozing Fasciitis) score. Understandably, they did not apply the criterion standard test, surgery, to all patients, and those with low scores that did not have surgery were assumed to be free of nectrotizing fasciitis. This is an example of **verification bias**. This bias is common in studies of diagnostic tests and in studies describing associations between clinical features and disease. Since application of an invasive criterion standard test to all participants may be ethically problematic, verification bias is often difficult to eliminate. Methods of minimizing it are to choose a low cost, non-invasive criterion standard test when available or to apply the criterion standard test to a random sample [4].

Chart reviews
Chart reviews are especially prone to bias. Many chart reviews are lacking in a description of their chart review methodology. If an investigator sets out to prove a hypothesis, bias can creep in as he discards charts and subjectively measures some variables. A classic article by Gilbert and Lowenstein described several techniques to minimize bias in chart reviews: explicit eligibility criteria, explicit variable definitions, standardized data collection, blinding of abstractors to the study hypothesis, and assessment of inter-rater reliability [5].

Confounding

Confounding is a special type of bias in which another variable, often unmeasured, causes changes in the dependent variable, but the independent variable of interest gets the credit or blame because it was associated with the causative variable. A classic example of confounding is the association between carrying matches and lung cancer. Match carrying is associated with lung cancer, but it is smoking, which is associated with carrying matches, that actually causes lung cancer. Thus, smoking confounds the association between match carrying and lung cancer.

One condition for confounding is an association with both the independent variable and the dependent variable. Another condition of confounding is that the variable must not be directly caused by the independent variable of interest; in other words, the potentially confounding variable must not be in a causal chain between the independent and dependent variables. In the example that opens this chapter, the father's illness was likely the confounding variable that caused him to go to the hospital and also to die. However, if going to the hospital led to a medical error or encounter with an evil physician that caused his death, then we would not consider this confounding [1, 2].

Strategies to minimize effects of confounding

When you plan your study, make a list of variables that are associated with your independent variable; make another list for your dependent variable. Do any variables show up on both lists? If so, there is potential for confounding by these variables.

You can minimize the biasing effects of confounding variables in the design stage by a variety of methods: you can exclude patients with that factor (*selection*), you can match patients by that factor (*matching*), or you can randomize them (*randomization*) in the hope that confounders will even out. Using the carrying of matches example, if you are concerned about smoking as a confounder, you could exclude smokers (*selection*), enroll a smoking match-carrier for every smoker who does not carry matches (*matching*), or randomize patients to carrying or not carrying a match.

You can also deal with confounding in the analysis stage. One way is by *stratification;* here, you analyze the association between your independent variable and your dependent variable in subgroups defined by the potential confounder. In the match carrying example, you could look at the association between match carrying and cancer in a subgroup of smokers and a subgroup of non-smokers. Another way to deal with confounding is *adjustment,* done using multivariable regression modeling to adjust for the independent effects of variables [2].

> In studying whether hydrocortisone has a beneficial effect in septic shock, there is a potential for bias in the application of the intervention. Physicians viewing steroids as beneficial may only provide them to their sickest patients, which would tend to bias toward showing no benefit or harm from steroids. In the CORTICUS trial, investigators used randomization to minimize this effect, randomizing patients to receive steroids or placebo in addition to standard care. In an observational study, one could adjust for severity of illness or use matching to minimize its biasing effect [6].

KEY POINT

- Bias and confounding are important threats to study validity. They can be minimized using thoughtful study design and data analysis.

References

1 Gordis, L. (2000) *Epidemiology,* 2nd edn. WB Saunders, Philadelphia, PA.
2 Hulley, S.B., Cummings, S.R., Browner W.S., *et al.* (2001) *Designing Clinical Research: An Epidemiologic Approach,* 2nd edn. Lippincott Williams & Wilkins, Philadelphia, PA.
3 Mower, W.R. (1999) Evaluating bias and variability in diagnostic test reports. *Ann Emerg Med,* 33:85–91.
4 Wong, C.H., Khin, L.W., Heng, K.S., *et al.* (2004) The LRINEC (Laboratory Risk Indicator for Necrotizing Fasciitis) score: A tool for distinguishing necrotizing fasciitis from other soft tissue infections. *Crit Care Med,* 32:1535–1541.
5 Gilbert, E.H., Lowenstein, S.R., Koziol-McLain, J., *et al.* (1996) Chart reviews in emergency medicine research: where are the methods? *Ann Emerg Med,* 27:305–308.
6 Sprung, C.L., Annane, D., Keh, D., *et al.* (2008) Hydrocortisone therapy for patients with septic shock. *N Engl J Med,* 358:111–124.

CHAPTER 11

How to design a study that everyone will believe: An overview of research studies and picking the right design

Julian Villar, Jennifer Lanning, and Robert Rodriguez

Department of Emergency Medicine, University of California San Francisco, San Francisco General Hospital, CA, USA

Introduction

It's midnight in your shop when a patient presents with a large shooter's abscess. The patient needs procedural sedation for the incision and drainage (I & D), and you decide to anesthetize with some good old ketamine. In spite of the lovely abscess smell, you are starving during the procedure and debate with your partner the best place for burrito delivery. When the patient emerges from sedation, the first thing he says is, "Doc, I'm so hungry! Where's a good place to get a burrito around here?"

At the end of your shift, you decide to explore the following research question: Can you use hypnotic suggestion during procedural sedation to promote a healthy change, such as smoking cessation?

In previous chapters you were sagely taught to pick an interesting question for clinical research. Now, we discuss the plan of attack! If choosing the right question is arguably the most important part of clinical research, then choosing the appropriate study design to answer that question runs a close second. Herein, a brief overview of the different primary research study designs is given, providing pearls of wisdom about choosing the correct design with some real world examples of such studies.

Overview of study designs

Firstly, let us briefly review the various categories of study designs, which are listed in order of the hierarchy of evidence they provide. In other words, a randomized controlled trial (RCT) is generally considered a stronger study design than a case series for evidence-based clinical decision making. But remember that each type of study has its own advantages and disadvantages, which are discussed in further detail her. Please refer to Table 11.1 as we proceed through the chapter.

Clinical research can generally be divided into *Experimental (Interventional)* versus *Observational* categories. In experimental research, you make an intervention and measure a response to that intervention. The classic example of an interventional study is the RCT. Observational studies can be further divided into *Analytic* and *Descriptive* studies. In analytic studies, the observed group of subjects has a comparison or control group. Examples of observational analytic designs include cohort and case–control studies. Conversely, in descriptive studies there is no comparison or control group. Examples of observational descriptive designs include cross-sectional studies and case series.

Randomized controlled trials

The gold standard of clinical research! The holy grail of evidence-based medicine! The ticket to fame, fortune and an oral presentation at a national or international conference! Not so fast, however! Let us first discuss what a RCT entails, then we will discuss the good, the bad, and the ugly (Box 11.1).

Doing Research in Emergency and Acute Care: Making Order Out of Chaos, First Edition. Edited by Michael P. Wilson, Kama Z. Guluma, and Stephen R. Hayden.

Table 11.1 Types of clinical research designs, organized by evidence hierarchy.

Study name	Type of design
Meta-analysis	Analytic
Randomized control trial	Experimental
Cohort	Observational analytic
Case–control	Observational analytic
Cross-sectional	Observational descriptive
Case series	Observational descriptive

Box 11.1 Features of randomized controlled trials.

Characteristics

- Two groups randomly assigned to intervention or control
- +/– Blinding

Good

- Minimize bias

Bad/Ugly

- Time, labor, money
- Hard for rare conditions
- May be unethical

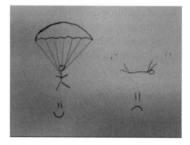

Figure 11.1 The gravity challenge.

In a RCT, an actual experiment is performed in the classic sense. An intervention is administered to a group of subjects and its efficacy or response is measured against the response in a control group (no intervention). As the name implies, in this type of study subjects are *randomized* to different treatments (randomly allocated to receive either the study intervention or a control treatment) in order to minimize bias. The best RCTs are also *blinded*, meaning that study participants, caregivers, and even researchers do not know which treatment is being administered. Because this study design reduces many kinds of bias, it generates (for the most part) the most solid and reliable form of scientific evidence.

So why are research journals not overflowing with RCTs? Well, conducting these trials can be a very time consuming, laborious, and expensive process. More importantly, there are many research questions that simply do not lend themselves to RCTs. For example, some disease processes are so rare that they cannot feasibly be studied prospectively. If the event you are after only happens once every three months and you need 240 events for adequate power (more on power and sample size is detailed in Chapter 28), it will take you at least 60 years to collect your data in a RCT! Additionally, there are some questions for which performing a RCT may be unethical – exposing a group of patients to unacceptable harm. We cannot deny patients potentially life-saving chest compressions during cardiac arrest, for example, even though there has never been a randomized trial demonstrating their efficacy as compared to no compressions. As Smith and Pell discuss in their *landmark* meta-analysis of the effectiveness of parachutes "to prevent death and major trauma related to gravitational challenge," some therapies (i.e., parachutes in skydiving) are so clearly effective, that denying their use to a control group in a RCT would be ludicrous [1] (Figure 11.1).

Box 11.2 Seminal observational study.

- NEXUS
  - Prospective
  - Observational
  - Widely accepted as valid

Data from *Hoffman et al.* [2]

Box 11.3 Example of a cohort study.

- Frequent enough disease process → prospective.
- Aim: to define risk factors → no intervention needed.
- Result → Prospective observational cohort study.

Data from Perry *et al.* [3]

Many doctors assume that *experimental* research designs are always the way to go, and that observational studies are not worth the paper (or Epub digital code) they are printed on. Nonsense! Many of the most seminal pieces of medical science have been pure *observational* studies. What it comes down to is choosing an optimal, feasible, ethical, and valid design that answers your question with the least amount of bias (Box 11.2).

Cohort studies

The next type of study is the non-interventional cohort study. Cohort studies are largely used to study risk factors for disease, or to develop decision guidelines and instruments for identifying a disease.

What's a cohort? The Merriam Webster dictionary defines it as "a group of individuals having a statistical factor in common in a demographic study" (http://www.merriam-webster.com). In order to determine whether there are any risk factors for or characteristics associated with a cohort, you need a comparison group. There are two ways to get this comparison group. You can look at people without the characteristic from the general population from which your cohort is drawn, or you can examine an entirely different group of people who were specifically not exposed to the risk factor under investigation.

Cohort studies can be performed either prospectively or retrospectively. *Prospective* means that patients are enrolled in real time as the events take place, while *retrospective* means the investigators look back at events that have occurred. Prospective studies are generally thought to carry greater weight on the evidence-based medicine scale than retrospective studies because they are less prone to selection and information biases (Chapter 10 gives more information on biases). However, practical concerns may make a retrospective study design a more appropriate choice. Rare diseases that you see only a few times in your career, for example, traumatic aortic injury, may not be feasible to study in a prospective manner. Looking back through years of records to identify cases retrospectively simply makes a lot more sense.

A good example of a cohort study is a paper from 2010 by Perry *et al.*, in which the investigators sought to define high risk clinical characteristics for subarachnoid hemorrhage (SAH) [3]. Because their aim was to determine risk factors for a somewhat unusually occurring disease, intervention was unnecessary (and impractical), making an observation cohort study the optimal choice. Prospectively enrolling adults with acute, non-traumatic headache over five years, they compared clinical characteristics of the 130 patients with confirmed SAH with those whose ultimate diagnosis was not SAH. The prospective design allowed them to minimize bias that would occur from retrospective chart review (inconsistent recording of patient characteristics and risk factors) and set the stage for the development of a predictive decision rule. This is a great example of the power and appropriate use of the cohort study design. (Box 11.3)

Case–control studies

Another example of an observational study is the case–control study, in which two groups of subjects with the outcome of interest (cases) are matched to unaffected controls, and factors that may have contributed to their outcome differences are then assessed. Wiebe *et al.* used a case–control study design to provide a great look at guns in the home as a risk factor for homicide or suicide [4]. These investigators reviewed 1720 homicide and suicide cases from a national homicide/suicide database and compared them to 8084 matched control subjects from a different database. Compared with adults in homes without guns, the adjusted odds ratio (OR) for homicide was 1.41. Similar analysis for the suicide sample produced an odds ratio of 3.44 (Box 11.4).

Case–control studies can produce causal inference, unlike cross-sectional studies (next section), but provide less strength of evidence than that arising from cohort or interventional studies. Of course, in this example, can you imagine an interventional study? Passing out guns to randomized groups of families and then determining the subsequent homicide and suicide rates!

Case–control studies are usually less expensive and are easier to implement than interventional studies, but have a number of drawbacks. The most important limitation is the difficulty of reliably confirming an individual's extent and duration of exposure – a type of recall bias.

Cross-sectional studies

What about cross-sectional studies? Use this design when your goal is to describe the characteristics of a population at a specific point(s) in time or over a specific block of time. Cross-sectional studies can be used to assess the prevalence of acute or chronic disease, to measure the results of medical intervention, or to give census-like data. Cross-sectional studies often rely on data originally collected for other purposes. The study by Korley *et al.*, in which the authors wanted to determine whether the use of advanced diagnostic imaging has changed in US emergency departments, provides an excellent example of the appropriate use of cross-sectional data [5]. The investigators used a large database (the National Hospital Ambulatory Medical Care Survey) to determine that from 1998 to 2007, the prevalence of CT or MRI use during ED visits for injury-related conditions increased significantly, without a corresponding increase in the prevalence of life-threatening conditions (Box 11.5).

Note that cross-sectional studies cannot attribute cause-effect, but rather they are intended to generate hypotheses. Testing of cross-sectional study-derived hypotheses requires further investigation with other study methods. Another disadvantage of cross-sectional study design is that it does not work well for studying rare diseases, because the number of affected individuals may be too low during a specific time frame.

Box 11.4 Example of a case–control study.

- Goal: is gun in home risk factor of suicide or homicide?
- Could carry out a RCT – randomize one group to guns and another to no guns? → Yes, but UNETHICAL.
- Could carry out a cohort study? → Thankfully suicide/homicide is infrequent event → Impractical.
- So – case–control study – Suicide and homicide victims matched to healthy controls.
- Odds of having guns in home in group with outcome was compared to odds of having guns in home in control.
- NOTE:
  ○ In case–control studies we measure the odds of the *risk factor*.
  ○ For rare events (which this is) this approximates the *relative risk of the outcome*.

Data from Wiebe 2003 [4]

Box 11.5 Example of cross-sectional study.

- Goal: to determine the incidence of advanced imaging at discrete points in time.
- Used database of frequency of use of CT or MRI in 1998 and 2007.
- Advantages:
  ○ Easier than prospective studies.
  ○ Often large volumes of data available.
- Disadvantages:
  ○ Cannot make causal inferences.

Data from Korley *et al.* 2010 [5]

Case series

Lowest on the evidence-based totem pole, but certainly an important type of research, is the case series study. Like cross-sectional studies, this is a *descriptive observational* design with no control or comparison group. A case series simply reports on the course and outcome of patients that have had a known similar exposure, disease or treatment. Case series may be prospective or retrospective and usually examine fewer patients than case–control studies. The findings from case series are greatly limited by many types of bias and by the fact that there is no control group available for comparison.

So what is the point of case series reports? Case series can be novel and can spark new areas of investigation. If you are an emergency department doctor and notice a new, interesting disease or find a novel method of treatment in your shop, a case series is the way to go. At UCLA, Levine *et al.* noted three patients presenting with bath salt intoxication and compartment syndrome [6]. They reported their series in a short but sweet 2013 *Annals of Emergency Medicine* paper to bring attention to this previously unrecognized complication of this drug abuse (Box 11.6).

Meta-analyses

Finally, what if you have a topic that has been studied a lot without clear answers from the various papers? In that case, a meta-analysis might be right for you. In a meta-analysis, the data from multiple studies are combined, assessed for bias, homogeneity, and validity, and re-analyzed as a single, larger data set in the hopes of arriving at a consensus answer or more accurate estimate of effect. In 2012, DeBacker *et al.* published a meta-analysis regarding the most commonly used vasopressors (dopamine and norepinephrine) in septic shock [7]. Through a systematic literature search, they found five observational studies and six RCTs addressing morbidity and mortality. After analyzing for bias and assimilating the data, they found a significant increase in mortality and arrhythmic events when dopamine was administered as compared to norepinephrine.

Conclusion

So now that you are an expert in picking the right clinical research design, which type of study will you use to investigate your ketamine hypnosis? Let us use Figure 11.2 to help guide us. Is procedural sedation a common event in the emergency department? Yes. Are we testing a new therapy? Yes. Therefore, a small RCT is likely the best choice to test the hypothesis that using suggestion during procedural sedation can improve smoking cessation.

Picking the right design for the question you are trying to answer is one of the most important things you can do to guarantee that people will believe your results. Remember that although practical or ethical considerations may preclude RCTs and other high level of evidence studies, important research can be produced with other appropriately chosen study designs. Use Figure 11.2 and consider feasibility and limiting bias as much as possible. When writing your manuscript, explain your thought process behind study design selection and candidly present your limitations. Your decision editor will love it!

Box 11.6 Example of case series.

- Goal: to report on a new clinical observation on a limited number of patients.
- Advantages:
  - May increase recognition of a previously unrecognized association (bath salts and compartment syndrome).
  - May herald the arrival of new epidemic.
- Disadvantages:
  - Limited by many types of bias, especially selection bias.
  - No control group.

Data Levin *et al.* 2013 [6]

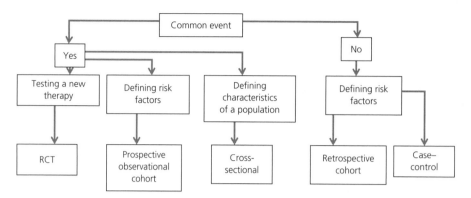

Figure 11.2 Flowchart, picking a study design.

KEY POINTS

- Choose a study design that will best allow you to answer your research question.
- Although randomized controlled trials have the least bias, they may not be practical or ethical.
- Cohort studies are useful for identifying risk factors for diseases.
- Case–control studies are a practical method to study unusual or rare diseases, but are prone to bias.
- Cross-sectional studies measure prevalence of a disease or characteristic at one point in time.
- Meta-analysis can be an excellent tool to summarize the evidence from smaller trials. When performed properly, it may provide the highest level of evidence on a topic.

References

1 Smith, G.C.S. and Pell, J.P. (2003) Parachute use to prevent death and major trauma related to gravitational challenge: systematic review of randomized controlled trials. *BMJ*, **327**(7429):1459–1461.
2 Hoffman, J.R., Mower, W.R., Wolfson, A.B., *et al.* (2000) Validity of a set of clinical criteria to rule out injury to the cervical spine in patients with blunt trauma. National Emergency X-Radiography Utilization Study Group. *N Engl J Med*, **343**:94–99.
3 Perry, J., Stiell, I.G., Sivilotti, M.L., *et al.* (2010) High risk clinical characteristics for subarachnoid hemorrhage in patients with acute headache: Prospective cohort study. *BMJ*, **341**:c5204.
4 Wiebe, D.J. (2003) Homicide and suicide risks associated with firearms in the home: A national case-control study. *Ann Emerg Med*, **41**(6):771–782.
5 Korley, F.K., Pham, J.C., and Kirsch, T.D. (2010) Use of advanced radiology during visits to US emergency departments for injury-related conditions, 1998–2007. *JAMA*, **304**(13):1465–1471.
6 Levine, M., Levitan, R., and Skolnik, A. (2013) Compartment syndrome after "bath salts" use: a case series. *Ann Emerg Med*, **61**(4):480–483.
7 DaBacker, D., Aldecoa, C., Njimi, H., and Vincent, J.L. (2012) Dopamine versus norepinephrine in the treatment of septic shock: A meta-analysis. *Crit Care Med*, **40**(3):725–730.

CHAPTER 12

How to design a study that everyone will believe: Random selection and allocation of patients to treatment conditions

Katie L. Tataris[1], Mary Mercer[2], and Prasanthi Govindarajan[3]

[1] Section of Emergency Medicine, University of Chicago, Chicago, IL, USA
[2] Department of Emergency Medicine, San Francisco General Hospital, San Francisco, CA, USA
[3] Stanford University Medical Center, Stanford, CA, USA

"A clinical trial is a powerful tool for studying the efficacy of an intervention. While the concept of clinical trial dates back to 1926, only in the past few decades has this emerged as the preferred method of evaluating medical interventions" [1].

> "Evidence based pride and observational prejudice".
>
> Smith et al., BMJ, 2003 [2]

The issue of BMJ from which the quote is taken states the importance of a randomized control trial (RCT) and how observational findings should often be verified through a well-planned and executed RCT before practice change is implemented.

Why conduct a randomized control trial?

> RCTs are prospectively designed studies that compare the effect of an intervention against a control group that is similar to the intervention group in every way except for the intervention being studied [1].

While other methods of study design exist, a well-designed, well-conducted RCT provides a better rationale for causality than observational designs. Observational studies are vulnerable to **confounding**, in which a false association could be shown when one fails to control for a variable related to the risk factor and outcome. For example, observational studies found evidence of lower rates of coronary heart disease (CHD) in postmenopausal women taking estrogen compared to women that not taking estrogen and advocated for use of hormone supplements in these women. However, follow up RCTs such as the Heart and Estrogen/progestin Replacement Study (HERS) and the Women's Health Initiative study showed hormone replacement increased the overall risk of CHD events in postmenopausal women with established coronary artery disease, demonstrating the pitfalls of observational data [3]. Often in an observational study, factors that are known to confound a causal association are controlled for in the design or analytical phase. RCTs are superior in that they control for unmeasured confounders by balancing the known and unknown baseline variables between the groups. For example, when studying the association between community characteristics and survival in out-of-hospital

Doing Research in Emergency and Acute Care: Making Order Out of Chaos, First Edition. Edited by Michael P. Wilson, Kama Z. Guluma, and Stephen R. Hayden.

cardiac arrest, there may be emergency medical services variables that could influence the outcome. In a RCT, these would be balanced between the intervention and control arm through the process of randomization, thereby eliminating their effect on the outcomes.

Planning a clinical trial

While several steps must occur before a Phase 3 trial is designed, this chapter describes a clinical trial that assesses the effectiveness of an intervention relevant to clinical practice in an acute care setting.

A well-planned and executed RCT can be carried out in the acute care environment. The key steps shown in Table 12.1 will help to design and execute the study, and in the writing up of the results according to the CONSORT guidelines. [4, 5]. CONSORT stands for Consolidated Standards of Reporting Trials and offers recommendations for reporting findings of RCTs.

The planning phase

There are several steps for laying the groundwork for a successful trial. These include planning and protocol design, sample size calculation, recruitment of participating sites, implementation, and execution of the trial.

Choosing the intervention and controls

RCTs have an experimental arm and a control arm. Patients in the experimental arm are assigned to the intervention and controls are most commonly assigned to the non-intervention or "standard of care" arm. This arm may include a placebo or existing treatments and active therapies. Since patients are selected to receive the intervention, equivalent treatment, or placebo, it is important that the different treatments being studied show clinical equipoise. It is unethical if clinical patients are treated with agents that are considered clinically superior or inferior at the start of the trial.

> **Ethical issues in selecting controls** When the Resuscitation Outcomes Consortium sought an RCT to study the effect of an impedance threshold device (ITD) on survival of patients with out-of-hospital cardiac arrest, the prior observational literature suggested that it might have some benefit [6]. Therefore, there was an initial concern that withholding this device from half of patients would be unethical, as many assumed superiority of the ITD. However, after institutional review board approval, a large RCT was conducted comparing outcomes for patients with out-of-hospital cardiac arrest who received standard CPR with use of an ITD and those who received standard CPR with a sham device [7].

Table 12.1 Phases of a clinical trial.

Phase	Core elements
Planning	Protocol design
	Choosing interventions and controls
	Choosing randomization techniques
	Selecting outcomes
	Measuring baseline variables in the study population
	Defining inclusion (and exclusion) criteria
	Institutional Review Board (IRB) approval
	Acquiring funding
Preparatory	Establishing oversight infrastructure
	Specifying operations (manual of operations)
	Standardizing and testing study documents
	Training for participant investigators
Recruitment	Deploying inclusion and exclusion criteria
	Utilizing informed consent process (or exception from informed consent, where applicable)
Patient follow-up and trial termination	Interval-based follow-up
	Specific protocol for termination
Analysis	Statistical analysis
	Manuscript writing

Selecting outcomes

The impact of the intervention on outcome is of utmost importance to the research community. There should be a single *primary* outcome for each research question, as RCTs are usually powered to examine the primary outcome only. Any remaining outcome variables are classified as secondary outcomes. While secondary outcomes are important and informative (especially with regards to the design of a potential follow-up trial), conclusions pertaining to them are limited due to the nature of the study design. Also, outcomes can be simple or composite. A simple outcome include all-cause mortality while a composite outcome includes all cardiovascular deaths, non-fatal heart attacks and emergency surgery related to the intervention. Further, an outcome may be a direct measure of clinical status, such as mortality, or may be a measure of something else (i.e., a surrogate outcome) that implies clinical status, such as viral load in HIV patients or peak expiratory flow rate in asthmatics [8].

Measuring baseline variables

Baseline variables are descriptive patient information and should be collected for patients in both arms of the study. Examples of baseline variables include age, gender, educational status, past medical conditions, and so on. Baseline variables that are known to influence outcome should definitely be recorded. For example, stroke severity is associated with functional status at the time of discharge. Therefore, the effect of an intervention on final outcome may be affected by stroke severity as measured by National Institute of Health Stroke Scale at the time of presentation. Therefore, having this as a baseline variable will help discover the true effect of the intervention on the outcome [9].

Participant selection

Patient selection is a requirement for meeting the study objectives and goals; it is accomplished objectively using the inclusion and exclusion criteria. Inclusion criteria are attributes that are present in a patient that qualify them to participate in a clinical trial. On the other hand, the presence of exclusion criteria disqualifies them from participating in a clinical trial. The advantages of having these criteria include reproducibility of patient enrollment at the different study sites, not subjecting patients at risk to the intervention and protecting the vulnerable population such as pregnant women, children, and so on [8].

Examples of inclusion criteria for a drug trial for Transient Ischemic Attack (TIA) would be a clinical diagnosis of TIA, objective criteria to stratify high risk TIA patients and minor stroke patients, and radiological confirmation of non-stroke causes. Exclusion criteria would include those with an allergy to the medication, those who may have risks such as bleeding or renal failure from the medication, those who cannot swallow pills, or those who cannot give informed consent.

While inclusion criteria help define the study population of interest, exclusions should be chosen sparingly in order to preserve the generalizability of a study's findings. The most important reasons to exclude patients are if the participants would be harmed by the intervention, if there is certainty that there will be no benefit to this group, if age or other factors prevent them from being able to provide truly informed consent, or if the treatment regimen cannot be applied to this group as stated in the protocol.

Randomization and blinding

Once patients are screened and found to meet the inclusion criteria, they are randomized to the intervention or control group. **Random allocation** means that all participants have a defined probability of assignment to a particular intervention. Random allocation allows the baseline variables to be distributed equally across the groups and thus allows for balancing of groups. Random assignment of study participants is a critical part of the study design and must be performed methodically [8].

Randomization methods

1 **Simple randomization** can be achieved by using the flip of a coin or a random number table or generator.
  - This is the easiest method to randomize patients in an equal ratio into each intervention group.
  - *Advantage*: easy to implement.
  - *Disadvantage*: at any point in the randomization there could be an imbalance between the two groups.
  - "Pseudorandomization" is a technique that assigns participants based on study entry on an even or odd day of the week, birth month, medical record number or other fixed patient/study characteristic. The problem with these methods is that the investigator knows in advance the group to which a particular patient will be assigned, which leads to selection bias and should be avoided.

2 **Blocked randomization** ensures an equal balance of patients in each arm of the study (stratifying by time).
- Balances patient characteristics over time.
- Divides potential patients into a number of groups or blocks; for example, for blocks of 4, 6, 8 there will be equal participation from each arm of the study (groups A and B) in each block.
- The order in which interventions are assigned in each block is randomized and the process is repeated for consecutive blocks until all participants are randomized.
- *Advantages*: The balance between the number of participants in each group is guaranteed during randomization, therefore increasing the power of the study. This is also useful with small sample sizes and if the trial is terminated before complete enrollment the groups will be balanced.
- *Disadvantages*: Assignments at the end of each block could be predicted and manipulated, but varying block size helps prevent this. Analysis of data may be more complicated, as many analytical methods assume simple randomization.
- Example: In a block size of four (Figure 12.1) there will be two control patients and two test patients. The order of the test and control patients will vary within the blocks but the number of patients is kept constant.

3 **Stratified randomization** allows organization of participants by characteristic (age, sex) and then assignment of treatment randomly to each strata (stratifying by factors other than time).
- If a single factor is used, it is divided by two or more subgroups or strata (example: age 0–5 years, 6–10 years, 11–15 years). If several factors are used, that is, gender and race, a stratum is formed by selecting one subgroup (non-Hispanic whites and females) from each of them. The total stratum number is the product of the different subgroups (see table below for details).
- How does the randomization work? Measure characteristics or factors among participants, assign appropriate strata and randomize within strata.
- Within each strata, most clinical trials use blocked randomization to keep the group numbers balanced
- *Advantage*: The power of the study can be increased by using stratification in the analysis, as it reduces variability between group comparisons.
- *Disadvantage*: Increased stratification in small studies can limit data and so only important stratifying variables should be used.
- Example: An investigator is looking at the effect of household smoking on childhood asthma and wants to stratify on age, sex, and household smoke (Table 12.2).
- This design has $3 \times 2 \times 3 = 18$ strata (Table 12.3).
- Participants between 0 and 5 years of age, male, and with no household smoke (stratum 1) would be assigned to groups A or B in the sequences ABBA, BABA, and so on.
- One variation on stratified randomization is **Cluster Randomized Trials** in which the group is randomized, not the individual. Examples would be hospitals, families, or towns. In some situations, the intervention can only be administered to one group for convenience or economic reasons, but are likely to randomize fewer groups and may have imbalance among group size.

Blinding is another important aspect of RCT. Concealing knowledge of the treatment assignments can help reduce bias. Physicians if not blinded to a weight loss drug intervention may consciously or unconsciously provide advice on lifestyle modification that is likely to influence the outcome. Similarly outcome assessors may show bias when abstracting outcomes from medical records if they are not blinded to the intervention.

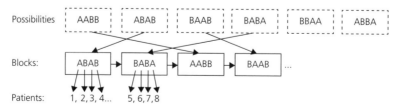

Figure 12.1 Blocked randomization example.

Table 12.2 Factors in study of the effect of household smoking on childhood asthma.

Age (years)	Sex	Household smoke
0–5	Male	None
6–10	Female	Occasional
11–15		Daily

Table 12.3 Strata in study of the effect of household smoking on childhood asthma.

Strata	Age (years)	Sex	Household smoke	Group assignment
1	0–5	M	None	ABBA, BABA, etc.
2	0–5	M	Occasional	
3	0–5	M	Daily	
4	0–5	F	None	
5	0–5	F	Occasional	
6	0–5	F	Daily	
7	6–10	M	None	
8	6–10	M	Occasional	
9	6–10	M	Daily	
10	6–10	F	None	
	etc.			

The preparatory phase

This is the first step in the operational phase and involves creating a manual of operations, organizational oversight policies, reporting structure, data monitoring committee, and communications between sites [10].

Recruitment phase

Strategies for recruitment vary based on the clinical question and the setting, but the overall goal of this phase is to recruit the appropriate number of patients in a timely manner. Some methods of recruiting patients for a clinic-based trial for epilepsy include fliers and posters in doctor's offices and support organizations for patients with seizure disorders. However, recruitment may not be possible for trials that include life threatening or time-sensitive conditions like seizures, acute intracranial hemorrhage, acute spinal cord injury, and so on. For these conditions, investigators inform the community about the ongoing trials through the process of community consultation and public disclosure, and patients who chose not to participate may opt out of these trials [11, 12].

The patient follow-up and termination phase

Patient follow-up entails a standardized protocol for follow-up intervals based on the study design and outcome measures, as well as a protocol for terminating patient involvement in the study. Follow up may be conducted in person, by phone, or by correspondence depending on the time intervals needed [8, 13]. Some examples of follow-up include 90-day in-person follow-up of functional status in a study evaluating early management of systolic blood pressure in acute intracranial hemorrhage. In addition to baseline variables, investigators should always record the name, phone number, and e-mail addresses of participants in order to maintain contact through the follow-up phase.

The analysis phase

The final phase of a study includes the tasks of statistical analysis and manuscript preparation. One needs to be familiar with the intent to treat and per protocol types of analysis. Intention-to-treat analysis is performed based on the study arm to which the patient was assigned and the treatment they were intended to have, regardless of whether they actually received that treatment. In per protocol analysis, statistical comparison of outcomes is based on what treatment the patient actually received rather than what was intended by the initial random assignment [8, 10]. Take, for example, a hypothetical study looking at the effectiveness of apple sauce in acute myocardial infarction. In an intention-to-treat analysis, a patient who was initially assigned to the apple sauce arm would still be included in the apple sauce cohort for outcomes analysis, even if he did not receive it. In a per protocol analysis, the same patient would be included in the non-apple sauce cohort for analysis based on the actual treatment they received. Intent-to-treat analysis is considered superior as it maintains the integrity of randomization.

Ethical aspects of research

The first step in any research process is to obtain an approval from the institutional review board (Chapter 8). The goal of any ethical review is to respect study participants through autonomy, minimize risks, maximize benefit, and ensure a fair selection of study patients [14]. A critical component of ethical principles is obtaining informed consent in research. However, there are situations that one may encounter in the emergency setting where informed consent may not be practically possible. This includes disease processes such as status epilepticus, traumatic brain injury and out-of-hospital cardiac arrest. Under these circumstances, FDA recommendations allow for exception from informed consent [12].

KEY POINTS

- A clinical trial is the clearest method of establishing the effect of an intervention on outcome.
- Inclusion should be broad and exclusions should be minimal if you want your results to be generalizable.
- Randomization can be simple, blocked, or stratified; the method chosen depends on the study to be performed.
- A double blinded design should be used when possible to avoid bias during data collection and assessment.
- Exception from informed consent may apply in research scenarios for some emergency conditions, but strict guidelines apply.

References

1 Friedman, L.M., Furberg, C.D., and Demets, D.L. (1998) *Fundamentals of Clinical Trials*, 3rd edn. Springer, NY.
2 Smith, G.C. and Pell, J.P. (2003) Parachute use to prevent death and major trauma related to gravitational challenge: a systematic review of randomized control trials. *BMJ*, **327**(7429):1459–1461.
3 Rossouw, J.E, Anderson, G.L., Prentice, R.L., *et al.* (2002) Risks and benefits of estrogen plus progestin in healthy postmenopausal women: principal results from the Women's Health Initiative randomized controlled trial. *JAMA*, **288**:321–333.
4 Hulley, S., Grady, D., Bush, T., *et al.* (1998) Randomized trial of estrogen plus progestin for secondary prevention of coronary heart disease in postmenopausal women. *JAMA*, **280**(7):605–613.
5 CONSORT (n.d.) The CONSORT flow diagram. http://www.consort-statement.org/consort-statement/flow-diagram0/ (last accessed (3 May 2015).
6 Thayne, R.C., Thomas, D.C., Neville, J.D., and Van Dellen, A. (2005) Use of an impedance threshold device improves short-term outcomes following out-of-hospital cardiac arrest. *Resuscitation*, **67**(1):103–108.
7 Aufderheide, T.M., Nichol, G., Rea, T.D., *et al.* (2011) A trial of an impedance threshold device in out-of-hospital cardiac arrest. *N Engl J Med*, **365**:798–806.
8 Hulley, S.B., Cummings, S.R., Browner, W.S., *et al.* (2013) *Designing Clinical Research*, 4th edn. Lippincott Williams & Wilkins, Philadelphia, PA.
9 Meinert, C.L. (1981) Organization of multicenter clinical trials. *Control Clin Trials*, **1**(4):305–312.

10 Klimt, C.R. (1981) The conduct and principles of randomized clinical trials. *Control Clin Trials*, **1**(4):283–293.

11 Prout, T.E. (1981) Patient recruitment techniques in clinical trials. *Control Clin Trials*, **1**(4): 313–318.

12 FDA (Food and Drug Administration) (2010) *Exception from Informed Consent for Studies Conducted in Emergency Settings: Regulatory Language and Excerpts from Preamble – Information Sheet. Guidance for Institutional Review Boards and Clinical Investigators.* http://www.fda.gov/RegulatoryInformation/Guidances/ucm126482.htm (3 May 2015).

13 Klimt, C.R. (1981) Terminating a long-term clinical trial. *Control Clin Trials*, **1**(4):319–325.

14 Prout, T.E. (1981) The ethics of informed consent. *Control Clin Trials*, **1**(4):429–434.

CHAPTER 13

How to design a study that everyone will believe: Surveys

Edward M. Castillo and Gary M. Vilke

Department of Emergency Medicine, University of California San Diego, San Diego, CA, USA

> *"A telephone survey says that 51% of college students drink until they pass out at least once a month. The other 49% didn't answer the phone."*
>
> Craig Kilborn

The time has come for you to develop a survey for a research project and you realize that you were never taught study survey design in medical school, or you simply used that time for much needed sleep. But how hard could it be? All you need to do put a few questions on a form, have people complete it, and then you are halfway to a conference in the Caribbean to present your results. Not so fast. There are a few things that you much consider prior to starting your survey journey. In this chapter, the planning that should go into a well-developed survey, survey methodology, issues about questions and wording, and the importance of the layout and design of a survey are described.

Surveys can be useful in acute care and emergency medicine. Although there are limitations when using surveys, they are a cheap and relatively quick method to collect study data. They are also a great tool for a variety of studies, including descriptive studies and analytic studies, and can be combined with other data sources. For example, in a prospective observational cohort study, a survey can be used to collect behavioral information at various time points and combined with physical examination data. They can also be useful to help develop clinical decision rules or to obtain descriptive baseline data for grant proposals. However, a little work needs to be done upfront so that you can collect useful and accurate data from a survey.

When thinking about developing your survey, you really need to have most of your study planned out, including your study design and analysis plan. What are the objectives of your study? Is there only a primary objective or do you also have one or more secondary objectives? How does your study fit in with the current literature and will your results be comparable? The timing of when data will be collected is another important consideration to avoid unnecessary bias. For example, does the survey have to be completed during care in the emergency department or can the patients be called after discharge? Once these questions have been clearly defined on paper, not just in your head, you can begin developing the survey.

Overview of survey methodology

When you have your research objectives well thought out, you can start thinking about the study design. There are a couple of general approaches that need to be considered when you start planning your study prior to developing your survey; specifically, will your survey be qualitative, quantitative or a mixed methods design? This will be largely dictated by your study objectives and the research questions you are trying to answer. Qualitative studies, or exploratory studies, are designed to provide an in-depth understanding of an issue by investigating *why* and *how*. These types of studies often consist of a relatively small focused sample group and less-defined questions with the

---

Doing Research in Emergency and Acute Care: Making Order Out of Chaos, First Edition. Edited by Michael P. Wilson, Kama Z. Guluma, and Stephen R. Hayden.

Box 13.1 Examples of qualitative and quantitative survey questions.

Qualitative Research Questions

Please tell me about your experience in the Emergency Department this afternoon.

Why did you choose to come to the Emergency Department today for your chronic condition?

Quantitative Research Questions

What is the likelihood of you returning for care in our Emergency Department if needed.

- Very Poor
- Poor
- Fair
- Good
- Very Good

Rate your pain on a scale from 0 to 10.

resulting data categorized into patterns. Quantitative studies, or descriptive and causal studies, are more common in clinical research and investigate the *what*, *where*, and *when* of an issue. These studies require larger random samples with data that are numbers and anything measureable. Mixed methods designs are a combination of both methods, with both exploratory and descriptive or causal objectives. Examples of qualitative and quantitative survey questions are shown in Box 13.1.

Administration

After you have decided whether you are going to take a qualitative, quantitative, or mixed method approach, it is time to consider how the survey will be administered. There are several different methods that can be used to collect surveys and all of them may impact the design of the survey. The main considerations when deciding the best method for administering your survey are the cost, feasibility, and potential completion rates for various methods, your timeline, and potential bias with each method.

Another main issue that must be considered when developing your project is non-responders, the Achilles heel of survey research. The non-response rate will vary based on a variety of issues, including the topic of the research, the method used to administer your survey, the clarity of the questions, how it is formatted, and the time it takes to complete the survey. This must be considered in the planning phases of your project, or you may be wasting your time.

So what does it matter if you have a low response rate, but still get the sample size you aimed for? Bias, bias, bias, and it is often difficult to estimate how non-responders are impacting your results, if at all. So what is a good response rate? It depends on a number of factors, including what you are researching and your sample population. Sometimes a response rate of 60% is not acceptable and at other times 10% can be considered a success. The most important thing is to understand how the response rate can impact your study prior to implementation so you can adequately plan to obtain the most ideal response rate.

Survey methods

Personal interviews

Personal interviews are common in emergency medicine survey studies, especially in departments with Research Associate programs (usually undergraduates volunteering on research projects). The benefits for this type of survey administration are that you can obtain in-depth information from the participant using a variety of question types and approaches. The questions can be interactive and the reviewer has some ability to limit unclear and non-responses. However, this method can also be time intensive and costly, especially if you are paying research staff to administer the surveys to a large population. Other potential issues are the possibility of interviewer and response bias as well as the lack of anonymity.

Telephone interview

Telephone interviews are a useful method for survey studies, especially for patient follow-up. Similar to personal interviews, telephone interviews can probe for detailed information, specific questions or responses can be clarified if needed, and they have a relatively quick turnaround compared to other methods. Also, similar to personal interviews, there a few limitations with telephone interviews that should be considered before picking up the telephone. In general these limitations are similar to personal interviews and include cost, interviewer and response bias as well as the lack of anonymity. In addition to these issues, you will need to consider your target population to ensure you do not bring in difficulties with your response rate and bias. For example, if targeting homeless patients or immigrants, they may not have a land line and they may use pay as you go phones with frequent phone number changes. Plus, nobody wants to answer a survey during dinner!

Mail surveys

Although mail surveys are common for information gathering for patient satisfaction or follow up, they are not as common for formal research studies. Mail surveys have a few benefits over personal and telephone interviews, including that they can decrease response bias because they can be anonymous, interview bias is eliminated, the surveys can use pictures and images, and they can be relatively inexpensive when compared to staff time. Unfortunately, studies utilizing mail surveys may need multiple mailings to get the desired response rate, which can significantly increase the data collection period for your study.

E-mail/Internet

The expansion of the Internet and e-mail has led to the development of companies such as SurveyMonkey, KwikSurveys, and Zoomerang that develop, customize and distribute surveys quickly and cost effectively. Another bonus over paper surveys is that they are already entered electronically and most can produce simple descriptive statistics. Although computer program requirements must be considered when using e-mail and Internet surveys, these programs are usually easy to use, but you may be limited to specific types of questions. The generalizability may also be an issue, as potential participant's electronic communication habits change. For example, e-mail is not always the primary source of communication. Additionally, response rates may be affected by files ending up in spam folders or quarantined by security programs. Actually, many university students communicate more often on other platforms, such as Facebook and Instagram. These trends, as well as e-mail fatigue, must be factored in when using these methods of survey distribution.

Technology and surveys

Technology is also helping the ease of data collection for surveys. Regardless of the survey approach used, tablets and touch screen laptops are making personal interviews relatively easy compared to paper methods that require the added step of data entry, which can lead to data entry errors. Data collection systems, such as REDCap (**R**esearch **E**lectronic **D**ata **Cap**ture) (http://www.project-redcap.org/), which is a consortium composed of nearly a thousand institutional partners in 75 countries, have increase the productivity and streamlining of research studies. These types of systems are secure web applications that are designed for building and managing on-line surveys and databases and can be used for personal interviews, data collection from paper forms, and on-line surveys. So when embarking on developing a survey, definitely determine how technology can help make your study successful, but keep in mind that there are still the underlying limitations for the survey design, type of administration and potentially using the actual technology.

Time to develop your survey

"You should approach a survey the same way you approach a patient … by first warming your hands so you don't make them jump."
Dr Gary Vilke

Regardless of the approach or type of survey administration, you must be sure that you have laid the groundwork for your study. As previously noted, at this point your primary and secondary objectives should be fully developed and your data management and analysis plan should also be finalized. This should include knowing your primary and secondary outcomes, what data are required for analysis, how the data should be formatted or reformatted after collection, and what will be the specific analysis to be performed on that data. If you need to record data as a continuous variable to be analyzed with a t-test for comparability to previous studies, then you want to be sure you do not include that variable on the survey as a Likert scale or other categorical format.

Survey questions

When you begin developing your questions, you should already know what you want to do with each response. Many survey studies have gone awry by asking additional unnecessary questions that are not relevant to the objectives of the study. Depending on the specific additional questions, they can mislead the respondent, incorporate additional and unnecessary bias, or even increase the incomplete or overall response rate. On the other hand, additional questions may be desired based on the answer given by the respondent to a particular question. Once a survey is complete and the subject is done, typically it is impossible to go back and ask additional questions. With a well-developed data analysis plan, you should already understand how the responses will be analyzed. Therefore, it is best to keep it short and simple, but complete for the required task at hand.

When developing your survey, it is a good idea to group related questions as much as possible. For example, put demographic related questions together (i.e., age, gender, etc.) and behavioral questions together (i.e., smoking and alcohol history, etc.). To avoid potentially making the respondent uncomfortable, ask general, interesting and non-threatening questions before more specific questions. Questions respondents may find uncomfortable or threatening include sexual history, history of drug abuse, and even education or income.

There are several types of questions that can be used in a survey. Structured, closed or fixed response questions have a predetermined set of answers for the respondent to choose from. These types of questions make data collection faster and data management and analysis easier, and are best used when you have a thorough understanding of the question and responses and when you are not trying to collect new ideas or thoughts from the participant. When developing these questions, you want to be sure that every possible answer is included and that the answers do not overlap (i.e., 0–10, 10–20, 20–30) to avoid non-responses and difficulty with the interpretation. Options of 0–10, 11–20, 21–30, and so on would be the better way to offer the possible responses. If there are potentially other answers that are not listed, then including "Other", "Not Applicable" or "Don't Know" would be appropriate and necessary.

Although you would think it is easy to develop structured questions, it can be more daunting than you think. For example, Likert scale and Likert-type questions are often used in survey research to get an overall measurement of a specific topic. Likert scale questions have opposing responses around a neutral response, such as Strongly Agree, Agree, Neutral, Disagree, and Strongly Disagree. Likert-type questions are similar, but do not have directly opposing responses. When including these types of questions in a survey, you must think about the value that the question has by itself (if at all) versus including it as a composite value from several questions and report results appropriately.

Unstructured, or open-ended questions, allow the respondent to complete the question in their own words and are useful when trying to get new ideas and thoughts about a subject. Unlike structured questions, these take longer to complete and analyze. Although these questions are useful when developing an all-inclusive set of answers is difficult, they should be minimized when you are trying to take a qualitative approach to your research. Otherwise, it may be necessary to review the literature further or do more preliminary work to get a better understanding of your research topic.

Question wording

When developing your survey, you must remember that specific wording can have an effect on how people respond. Avoid adjectives and adverbs with unclear or highly variable meaning such as usually, often, sometimes, occasionally, seldom, rarely, most, numerous, and several. These words often have different meaning to different people, so it is important to be as precise as possible. When possible, also avoid the use of "and/or", for example, "Do you feel your injury risk is increased in your home and/or work?" This makes it difficult to determine if a positive response is related to home or work or both.

As mentioned, include "Other" or "I don't know" answers where appropriate because respondents often do not respond to a question if the available answers are not directly applicable to them, and the reason for a non-response

Box 13.2 Examples of good and bad survey questions and answers.

Bad Survey Question	How many times in the last year have you seen your primary care provider or been admitted to the emergency department?
	• 0 times
	• 1 time
	• 2 times
	• 3 times
	• 4 or more times
Good Survey Questions	How many times in the last year have you seen your *primary care provider*?
	• 0 times
	• 1 time
	• 2 times
	• 3 or more times
	How many times in the last year have been *admitted to the emergency department*?
	• 0 times
	• 1 time
	• 2 times
	• 3 or more times
Bad Survey Answers	How many times in the last year have you seen your *primary care provider*?
	• 0–1 times
	• 1–2 times
	• 2–3 times
	• 3 or more times
Good Survey Answers	How many times in the past twelve months have you seen your *primary care provider*?
	• 0–1 times
	• 2–3 times
	• 4–5 times
	• 6 or more times

is difficult to interpret. Similarly, the available responses should be relevant to the survey to avoid distraction. Another important thing to keep in mind is that you need to know your target population. Avoid using slang, jargon, or acronyms and verify that the meaning of all words utilized is clear. Use language that is appropriate for the knowledge and education level of your subject. Asking a lay or high school educated person if they ever had a myocardial infarction might not get you the response you desire compared with if you asked them if they ever had a heart attack. Lastly, be as specific as possible when asking about a specific time period. For example, use "in the last 7 days", "12 months", AND SO ON rather than an open-ended time period. Examples of good and bad survey questions and answers are illustrated in Box 13.2.

Survey layout and respondent interaction

As with anything you are presenting to a potential participant, make the survey look professional. Use a standard format that is easy to follow and understand. For this, electronic forms are helpful because skip patterns can be built in and are hidden when not needed. If paper is required, be sure to format it so it is as obvious as possible for both the respondent and interviewer to see and understand; use different fonts and/or formats such as bold, italics, and so on. In general, a vertical layout is easier to read and follow than a horizontal layout. Also, using anything lower than a 12 point font or condensing your survey onto one page is not necessary and often makes it difficult to follow. If you have unstructured questions, allow for enough room for the participant to fully respond. A simple thing like numbering can also go a long way.

The more comfortable a potential respondent is with you the more likely they will complete the survey. Make them feel good. Regardless of the method of administration you decide on using, tell them why you need their help and the importance of your project with them and potentially future patients. And, of course, thank them for their time when they are done.

Final steps

Now that you have developed your primary and secondary objectives, determined if you want to use a qualitative, quantitative or mixed methods approach, have determined the most appropriate administration process, and have painstakingly gone over all of your questions, you are ready to begin, right? Again, not so fast! It is always a good idea to make sure your survey is reliable and valid. Reliability is important when you are developing a score measure; it is when your survey produces consistent results among the same person or similar types of people. Reliability can be measured with a variety of statistical methods, including Cronbach's α, which are available in most statistics software packages.

Validation is the process of ensuring your survey is truly measuring what you think it measures. There are several types of validation and how you validate your survey will depend on your survey. The most important thing is that you pilot your survey to verify that the questions you are asking are understood and mean the same to the respondents, and to make sure the format and questions are appropriate for the method of administration. Have some of the people who you are planning to administer the survey (if not a mailing or on-line survey) practice using the survey tool. Often, vague questions or missing responses will be captured at this time and can then be adjusted and incorporated into the survey prior to initiating the study. Similarly, beta-testing the tool with a few sample subjects may also find some questions or answers that need to be clarified before the study is formally started. Colleagues can also be helpful, but you will get the most benefit from piloting your survey with your target population.

KEY POINTS

- Planning is key. Your objectives, research questions, and analysis plan should be completed prior to developing a survey.
- Different methods of survey administration have various benefits and limitations. Know and understand what these are.
- Technology can be a great way to make your survey a success.
- Keep your survey simple and relevant to your research questions.
- Make sure your survey is reliable and valid.

Further reading

1 Andres, L. (2012) *Designing and Doing Survey Research*. Sage Publications Ltd.
2 Fink, A. (2013) *How to Conduct Surveys: A Step-by-Step Guide*. Sage Publications Ltd.
3 Fowler, F.J. (2013) *Survey Research Methods (Applied Social Research Methods)*, 5th edn. Sage Publications Ltd.

CHAPTER 14

How to design a study that everyone will believe: Retrospective reviews

Jonathan Auten[1] and Paul Ishimine[2]

[1] F Hebert School of Medicine, Uniformed Services University of Health Sciences, Bethesda, MD, USA
[2] Department of Emergency Medicine, UC San Diego Health System, San Diego, CA, USA

> *"Understand and accept your study's limitations before collecting any forms of data."*
>
> Richard Clark, MD

I can still recall the overwhelming sense of frustration generated by my first research project, a retrospective review of a poison control center database. The senior researcher carefully reviewed the protocol guidelines for abstraction, went over the data forms, and gave the junior researchers practice charts for review. I went into the project feeling well prepared, but, several days later, after reviewing hundreds of charts, I felt utterly defeated. Despite my best efforts and attention to detail, many abstraction sheets did not have full sets of variables and many charts were limited by incomplete follow-up. My mentor noticed my frustration and handed me an article by RS Hoffman titled, "Understanding the limitations of retrospective analyses of poison center data" [1]. In this article, the author explained, in an almost accepting and even-handed tone, that the barriers that I had experienced were common difficulties with conducting a retrospective review. The ability to understand these limitations offers a certain degree of confidence as you take a structured approach to designing and eventually interpreting a retrospective study. It is our hope that this chapter provides clarity on the strengths of retrospective reviews and the importance of understanding and accepting the limitations before moving forward.

Why are retrospective reviews held in a negative light?

You may have read a meta-analysis, participated in a journal club or been part of an academic discussion in which the merits of retrospective chart reviews are marginalized and dismissed. Someone will cite poor methodology, researcher bias and incomplete databases as reasons to avoid retrospective studies. However, those same clinicians will recommend HIV postexposure prophylaxis for a high-risk needle stick exposure, even though the initial evidence for these recommendations came from a case–control study [2]. Similarly, you may also find those same colleagues counseling a patient against smoking tobacco, even though the initial research regarding the deleterious health effects of smoking came from retrospective studies [3]. A quick glance at the venerable research pyramid shows that, while not at the apex, retrospective case control and cohort studies are part of the foundation of the current paradigm (Figure 14.1). A thoughtfully conceived and designed retrospective review can not only be believable, but may add significant value to the acute care and emergency medicine literature.

The starting point for designing a good retrospective study is to first understand the pitfalls of chart review. A 1996 study found close to one quarter of all emergency medicine research to be retrospective [4]. The authors of this manuscript reviewed 244 articles published in three major emergency medicine journals for eight key criteria of high-quality chart reviews and found inconsistent methods throughout these articles. They found little standardization of abstractor training, monitoring, or blinding. Inter-rater reliability was rarely mentioned and tested less than 1% of the time [4]. Changes to chart review methodology was suggested and adopted by at least one major emergency medicine journal [5]. Nearly a decade later, two separate articles followed up this sentinel review to ascertain the effect that greater awareness had on improvement of methodological flaws of chart review studies. Both articles found that

---

Doing Research in Emergency and Acute Care: Making Order Out of Chaos, First Edition. Edited by Michael P. Wilson, Kama Z. Guluma, and Stephen R. Hayden.

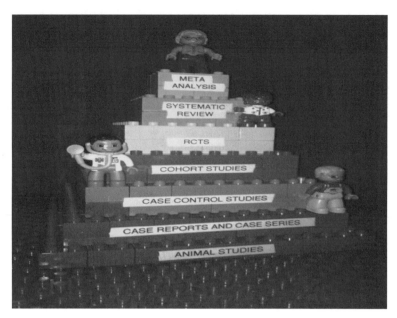

Figure 14.1 Research pyramid (Source: Courtesy of Dylan Auten, 4 years old).

within the international emergency medicine literature, only marginal improvements had been made [6, 7]. Abstractor training, meetings, monitoring, and blinding were still poor. Inter-rater reliability testing occurred in less than 15% of papers and descriptions of sampling methods and missing data management were often omitted.

With the existing bias against chart reviews, why spend the time?

Retrospective studies offer unique advantages to the researcher. Every researcher should go through the "FINER" (Feasible, Interesting, Novel, Ethical, Relevant) mnemonic when generating a research question (Chapter 3). A working knowledge of the strengths of retrospective design can assist you in picking the right project, as certain types of research questions are particularly well suited to this type of study (Box 14.1) [8]. Chart reviews do not require patients to be followed into the future, as events have already taken place. Retrospective studies also offer the distinct advantage of requiring less infrastructure and time to complete than prospective studies. You generally only need time, a well-designed concept, solid patient database, and fundamental understanding of the limitations and advantages of such research. A retrospective study may be the only ethical method for studying harmful treatments or bad outcomes. These types of studies are alluring to some, as they are generally less likely to be biased by outside sources like the pharmaceutical or medical device industry (Box 14.1).

Box 14.1 Retrospective design concepts.

- Description of disease process
- Diagnostic test performance
- Clinical–pathologic correlations
- Quality audits, including adherence to clinical guidelines
- Derivation and validation of clinical prediction rules
- Analyses of the costs of care
- Hypothesis generation

Source: Lowenstein, 2005 [8]. Reproduced with permission of Elsevier.

Box 14.2 Advantages to retrospective design.

- Relatively inexpensive
- Readily accessible existing data
- Long latency between exposures and disease
- Allows the study of rare occurrences
- Generation of hypotheses that can be tested prospectively
- May be the only ethical method for evaluating harmful treatments or bad outcomes

There are several key advantages to retrospective design that can assist you in balancing the limitations of design and deciding whether your investment of time can generate believable results (Box 14.2). If the outcome of interest is uncommon, a prospective investigation would typically be too large to be feasible and favored measures of association, such as absolute risk reduction or number needed to treat, cannot be generated. However, if proper methodology is applied, retrospective research can be reported in terms of odds ratios or an estimate of relative risk [9].

What are the limitations to retrospective review?

"You are only going to get out of a chart review at the end what you put into it at the beginning."

David Tanen, MD, FAAMT

Medical record reviews will rarely provide "the answer" or "the best treatment," but they can offer unique perspectives that are limited in prospective studies. Furthermore, they can lead to prospective validation studies that generate more impactful answers; it is in this manner that retrospective research can add to the medical literature, by generating ideas or creating steps up the research pyramid.

The main question you should ask yourself is the same that your readership should ask: "Do I believe in the methodology of this study?" A study does not have to be perfect, but the researcher must understand the limitations and common errors associated with retrospective design (Boxes 14.3 and 14.4; Chapter 10).

The single largest limitation to medical record reviews is that documentation contained within the record is frequently incomplete or missing for the needs of record review for research [10]. This chapter began with a discussion on a retrospective poison center chart review. It was not uncommon during review to encounter ambiguous entries, such as, "the patient was hypertensive," "CXR normal, "not sure of method of exposure"or "patient is altered." There is no systematic method for recording chief complaints, capturing a full set of vitals or laboratory studies, conducting diagnostic workups, administering treatments, or assessing outcomes. This may be adequate for real-time patient care, but may be inadequate for study data collection. This problem is not limited to reviews in the emergency medicine and acute care literature, and may be further compounded by the advent of the electronic medical record, where greater room of transcription error is present [11]. The first limitation that you must accept and report is that almost all variables in a medical record (histories, physical findings, test results, discharge diagnoses, and outcomes) depend on how physicians chart their observations and synthesize findings.

The second most significant limitation is the degree of bias in a study. This directly affects the validity or generalizability of the study and occurs in addition to random error or chance [9, 12]. The best way to avoid bias is to understand how it can affect the outcome of a study. One of the best historical lessons on selection bias was presented in an article, titled "Coffee and Cancer of the Pancreas," in 1981 in the *New England Journal of Medicine* [13]. The authors performed a case–control study of histologically confirmed pancreatic cancer from 11 Boston and Rhode Island hospitals. Study controls were selected from a group of patients without pancreatic cancer that were admitted by the same doctor at the same hospital as the study cases. However, these controls were selected from the gastroenterology doctor's clinic and carried pre-existing conditions such as peptic ulcers that preselected them to be non-coffee drinkers. This selection bias created a control group that was not representative of the general population. The apparent association between coffee and pancreatic cancer has failed to be proven in subsequent prospective studies. In addition to selection bias, the absence of rules for abstraction, coding, review, and oversight creates a large degree of bias that influences the abstraction itself [4, 14] Creation and adherence to protocols, training, performance monitoring and performance review are the best

Box 14.3 Limitations to retrospective research.

- Internal validity
- Confounding
- History
- Regression toward the mean
- Instrumentation change
- Differential attrition
- External validity

Box 14.4 Common sources of errors.

- Researcher bias
- Abstractor bias
- Case selection bias
- Missing variables
- Incomplete charts
- Absent inter-rater reliability measures

ways to minimize this bias. The single greatest flaw in most retrospective research is the failure to control for this form of bias. Left uncontrolled, the results are difficult or impossible to interpret.

Missing variables are another source of error in these studies. Deletions of the cases or categories introduce additional bias into the study and need to be clearly addressed in the results and limitations sections of your paper. Sampling and measuring reliability are remaining sources of bias. If possible, chart abstractions should be performed between two and four people and inter-rater reliability should be measured (e.g., calculation of a kappa statistic). You should also clearly state within your methods how you arrived at your sample size. Was it a convenience sample or derived with the assistance of a statistician targeting a specific confidence interval?

Designing a believable retrospective study

Once you have generated your idea, performed a thorough literature search and further refined your research question, you will begin to consider your methodology. Carefully weighing the pro's and con's, you have decided to move forward with you research idea. For some of the reasons highlighted above you have chosen a retrospective study design. Now what? Firstly, consider what type of retrospective study fits your available data set. Retrospective studies are categorized into two types: non-analytical and analytical. Non-analytic retrospective studies can broadly be classified as descriptive studies. These studies do not try to determine any quantitative relationships but try to give us a picture of what is happening in a population. Types of non-analytic studies include case reports and case series. Some measures of association can be determined from these types of studies. Analytic studies utilize a comparison group as well as the intervention or exposed group [15]. These include case–control, matched case–control, and retrospective observational cohort studies. The difference between a case–control and a matched case–control study design is that the latter control subjects are selected so they resemble cases (Boxes 14.5 and 14.6). A retrospective cohort study can evaluate two groups, with and without a high risk exposure, to find associated disease or outcomes of interest (Figure 14.2). The opposite is true of case–control studies (Figure 14.3), where you start with the disease or outcome and look backwards for the exposure of interest. A case–control study will allow you to calculate an odds ratio to describe the observed measure of association. Retrospective cohort studies allow us to calculate further measures of association, like the relative risk.

Once you have decided between a non-analytical or analytical design you will need to design a method for record abstraction. There are clear published recommendations that assist in controlling for bias (Box 14.7) [4, 16]. In addition to these two separate guidelines, the STROBE statement represents an international initiative of epidemiologists, methodologists, statisticians, researchers and journal editors aiming to strengthening observational studies in the medical literature. The resources which can be found on their web site (http://www.strobe-statement.org/index. php?id=available-checklists) contains checklists for various types of retrospective studies [17–20]. As you move forward, acknowledge imperfections and limitations, control for obvious sources of bias external to the data set, and adhere to one of these guidelines. Your study may not be featured on your favorite podcast, but perhaps it can serve as the building block for some yet unproven advance in the practice of medicine.

Box 14.5 Features of case–control studies.

- Usually retrospective
- Start out with the disease and measured exposures
- Controls are selected for not having the outcome
- Good for rare outcomes
- Relatively inexpensive
- Smaller numbers required
- Quicker to complete
- Prone to selection bias
- Recall/retrospective bias
- Can calculate odds ratios

Box 14.6 Features of retrospective cohort studies.

- More prone to bias than prospective cohort
- Start with the exposure and measure the disease
- Can study several different disease processes from a single exposure
- Best for common outcomes
- Requires large numbers and expensive
- Takes a long time to complete
- Prone to attrition bias and change in methods over time
- Can calculate odds ratios and relative risk

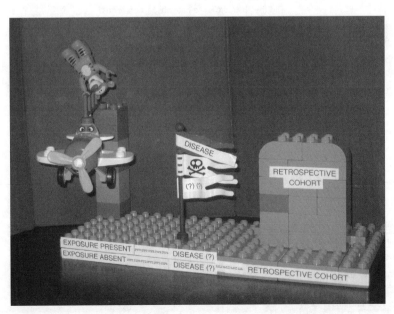

Figure 14.2 Retrospective cohort (start with exposure to find disease) (Source: Courtesy of Lucas Auten, 3 years old).

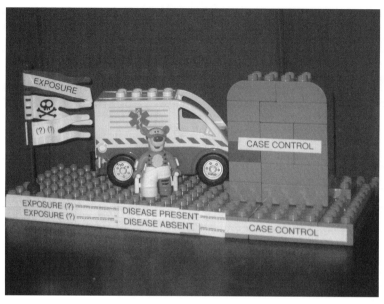

Figure 14.3 Case–control (start with disease to find exposure) (Source: Courtesy of Lucas Auten, 3 years old).

Box 14.7 Retrospective review method.

1. Training	Were the abstractors trained before the data collection?
2. Case selection	Were the inclusion and exclusion criteria for case selection defined?
	Was the method of sampling described?
3. Variable definition	Were the variables defined?
4. Abstraction forms	Did the abstractors use data abstraction forms?
	Was the statistical management of missing data described?
5. Performance monitored	Were the abstractors' performances monitored?
6. Blind to hypothesis	Were the abstractors blinded to the hypothesis/study objectives?
7. Inter-rater reliability (IRR) mentioned	Was the interobserver reliability discussed?
8. Inter-rater reliability (IRR) tested	Was the interobserver reliability tested?

Source: Gilbert *et al.* 1996 [4]. Reproduced with permission of Elsevier.

KEY POINTS

- Adopt one of several published retrospective design methodologies.
- Understand the limitations of chart review and your data set.
- Have a plan to mitigate potential forms of bias before your start to abstract.
- Work to the strengths of the design: hypothesis generation, disease description, and the study of the occurrence of rare diseases.
- Do not over state your findings!

References

1 Hoffman, R.S. (2007) Understanding the limitations of retrospective analyses of poison center data. *Clin Toxicology*, **45**(8):943–945.

2 Cardo, D.M., Culver, D.H., Ciesielski, C.A., *et al.* (1997) A case-control study of HIV seroconversion in health care workers after percutaneous exposure. *N Engl J Med*, **337**(21):1485–1490.

3 Doll, R. and Hill, A.B. (1950) Smoking and carcinoma of the lung. *Br Med J*, **2**(4682):739–748.

4 Gilbert, E.H., Lowenstein, S.R., Kozoil-McLain, J., *et al.* (1996) Chart reviews in emergency medicine research: where are the methods? *Ann Emerg Med*, **27**:305–308.

5 Anon (nd) Instructions for Authors: Chart Reviews. *Ann Emerg Med*. http://www.annemergmed.com/content/designs#chart; last accessed 7 May 2015.

6 Badcock, D.B., Kelly, A., Kerr, D., and Reade, T. (2005) The quality of medical record review studies in the international emergency medicine literature. *Ann Emerg Med*, **45**(4):444–447.

7 Worster, A., Bledsoe, R.D., Cleve, P., *et al.* (2005) Reassessing the methods of medical record review studies in emergency medicine research. *Ann Emerg Med*, **45**(4):448–451.

8 Lowenstein, S.R. (2005) Medical record reviews in emergency medicine: The blessing and the curse. *Ann Emerg Med*, **45**(4). 452–455.

9 Guyatt, G., Jaeschke, R., and Meade, M. (2008) Why study results mislead: Bias and random error. In: G. Guyatt, D. Rennie, M. Meade, and D. Cook (eds) *User's Guide To The Medical Literature: Essentials of Evidence Based Clinical Practice*, 2nd edn. McGraw-Hill Professional, pp. 77–84.

10 Schwartz, R.J., Boiseneau, D., and Jacobs, L.M. (1995) The quantity of cause-of-injury information documented on the medical record: An appeal for injury prevention. *Acad Emerg Med*, **2**:98–103.

11 Burnum, J.F. (1989) The misinformation era: The fall of the medical record. *Ann Intern Med*, **110**:482–484.

12 Worster, A. and Haines, T. (2004) Advanced statistics: understanding medical record review studies. *Acad Emerg Med*, **11**:187–192.

13 MacMahon, B., Yen, S., Trichopoulos, D., *et al.* (1981) Coffee and cancer of the pancreas. *N Engl J Med*, **304**(11):630–633.

14 Hess, D.R. (2004) Retrospective studies and chart reviews. *Respir Care*, **49**(10):1171–1174.

15 Mann, C.J. (2003) Observational research methods. Research design II: cohort, cross sectional, and case-control studies. *Emerg Med J*, **20**:54–60.

16 Gearing, R., Mian, I., Barber, J., and Ickowicz, A. (2006) A methodology for conducting retrospective chart review research in child and adolescent psychiatry. *J Can Acad Child Adolesc Psychiatry*, **15**(3):126–134.

17 Gregory, B.H., VanHorn, C., and Kaprielian, V. (2008) 8 steps to a chart audit for quality. *Fam Pract Manag*, **15**(7):A3–A8.

18 Lerner, E.B., Zachariah, B.S., and White, L.J. (2002) Conducting retrospective emergency medical services research. *Prehosp Emerg Care*, **6**(2 Suppl):S48–S51.

19 Rangel, S.J., Kelsey, J., Colby, C.E., *et al.* (2003) Development of a quality assessment scale for retrospective clinical studies in pediatric surgery. *J Pediatr Surg*, **38**:390–396.

20 STROBE Statement (2009) STROBE Checklists. http://www.strobe-statement.org/index.php?id=available-checklists; last accessed 7 May 2015.

CHAPTER 15

How to design a study that everyone will believe: Prehospital studies

Christopher Kahn

Division of Emergency Medical Services and Disaster Medicine, Department of Emergency Medicine, University of California, San Diego, CA, USA

"If you've seen one EMS system, you've seen one EMS system."

Origins unknown

Congratulations on your desire to pursue research in emergency medical services! It is a field with many exciting research opportunities, but perhaps more than its share of challenges. As pointed out in a 2009 editorial of the same name as the above quote, "In few other areas of medicine are such profound differences in practice, equipment, and outcomes accepted or even observed." [1] While the historical context that led to this is complex and interesting, at least if you are an emergency medical services (EMS) physician, the need for high-quality research to help provide a means for greater standardization and a decrease in regional disparities is great – and that is where you come in.

To make sure that your EMS research project is believable, you will need to address the following issues:

- External validity
- Sample size (power)
- Methodology
- Informed consent
- Patient outcomes
- Relevance of the specific topic under study.

External validity

As indicated, there is tremendous variability in EMS systems. While there are certainly some national differences, such as prevalence of volunteer systems in some parts of the country and transport time differences in urban versus rural systems, the differences from one locality to the next can be pretty striking, too. If your system consists of an urban/suburban community served by a fire-based tiered EMS system that uses a combination of first responder fire units and paramedic ambulances, it might be hard to convince the medical director of a rural community served by a single paramedic ambulance and police first responders that your findings are applicable to his or her system. Even in systems that look fairly similar at first glance, there are often major differences in protocols and skills utilization that make it hard to compare one to the other. For example, there is a lot of variation in how paramedics approach prehospital airway management. Should you stay on scene to manage an airway instead of rapidly going to the closest emergency department? Should you use rapid sequence intubation medications? Should you intubate children? Should you intubate anybody?

Fortunately for you, you are not the first EMS researcher that has ever had to deal with this. Any person reading through the EMS research literature with a critical eye and an interest in seeing what might be of value to their system knows what their own system is like, and that absolves you of the need to find a way to make your results generalizable

---

Doing Research in Emergency and Acute Care: Making Order Out of Chaos, First Edition. Edited by Michael P. Wilson, Kama Z. Guluma, and Stephen R. Hayden.

to every system (don't worry, they won't be). The most important step you can take to ensure that your research project has maximal external validity is to be specific in describing your system when you discuss your methodology. Make sure you detail items such as:

- System type (fire-based, third system, public utility model, etc.).
- Who responds to calls.
  ○ In systems where different calls get different responses, include the dispatch method used and the different response levels.
- Which medications, equipment, and protocols exist in your system that are relevant to your project.
  If you do not know this information, your local EMS medical director will.

Sample size (Power)

Given the variability in EMS systems, many researchers assume it is too difficult to look at questions across more than one system. After all, it is important to make sure that your data are being collected in the same way, and that they are comparable across every system you are looking at. Unfortunately, while limiting your study to one system is undoubtedly easier – and a lot quicker if you are trying to get your study done in a hurry – you are going to be limited to whatever cases are present in your locality. For questions related to common problems such as minor trauma and some respiratory complaints, or for more general concerns such as response times and charting compliance, this may not be an issue. However, for questions related to some of the more critical but rarer concerns such as cardiac arrest, neonatal emergencies, and mass casualty incidents, you are going to spend a long time waiting for enough data to come through your system to make it worth reporting. To figure out whether this is the case, it is important to run a sample size calculation during the design phase of your study (Chapter 28).

One solution is to combine forces with other researchers. There are some large, government-funded multicenter research groups such as the Resuscitation Outcomes Consortium and the Neurological Emergencies Treatment Trials group. However, while these are great for people already in the network, privacy laws, grant requirements, and other concerns often make it difficult to approach these groups as an outsider and access their data. Instead, consider finding other people in your region that share an interest in the research question you have brought up and see if you can work together to get access to data from each of your systems (Chapter 26 has a discussion on figuring out authorship and division of work questions). Your local EMS medical director and (if you have a local academic program) EMS fellowship director or emergency medicine program director will likely have some idea of whom you might wish to contact. Not only will you have more data to power your study, you also just might create a network of colleagues that you can access again for future studies.

Another approach is to carry out a well-designed retrospective look at a reliable data set (Chapter 14). EMS is fortunate to have a national data set that is designed (in part) to be available for research questions: the National EMS Information System (NEMSIS). NEMSIS has its roots in the 1990s efforts by the National Highway Traffic Safety Administration (NHTSA) and other stakeholders to develop a uniform prehospital data set and allow national reporting of information. Although it was officially founded in 2001, it took another few years for NEMSIS to realize the vision of being a national repository for EMS information. Local agencies submit a subset of their data to their state, which, in turn, submits a smaller core subset to NEMSIS. The de-identified national data are available for on-line reporting at the NEMSIS web site.

Other data sets to consider looking at include your state's EMS data repository and your state or local trauma registry.

Methodology

Although other chapters in this book go into more detail on appropriate study design (such as Chapter 11), it is worth emphasizing that, given the other difficulties inherent in EMS research, you must ensure that your methodology is sound and uniformly applied. A study that is otherwise flawless will become essentially worthless if you cannot trust that the data are accurate and unbiased. For prospective studies, pay close attention to blinding, randomization, and the Hawthorne effect. For retrospective studies, use an appropriate guideline to ensure that data are retrieved, reviewed, and analyzed in a consistent fashion (Chapter 14).

For all EMS studies, it is a great idea to have somebody on your team who actually works in the practice setting you are studying. If you are looking at dispatch protocols, you need somebody to help you know what is going on in the dispatch world. Similarly, it is hard to accurately design a study that can be carried out successfully in the back of an ambulance if you do not have any prehospital field personnel helping you with the design. Not only will this add credibility to your results, it will make the entire process of designing the study, collecting the data, and discussing your results much richer.

Informed consent

Informed consent procedures are a wonderful use of research associate time (see Chapters 7, 8, and 16 on informed consent, and Chapter 25 on research associate programs). However, it is rarely practical to have research associates riding in the back of an ambulance with the prehospital team to consent patients; not only would you need an unwieldy number of associates to cover all units at all times of the day, but you would likely find that they got in the way of patient care. Further, unless your system only has one hospital, you are going to find that your research associates are generally not permitted to do anything in other hospitals.

This leaves the informed consent process as a trouble spot for EMS research. Although it usually is not a problem to obtain waivers of informed consent and Health Insurance Portability and Accountability Act (HIPAA) authorization for retrospective reviews, prospective studies will likely require a whole lot of work if they involve any kind of intervention or privacy risk and, therefore, are not exempt from review. Some of the informed consent methods that have worked for EMS researchers in the past include:

- *Community consent.* Emergency research that does not practically allow for the time it takes to appropriately give information and obtain consent can undergo a community consent process. This is expensive and time consuming, and is generally reserved for things such as prospective trials of prehospital cardiac arrest interventions.
- *Consent by site investigators.* If your system consists of hospitals that have collaborative relationships with each other, you may be able to have one or two people at each site that can be contacted to obtain informed consent from your patients upon their arrival at the emergency department. While easier than community consent, it would be unethical to do this for studies that require an intervention prior to arrival at the emergency department and opportunity for consent.
- *Remote consent.* Your institutional review board (IRB) may allow you to be in telephone contact with the patient to answer any questions and obtain consent. The prehospital personnel would be witnesses to the consent process. This can still be unwieldy, but does centralize the consent process to the research team. However, this requires transport times long enough to allow for consent without interfering with patient care, as well as the cooperation of your local EMS agency in allowing their paramedics to witness consent (and perhaps footing the phone bill, too).
- *Consent by prehospital personnel.* This is workable if your IRB permits it, but would likely require that each paramedic and/or EMT has completed research training through your institution to qualify him or her to provide information for the consent process, along with the liability concerns that the EMS agency may have.
- *Do a study that does not require consent.* While it is cheating to list this here, it is reasonable to design studies specifically to avoid the need for consent. This, naturally, cannot work for studies with interventions that could reasonably produce any risk to a patient. However, if you are aware that your EMS system will be implementing a process, protocol, equipment, medication, or other change, there is a natural opportunity to look at patient outcomes before and after the change without actually being responsible for the change itself.

Patient outcomes

Speaking of patient outcomes, your study should focus on outcomes that people care about. Roughly 20 years ago, the NHTSA sponsored a workshop on EMS morbidity outcomes [2]. A list of high-value patient outcomes was developed, known as the "six Ds" (Box 15.1), that was described more comprehensively as part of the EMS Outcomes Project [3]. Your research will likely be regarded more highly if it focuses on outcome measures from this list.

Relevance

Another way to help improve external validity is to choose a research question that focuses on issues of more general concern to the EMS community, rather than issues that are specific to the intricacies of your system. Although it is important to look at system-specific issues in the context of quality assurance and continuous quality improvement,

Box 15.1 High-value patient outcomes.

- Death (mortality directly attributable to the condition).
- Disease (objectively measurable signs of altered physiology).
- Disability (a change in the functional status of the patient in terms of ability to live independently and go about their daily lives at home, work, or recreation).
- Discomfort (uncomfortable symptoms such as pain, nausea, vertigo, or shortness of breath).
- Dissatisfaction (expectations of patients and families are met by services provided).
- Destitution (the financial consequences of health care to the patient and society).

Source: Maio *et al.* 1993 [3]. Reproduced with permission of American College of Emergency Physicians.

you may find that this is less useful (or at least more frustrating) when it comes to peer review and scientific publication. There are several ways to get an idea of which topics might be more generalizable:

- Keep abreast of the EMS literature to see which topics are frequently discussed.
- Attend regional or national EMS meetings (both scientific and administrative) to get a feel for what some of the topics of concern are.
- Speak with your local EMS medical director.

Alternatively, when you come across a research question that intrigues you, discreetly ask a few people in other EMS systems if it is an issue for them, as well. If none of your contacts in other systems have any concerns with the topic you have identified, it may be difficult to find peer reviewers that feel otherwise.

A few parting thoughts

EMS research has a long and rich history of not being widely believed. A 1997 study reviewed 5842 MEDLINE publications focusing on prehospital care between 1985 and 1997, and found precisely one that was determined to have the ability to evaluate the efficacy of EMS. Fifty-four randomized controlled trials were found, but only seven showed an uncontradicted positive outcome, and only one of those focused on a major outcome such as survival [4]. There has certainly been progress since that rather dismal showing, but even today there is often a perception that EMS research is not of sufficient quality to inform our clinical practice. Your EMS research will hopefully avoid this concern by addressing the points mentioned in this chapter.

KEY POINTS

- Maximize external validity by carefully choosing your research question and giving enough detail for other EMS physicians to determine how their systems compare to yours.
- Harness the power of multiple investigators to increase sample size and further enhance external validity.
- Ensure that your research team includes people with specific experience in the topic and practice setting you are studying.
- Address informed consent issues early in the study design process.
- Focus on patient outcomes that matter.

References

1 O'Connor, R.E. and Cone, D.C. (2009) If you've seen one EMS system, you've seen one EMS system. *Acad Emerg Med*, **16**(12): 1331–1332.
2 National Highway Traffic Safety Administration (NHTSA) (1994) EMS outcomes evaluation: Key issues and future directions. Paper presented at the NHTSA workshop on methodologies for measuring morbidity outcomes in EMS, 11–12 April 1994, Washington, DC.
3 Maio, R.F., Garrison, H.G., Spaite, D.W., *et al.* (1999) Emergency medical services outcomes project I (EMSOP I): prioritizing conditions for outcomes research. *Ann Emerg Med*, **33**(4):423–432.
4 Callaham, M. (1997) Quantifying the scanty science of prehospital emergency care. *Ann Emerg Med*, **30**(6):785–790.

CHAPTER 16

How to design a study that everyone will believe: Ethical concepts for special populations in emergency research

Kimberly Nordstrom

Psychiatric Emergency Services, Denver Health Medical Center, Denver, CO, USA

Introduction

> *"Treat others as you want to be treated.*
> *Do no harm."*

Yes, yes, both statements come from ancient texts and may be considered outdated. But are they? When you became a physician was your goal to have the biggest name in research or to help (not harm) people? Even though these tenets seem obvious there have been several examples in which physicians, in the name of research, chose to ignore them. For instance, there were some Nazis in Germany in World War II and some physician-scientists working with the Tuskegee Institute. They did not do any real harm did they? Well, not only did they have a direct negative effect on the patients, they have profoundly affected people's trust in clinical research to today.

According to the National Hospital Ambulatory Medical Care Survey, cited by the Centers for Disease Control, there were 129.8 million visits to emergency departments (EDs) in 2010 [1]. With the vast numbers of patients and diverse presentations from emergent to urgent to even ordinary care, the ED allows for the capture of a breadth of information not to be found elsewhere. In the same vein, because the ED is the "front door" and not a specialty clinic, all diagnostic categories and disease types make an appearance. So, why is not more research done in this setting, if there is such a wealth of information? If you have ever stopped long enough and looked around, you will find people hustling from one patient to the next, saving lives. Is there really room for research in such an environment? My guess is that there is, or you would not be reading this. So, what gets in the way and what can we do to get over some of these hurdles?

There are several issues that come up when discussing research in the emergency setting, none bigger than ethical concerns, especially around informed consent. The purpose of this chapter is to delve deeper into research with special (protected) populations found in the acute care environment, and help you navigate the murky waters.

Primer on ethics

A detailed discussion of ethics in acute care and emergency department research can be found in Chapter 8 of this book, but the issue of ethics becomes especially important when it comes to special populations, so the following is a specific orientation towards these populations. What are the special populations found in acute care? They are the young, or not yet born, pregnant, intoxicated, and incapacitated patients. One may even consider homeless patients as a special population that needs additional consideration.

Doing Research in Emergency and Acute Care: Making Order Out of Chaos, First Edition. Edited by Michael P. Wilson, Kama Z. Guluma, and Stephen R. Hayden.

Firstly, let us review the main ethical principles. Then we will review regulations that pertain to these populations. Lastly, we will look at case examples and apply the fundamentals.

There has been discussion on ethics in medicine since the beginning of time but only after the atrocities mentioned above were the basic elements codified. You may have heard of the Nuremburg Code and the Declaration of Helsinki. Countries have gone further than these early beginnings in codifying ethical principles. In the United States, the National Commission for the Protection of Subjects of Biomedical and Behavioral Research developed the Belmont Report (1979) [2]. Rather than being a strict rule book, this report created an overarching framework to be used to guide researchers in the area of ethics. There are also international guidelines to help direct researchers in this area [3].

Belmont has you consider a few fundamental principles: respect for the individual (this is where you find the idea of informed consent), beneficence and justice. Beneficence usually refers to the costs to the individual and the gain to society; justice is more specific to the idea of not allowing an inequality of those shouldering the burden. An example of justice is not singling out a specific race when testing something that would affect the larger society.

Informed consent

This sounds simple but actually requires a few things (Box 16.1); for example, the patient needs to have "capacity" to be informed, the person must understand what is being requested and what the effect will be on him/her (this could be physical, emotional, or other costs such as time commitment), the person must actually agree (imagine that!) and consent must be achieved without coercion. Ah … new question. What is coercion? Coercion can be in the form of a threat but tends to more likely come in the form of money. Most review boards agree that a small amount of money for the participant's time and efforts is alright, which is why you may see on research advertisements "$5 for each blood draw."

Key Concept: Informed Consent

For patients' who are mentally ill, delirious, inebriated, minors, or even fetuses – does the subject have capacity to make the decisions to be a part of research; how can you figure this out; can you use a surrogate; any particular rules for emergency research?

Key Concept: Coercion

For the *homeless* participant, the need for money may be greater than consideration of risk. How do you get past that issue? For the *infant/child*: is the parent going to receive a benefit for signing up the child?

Beneficence

In research, beneficence incorporates the idea of giving the participant maximum benefit with the goal of minimizing harm. If you read up on beneficence, you will see that another term tends to show up, "non-malfeasance." This is the act of not doing harm. Doing no harm does not equal doing good. In fact, sometimes these principles are in conflict.

Box 16.1 Important aspects of the consent process.

- Written in plain language
  - Language is the primary language of the patient
  - Explains the study
  - Explains all known and suspected risks
  - Explains commitment level
  - Explains basic benefits to patient and society
- Voluntary, without any form of coercion
  - Consenter (ideally) not treating clinician
- Consenter able to assess capacity

Imagine that you are researching a medicine that helps reduce pain for terminal patients. This medicine, though, hastens death. Your goal is to reduce pain but you are studying a medicine that will shorten the person's lifespan. In this, you are doing good (reducing pain) and doing harm (hastening death).

> **Key Concept: Beneficence**
>
> Pregnancy: You need to consider both the mother and the fetus regarding benefit and risk of harm in the research.

Justice

The concept of justice is that there should not be inequality in the shouldering of risks versus the benefits. An example of this is use of minority populations for research that benefits society as a whole. The American Medical Association has weighed the concept of justice with that of the fact that some vulnerable populations (chronically ill and socioeconomically disadvantaged) may seek out research for altruistic reasons. The opinion from the Council on Ethical and Judicious Affairs is that research should not burden socioeconomically disadvantaged populations in a disproportionate manner but they should not be categorically excluded or discouraged from research, either. The inclusion or exclusion of particular populations should be decided based on sound scientific principles [4].

Clear as mud? This basically means that you cannot use only one subset of patients when creating your study unless there is a scientific reason for doing so. It may be that all of those suffering from X disease also are economically disadvantaged. You are not purposefully trying to find economically disadvantaged subjects to understand a larger population and, after reading the fine print above, you now understand, you don't want to exclude them *just because* they are economically disadvantaged.

> **Key Concept: Justice**
>
> Use of only mentally ill adult subjects in research--do you need to have only mentally ill subjects to answer the question or could the question be answered with research on any adults? Conversely, is there an actual reason to 'exclude' mentally ill patients from the study?

Specific patient populations

There are special provisions within the Code of Federal Regulations for pregnant women or fetuses, prisoners and children; subparts B, C, and D, respectively [5]. In fact, institutional review boards (IRBs) are to ensure that additional safeguards are included in all studies that include vulnerable populations, defined as "children, prisoners, pregnant women, mentally disabled persons, or economically or educationally disadvantaged persons" [6]. In the Department of Health and Human Services' IRB Guidebook [7], they also refer to the terminally ill as a vulnerable population that requires additional safeguards. Why does this matter to the research based out of an ED? Who comes into an ED? All of the above. Rarely do you find the adult, non-minority, non-mentally ill, non-economically nor educationally disadvantaged person in the typical ED. Meaning, most patients have something that might place them into a vulnerable population designation. With this said, it is important to recognize your patient population and make sure that there are safeguards in place to cover all vulnerable populations. If you purposefully focus on one population (either excluding or including) the scientific rationale will need to be stated. Also, if your protocol and IRB approval does not *specify* the inclusion of specific vulnerable populations, then they are not included.

Let us look at each of these "special" populations to better understand where we stand on our ability to use them in research studies.

Pregnancy

Who are the 'special populations' in pregnancy? The law has clear rules for the fetus, the pregnant mother, and specific guidelines for the pregnant teenager.

Rules around research that may affect a fetus are relatively strict. If the fetus is *in utero*, individual regulations regarding pregnant women and fetus apply. The researcher will need to show that the study has been performed on animal models, or, if able, non-pregnant women, and this initial research should be the basis of the risk–benefit analysis going forward. Research is generally allowed if the risk is considered not more than minimal. If greater than minimal, the research must confer an anticipated benefit to the health of the mother or fetus. Also, the consent of the mother and father on behalf of the fetus is necessary. There are a few exceptions regarding the consent of the father: identity or whereabouts unknown, not reasonably available, or if the pregnancy resulted from rape [8]. If these exceptions are not met, there is quite a hurdle to overcome if researching pregnant women in the ED setting.

For the pregnant mother, the research activities have to either meet the health needs of the mother and place the fetus at only the minimal necessary risk or the risk to the fetus is minimal (such as an ultrasound or a maternal diet change). As noted above, consent must be given for the fetus participation [9].

Pregnant teenagers
This is a tough one because laws around emancipation are different in each state. It is important to be familiar with the "age of majority" for your state, as this will determine whether one or both parents need to consent or if the teenager is able to do so on her own.

The World Health Organization created guidelines for adolescent research involving reproductive health. The themes include that the research was specific to the population – could not otherwise be done on adults – there is a relevant need for the research, and it is low risk with maximized benefit. Sound familiar – basic ethical tenets. The guidelines also stress the need for confidentiality [10].

Children
Research involving children usually requires assent (instead of consent) of the child/minor and permission by the parents. Similar to the pregnant teenager, there may be state law that is more restrictive/informative on this matter. Research has to comply with both state law and federal regulation.

Cognitively impaired persons (mentally ill/organic impairment/developmental disorder)
Even though these three groups are separate clinical populations, they have very similar ethical concerns. With cognitive impairment, there are concerns regarding capacity. This comes down to being able to give informed consent that is free of coercion. There are also concerns that these populations could be targeted by the unscrupulous researcher for studies that are not specific to the population and are otherwise onerous (experimental drugs/surgeries that have high risk and little benefit). Interestingly, the US Department of Health and Human Services and the Food and Drug Administration (FDA) only require that someone who is familiar with working with these subjects is on the IRB. There are no particular requirements regarding the research. That said, there is plenty written on the matter. Generally, a prudent researcher would need to show that there is some relationship between the condition being studied and the target population, especially if the population is considered cognitively impaired.

Subjects with "cognitive impairment" may have capacity. This would need to be determined prior to the outset. In the case of delirium or active mental illness, capacity may change over a period of time. So, if research is being done in this subgroup, measures should be in place to follow capacity. For those who will never have capacity, there are no specific regulations to guide behavior but ethics would suggest that the patient's guardian/medical decision maker give consent, that the study would benefit the population with minimal risks and that the research actually requires the specific population in order to benefit the population. In the ED setting, you are generally safe if you follow guidelines set for "waiver of informed consent" (see below).

Forensic (jail/prison population)
Firstly, it must be shown that this population is being targeted in the research for some reason other than convenience. The major concern of using prisoners in research is whether a prisoner can make an informed decision that is free of coercion. If the benefits of participating in the research (being able to be on a special unit, staying in a hospital for a longer period than just an ED stay, etc.) get in the way of a true risk/benefit analysis, this would be considered coercive. Also, in terms of justice, one would need to consider if the prisoner is having an unfair "burden"; that is, unless the research was for a particular issue surrounding prisoners, to only use inmates would not be considered ethically just. The regulations in place speak exactly to those principals. Researching this population is limited to having a valid reason for involving this specific population (conditions that affect prisoners, causes of criminal behavior, prisons as institutional structures, etc.) [11].

Traumatized or comatose patients
This brings up the *waiver of informed consent*. In the ED, there may be subjects who cannot give informed consent. This would include those patients who arrive confused, frankly delirious, or even unconscious. Regulators understand that research on this patient population is necessary to forward medical techniques that may save lives in the future.

They also understand that experimental techniques can lead to a life saved during a study. The waiver of informed consent was to help aid researchers in EDs in studying these techniques. Even though these concepts are understood, the waiver of informed consent is complicated by stricter state laws. Federal policy allows a waiver of informed consent only in those instances where there is no more than minimal risk to the patient [12]. The FDA expands this somewhat in recognizing that in the emergency department there may be life-threatening situations with no approved therapy available and that the research is more likely to save a person's life. The statute speaks to an equal or greater likelihood of saving a life with the therapy being studied [13]. There may be more restrictions placed by your state, so make sure to look into any state statutes that might pertain to this prior to IRB submission. Another useful tool is "deferred consent." Similar to the waiver of informed consent, this needs to be written into the IRB protocol and the procedure needs to be clear. The basics of deferred consent, is that it allows the researcher to initiate the research and get consent as soon as is possible from either the patient (capacity restored) or a proxy. If consent is not obtained, the information needs to be destroyed and not used in the research findings.

Application of concepts

So, now you have most of the theory, rules, policies and regulations. How do you apply it? Let us practice with a few case scenarios.

Case 1

You want to know whether, in patients intoxicated with alcohol, if using intramuscular olanzapine might affect oxygen saturation. You read a retrospective analysis and now want to study it prospectively. In your particular ED, intramuscular olanzapine is used regularly on agitated intoxicated patients; oxygen saturation just has not been followed. So, this is "normal" treatment in the ED with the plan of following a particular measure.

Let us talk about the main ethical principles. Beneficence: maximizing benefit with least amount of harm. In this case, it is treatment as usual. The only difference is measuring pulse oximetry at specific intervals. This would be considered as very little to no harm caused by the research. Justice: Uh oh! You are focusing on a population of intoxicated people. Actually, in this case it is okay, as you are trying to understand something within this population. It would be problematic if you were only doing this research on African American males and extrapolating the findings to all intoxicated persons. Also, you may exclude certain populations (children, etc.) because intramuscular olanzapine is not FDA approved for the population or may cause harm. Last but not least … informed consent. This is a little trickier and may come down to how intoxication is being defined. A person may be "clinically sober" but have a blood alcohol of 0.10. If you define intoxication by a number, you may be able to speak to the fact that some of the participants will have capacity. Otherwise, this would be one of those research protocols that ask for a waiver of informed consent. Remember, federal authorities are generally okay with using the waiver if there is minimal risk to the patient.

Case 2

You are interested in pharmaceutical research and want to know if a particular new medicine that is supposed to treat arrhythmias works in elderly patients. You want to study all patients ages 65 and up who come through the ED.

Hmmm … can you imagine some issues with this one? It seems that it would be okay to take "all comers" of a certain age because you are not discriminating. Right? Actually, it may be difficult to include "all" seniors – you will be hitting some special classes: the incapacitated, demented patient or inebriated patient, possibly an elderly prisoner. In these cases, you need to talk specifically of why you are including or excluding these subclasses. Is there a reason that the medication would work differently on someone incapacitated or in the penal system? Probably not – so you would need to add these populations to exclusion criteria. In both cases, informed consent would be the main principal – in the first instance, capacity to make the decision and, in the second, possibly coercion.

Case 3

You want to test a new coagulant reversal agent on patients with massive intracranial bleeds. The agent needs to be given within two hours of the bleed to be effective. You understand that many patients will not have capacity on presentation and there will be times when the patient-subjects arrive without family members.

Of course, the main concern is informed consent. This appears to be a perfect case for the "waiver of informed consent." You will need to show only a minimal risk (not likely) or that there is not a proven therapy already in place for this life-threatening emergency. What happens if there is already a "proven" therapy? Well, if that therapy is believed to have more risks than the new therapy and if the proven therapy could be given at some point after the newer treatment (after "failure"), the IRB may allow the waiver.

Case 4

You want to study factors in fetal demise with teenager pregnancy. You will need each teenager to have an ultrasound and several blood tests. The ultrasound would be a standard test performed in such situations but some of the ordered blood tests would be extra and only for research purposes. Factors that you hypothesize to be related to fetal demise in teenagers include drug use, mental illness, and inappropriate prenatal care. Wow! This brings up several issues. Firstly, focus on the obvious issue of the pregnant teenager. Can the teenager consent (without a parent) or assent with parental permission? You need to look to state law on this around emancipation. Since you want to follow all cases that come into the ED (teenagers of all ages), you will have to note the law and how you plan to deal with it. What about the case of the pregnant teenager who wants to participate with a parent that is solidly against the research? Again, there are clear rules on emancipation but there are "subgroups" that may still be considered to not have capacity – very young teenagers and those with chronic cognitive impairment.

The hypotheses of the research lead to subpopulations: the teenager who comes into the ED intoxicated on alcohol or drugs, the mentally ill teenager, and possibly the economically disadvantaged teenager. The intoxicated teenager may not have capacity due to the intoxication. A capacity tool can be used to help determine this. The mentally ill teenager – again, does the subject have capacity, did the subject intentionally harm the child? Is having mentally ill pregnant teenagers necessary to answer the question? To exclude them may negatively affect this special population in the long run by not collecting this important information (think "Justice" here). Lastly, the economically disadvantaged teenager may be coerced to enter into the research if there are monetary inducements. As noted earlier, IRBs do not tend to find minimal payments for procedures to be coercive.

In truth, other than making sure that subjects can consent, this study follows standard care, with the only exception of extra blood draws, which would be considered minimal risk. Also the study does not "target" the subpopulations listed in the hypothesis list. These are all advantages and should ease its approval with the IRB. A word to the wise: your proposal needs to clearly spell out state laws on age of majority/emancipation and exactly how capacity is determined.

Conclusion

The point of this chapter was to help remind you of ethical principles that we sometimes take for granted and to apply these principles to special populations. It is easy to get very excited about a research topic and lose sight of the cost to the individual. Emergency medical and psychiatric research is important and can answer questions that cannot be answered in other treatment settings. Do not be daunted by the ethics; become familiar with them and allow them to help guide your research plan. Remember … it is all about the karma. Good luck.

> **KEY POINTS**
>
> - When dealing with special populations in research, it is first important to understand which populations receive extra protection.
> - When crafting your Institutional Review Board proposal, do not exclude special populations, unless you are able to explain why you are going to do so (particular harm without much benefit to the specific population and person).
> - Do not forget about the "waiver of informed consent" when researching emergent, life-threatening conditions.

References

1 Ambulatory and Hospital Care Statistics Branch. *National Hospital Ambulatory Medical Care Survey: 2010 Emergency Department Summary Tables.* http://www.cdc.gov/nchs/data/ahcd/nhamcs_emergency/2010_ed_web_tables.pdf (last accessed 7 May 2015).
2 US DHSS (1979) *The Belmont Report: Ethical Principles and Guidelines for the Protection of Human Subjects of Research.* http://www.hhs.gov/ohrp/humansubjects/guidance/belmont.html (last accessed 23 May 2015).

3 Council for International Organizations of Medical Sciences (2002) *International Ethical Guidelines for Biomedical Research Involving Human Subjects*. http://www.cioms.ch/publications/layout_guide2002.pdf (last accessed 8 May 2015).

4 American Medical Association (1998) Opinion 2.071 – Subject Selection for Clinical Trials. http://www.ama-assn.org/ama/pub/physician-resources/medical-ethics/code-medical-ethics/opinion2071.page? (last accessed 8 May 2015).

5 US DHSS (2009) *Code of Federal Regulations:* 45 CFR 46. http://www.hhs.gov/ohrp/humansubjects/guidance/45cfr46.html (last accessed 8 May 2015).

6 US DHSS (2009) *Code of Federal Regulations*: 45 CFR 46.111(b). http://www.hhs.gov/ohrp/humansubjects/guidance/45cfr46.html#46.111 (last accessed 8 May 2015).

7 US DHSS (1993) *Institutional Review Board Guidebook*. Chapter VI: Special Classes of Subjects; (G) Terminally Ill Patients. http://www.hhs.gov/ohrp/archive/irb/irb_chapter6ii.htm#g8 (last accessed 8 May 2015).

8 US DHSS (2009) *Code of Federal Regulations: 45 CFR 46.107(b) and 45 CFR 46.208* (b). http://www.hhs.gov/ohrp/humansubjects/guidance/45cfr46.html#46.107 and http://www.hhs.gov/ohrp/humansubjects/guidance/45cfr46.html#46.208 (last accessed 8 May 2015).

9 US DHSS (2009) *Code of Federal Regulations:* 45 CFR 46.207. http://www.hhs.gov/ohrp/humansubjects/guidance/45cfr46.html#46.207 (last accessed 8 May 2015).

10 World Health Organization (nd) *Ethical issues, Scientific and Ethical Review Group: Reproductive Health Involving Adolescents*. http://www.who.int/reproductivehealth/topics/ethics/adolescents_guide_serg/en/ (last accessed 8 May 2015).

11 US DHSS (2009) *Code of Federal Regulations:* 45 CFR 46.305. http://www.hhs.gov/ohrp/humansubjects/guidance/45cfr46.html#46.305 (last accessed 8 May 2015).

12 US DHSS (2009) *Code of Federal Regulations*: 45 CFR 46.116(d). *General Requirements of Informed Consent*. http://www.hhs.gov/ohrp/humansubjects/guidance/45cfr46.html#46.116 (last accessed 8 May 2015).

13 US Food and Drug Administration (2014) *Code of Federal Regulations Title* 21: 21CFR50.23 – Exception from general requirements. http://www.accessdata.fda.gov/scripts/cdrh/cfdocs/cfcfr/CFRSearch.cfm?fr=50.23 (last accessed 8 May 2015).

How to design a study that everyone will believe: Industry studies

Richard F. Clark and Alicia B. Minns

Division of Medical Toxicology, UCSD Medical Center, San Diego, CA, USA

Introduction

You are working in a community Emergency Department at 1 o'clock in the morning on Saturday night. The local ambulance company has just delivered your next patient with a history of ethylene glycol poisoning into a major treatment room. On physical examination, the patient has normal vital signs but appears intoxicated. He admits to having consumed half a bottle of antifreeze because it tasted good and he had run out of malt liquor. You order basic chemistry panels, serum osmolarity, and laboratory testing for ethylene glycol, methanol, and ethanol. You are not certain whether your pharmacy stocks an antidote for this poisoning or if it is even indicated. You are also not certain if dialysis is the best way to manage this patient or if you can get a nephrologist to see the patient at this time of the morning.

Performing research on under-represented patient populations like this is challenging. The National Institutes of Health is unlikely to have much interest in contributing to research in areas such as toxic alcohols. However, for some diseases with which there is a potential to have an effective and marketable antidote, antivenom, or other therapy, a pharmaceutical or device manufacturing company may be the answer. Capitalism spawns innovation; the potential for innovation fuels the pharmaceutical and medical device industries; and the clinical researcher is vital to the success of both of these industries.

Conducting an industry study in an acute care setting such as the emergency department (ED) can be an adventure. In this setting, we depend on "enrollable" patients walking into our ED, often unsolicited. They could come in at all hours, when both the principal investigator and research staff are absent. In addition, guidelines adopted at many institutions in the past decade have altered the incentives for researchers in these areas. Finally, stricter and more frequently changing rules regarding informed consent have excluded some potential areas of acute care research where intellectual capacity is of question.

Several years ago your authors experienced first-hand the problems with ED enrollment of patients with rare disorders in an industry-funded study. We became part of a clinical trial examining the use of fomepizole for patients with toxic alcohol poisoning [1]. Many of the leading research institutions in toxicology were involved, and both the lead investigator and the pharmaceutical company funding the study knew that the incidence of toxic alcohol poisonings in this country is rare. In order to accrue enough subjects, they enlisted multiple sites in the clinical trial. Getting the study approved by our institutional review board (IRB) was difficult, but typical of such a study where the ability of the subject to give informed consent could be limited. However, many site investigators like us trod through the process and gradually were granted approval and received the study drug. Unfortunately, even with all the time and effort devoted to the study, quite a few institutions were unable to enroll a single subject during the study period. In the end, only sites who contributed cases were granted co-authorship. Many investigators were disappointed that their efforts failed to result in a scholarly work simply because not even one case had come through their ED doors.

Unpredictability aside, however, participating in industry studies can be rewarding in many ways. We will try to outline special aspects of this type of research.

Doing Research in Emergency and Acute Care: Making Order Out of Chaos, First Edition. Edited by Michael P. Wilson, Kama Z. Guluma, and Stephen R. Hayden.

Coming up with a question

Coming up with a research question for an industry-sponsored study can be approached in two ways (Chapter 3). In many cases, pharmaceutical or other medical companies will reach out to investigators to seek sites for enrollment [2, 3]. Most of these studies will be multicentered, with numerous investigators and institutions involved. Industry sponsors may identify potential sites through responses to advertisements, referrals by word of mouth, or by the sponsor personally seeking out known and proven investigators. These studies will usually fall into the categories of phase 2 or phase 3 trials (see the later section Types of industry studies or clinical trials) and often will not offer co-authorship for most investigators.

A second category of industry research involves the investigator developing a biological agent, technique, or device that attracts sponsorship from an industry partner. The process of research and development of a drug or device can be costly and often requires the backing of a company or investment group. However, smaller investigator-initiated studies are also possible. For example, several years ago when ondansetron was first marketed as an antiemetic, its indications initially included only postoperative and chemotherapy-induced nausea. We believed ondansetron could be effective in treating drug overdose-related emesis [4]. We generated a proposal to use ondansetron in such cases and formulated a budget to perform a pilot study of our hypothesis. Realizing the cost of ondansetron at the time would be a limiting factor in instituting our study, we contacted the pharmaceutical company marketing ondansetron and solicited a donation of drug. The company donated the drug for our study based on our proposal [5]. Since our study was investigator-initiated and meant not changing the package insert, it was not subject to the same IRB scrutiny or cost of a true industry-funded clinical trial. For example, since we did not intend to modify the original drug package insert and our drug (or device) was already approved by the FDA, an IND (investigational new drug) application was not required (Chapter 23 provides more details about INDs). This saved us time and resources in the approval process for our study. Drug acquisition costs are often the largest part of budgets for investigator-initiated studies, but companies are frequently willing to donate medications or supplies for local trials that may enhance the utility of their agent [6–10].

Types of industry studies or clinical trials

Some medical industries will sponsor animal or bench research at outside institutions [6]. However, much of this part of pharmaceutical and device development is now internal at laboratories and vivariums funded by the manufacturer. Academic institutional animal and bench research is largely funded by a mixture of governmental organizations, such as the National Institutes of Health, local, regional or institutional seed grants, or by the increasingly common partnership and contracting between private industry and academic institutions such as schools of medicine or pharmacy [7, 8].

Industry-sponsored studies or clinical trials in humans have traditionally fallen into three categories (Table 17.1). Phase 1 studies or trials usually involve studying the pharmacokinetics and initial safety of the product. Phase 1 studies are generally small studies with few participants and a lesser budget with a shorter timeline. Participants are often healthy volunteers testing the effects and doses of a product on the body, or affected individuals in small numbers [11].

Phase 2 studies or trials are usually designed more for dose finding. Groups of participants who usually are affected by the illness or disorder targeted by the study drug are given varying doses to determine an efficacious dose range. Safety is also considered in Phase 2 trials, but some may not be powered to detect small differences in outcomes. Placebos are often employed in Phase 2 trials [2].

Phase 3 studies or trials are usually prospective, multicentered, double-blinded studies involving large numbers of patients. Power analyses are important in setting up the needed number of subjects in each group to adequately compare efficacy and safety of the drug or device. Multiple institutions are usually required to get the desired number of subjects needed. Due to growing pressure to fully assess toxicity and efficacy of a product prior to release on the market, there is more scrutiny of results by agencies, leading to an increased cost to conduct a Phase 3 trial [3, 12].

Investigators can have different expectations of remuneration in the above studies based on the type of study, the company, and other factors. In Phase 3 trials, for example, investigators are often compensated for the time and effort in getting IRB approval and for entering a certain number of patients. However, large multicenter Phase 3 trials, in which there may be a large number of co-investigators, rarely reward individual investigators with authorship on publications unless the investigator was instrumental in the planning stages of the study or a limited numbers of institutions take part.

Table 17.1 Phases of clinical trials in industry studies.

Phase of study	Purpose	Number of investigators; patients	Type of volunteers
1	Safety, pharmacokinetics	One or small number of investigators; small number of patients	Often healthy, without disease
2	Safety, dose finding	Limited number of investigators; number of patients often powered to detect difference in dose and effect	Patients with disease or disorder being studied
3	Efficacy, safety	Large number of sites and investigators; large number of patients powered to detect meaningful difference in outcome	Patients with disease or disorder being studied

Developing methods

When a drug or device manufacturer sponsors a study, it will often request to approve the methodology used by the investigator prior to funding. The more resources the sponsor is asked to contribute, the more involved it will generally be in how the study is performed. This can be of benefit to the investigator, since statisticians employed by an industry sponsor can be helpful in planning sample sizes, analyzing data, and even planning the project design. Phase 3 trials that seek to judge efficacy will require a power analysis to calculate the minimum number of patients that must be included. In Phase 1 trials that we have worked on with industry, the sponsor may be more "hands off" with the proposed design, as long as the testing is done in a verified manner at a reputable laboratory [11].

There are two potential pitfalls in the proposal of methods to an industry sponsor. Firstly, in some early or Phase 1 proposals, industry sponsors have asked for more elaborate designs requiring higher costs. If the company is willing to fund the enhanced version, this can work out well for the investigator and the institution. However, the investigator must be certain that the augmented proposal can reasonably be finished with the resources offered by the company. More and more academic institutions are employing development and clinical trials offices that can assist investigators in these negotiations and at times provide leverage to the investigator.

The second potential pitfall is that when an investigator submits a proposal to industry for an extensive project, the company may either turn down or delay approval of the project based on the cost. This second situation is more often encountered by experienced researchers who have realized that industry often will seek to study an outcome for the least amount of research and design dollars. The economics are clear in that research and design costs erode eventual profit, especially when many agents or devices are never marketed. Therefore, companies will often negotiate the lowest cost methodology design until profit from the proposed device or drug becomes inevitable. Your authors have been forced to walk away from research funding proposals from industry in which they would not be able to obtain meaningful results with the resources being offered. It should be kept in mind that research with methodological flaws caused by funding limitations is almost never worth the effort. Institutions know this also and have, therefore, become much more involved in these processes as they also cannot afford the cost or liability issues resulting from poorly-funded trials.

Getting started with industry-sponsored research funding

After a clinician develops a question or hypothesis worthy of a clinical study and has developed a sound methodology, including analysis of results, the next step is to establish funding. If the research is aimed at a specific drug or device, the most likely source of funding is the pharmaceutical or device manufacturer of the drug or device, or a sponsor with the *potential* to have some financial gain from the proposed research. We have seen companies desire to assist in clinical research in several ways, either intimately involved in the process or at a distance. Often the sponsors will gauge their potential gain from the proposed research as a way of determining the investment. Perhaps the simplest and least "strings-attached" approach by an investigator is to seek a "donation" of a drug or device to perform the research. Industry sponsors often have excess stock or even almost-expired product that they are frequently willing to donate on behalf of research. Small studies using donated stocks, if well performed, can often convince industry sponsors that further research from the investigator or the institution may be worthwhile, and lead to more significant funding. The other way we have approached seed funding from industry is to identify and directly contact the company representative responsible for research and development. The person is often a clinician or former clinician and is frequently helpful in quickly assessing the viability of obtaining resources from the sponsor. The representative can then assist in giving details on how and where to submit proposals to the sponsor.

Another way of getting started with funding for industry research is to obtain a small seed grant from a local institution, such as a university academic senate, or from national organization, such as the Emergency Medicine Foundation. Usually, the organization providing the seed funding will assess the grant proposal for likelihood of further grant funding if results are positive. These preliminary results can then be used as part of a larger proposal to the device or pharmaceutical manufacturer.

Data safety monitoring boards

Most industry-sponsored studies with Phase 3 implications will require a data safety monitoring board (DSMB) to oversee the study. The DSMB is usually a panel of respected researchers not involved in the current trial but who have some knowledge of research about the specific drug or device being studied. The DSMB will review the methods being used prior to the study and review the results as they are collected. The main purpose of a DSMB is to insure a non-biased overview of the safety of a study, as there is a belief that some investigators can develop a bias to continue a project even in the face of undesirable outcomes. The DSMB will review all expected and unexpected adverse outcomes to ensure subject safety. For the investigator, this means more scrutiny over study results and methods, but this greater level of safety has proved to be the standard for large trials. Some IRBs will not approve certain clinical trials without a DSMB in place.

Material safety transfer agreements

A material safety transfer agreement is a legal contract that establishes the conditions and terms of transferring "tangible" research material between a provider, such as a principal investigator, and a recipient, such as a pharmaceutical company. It is meant to protect the rights of both parties while documenting the transfer. This would include blood or tissue collected as part of a study from patients at an academic institution, and would protect these samples from indiscriminant use by the receiving entity. This has become more important in recent years, as stem cell transfers have increased between institutions for oncology and other research involving cell lines. Many of these cell lines have potential proprietary value. These agreements outline the use of the transferred material and specify the criteria by which scientific publications can be produced from work involving the transferred resources. Without an agreement in place, both parties have potential legal liability arising from the study or published results. Examples of material often requiring material safety transfer agreements include blood, tissue, vectors, plasmids, databases, devices, and software. However, a material safety transfer agreement is usually not required when blood or tissue is being transferred or shipped for routine testing in connection with a clinical trial. Many institutions have differing interpretations of when a material safety transfer agreement is needed and there is usually an institutional office at most academic centers dedicated specifically to helping investigators with this process.

Compensation

Various forms of compensation exist for industry-sponsored research. The most important compensation for institutions and investigators is either monetary support or the opportunity to co-author scholarly works resulting from the study. Both of these goals are cherished by academic institutions as well; although monetary support for research has somewhat surpassed the name recognition in some areas.

Industry can financially support a project in several ways. Most obviously, the study could be funded to cover part of the salary or benefits of the faculty or associates required to perform it. Research nurses or assistants, statisticians, laboratory workers, and others within the institution can receive funding for clinical trials or bench studies. Once the research team is funded and in place, they can work together to secure more and future funding from other sources. Institutions have guidelines for salary support and a clinical trials office can assist in the set-up of a budget that will cover all salary and benefit needs. In addition to salary and benefits, institutions will usually require compensation for the services of the clinical trials office and IRB. These fees are generally covered either by specific costs that are added as line items in the budget at the time of negotiation or included as "overhead" in the negotiating process.

Overhead costs have fluctuated over the years, but have usually increased as the institutional overhead costs have increased. Overhead for government-sponsored studies has been around 50% or greater of the total cost of study for academic institutions. However, industry sponsors will often refuse extensive overhead charges, and at times have been willing to shift funding to institutions or investigators with lower fees. Each investigator will need to work with their clinical trials office when overhead fees are discussed in order to keep costs in ranges that industry sponsors require, without sacrificing the quality of the methods or necessary investigator support. We have again found that allowing a clinical trials office to assist in this process can be quite helpful. The clinical trials office staff are often versed in what an industry sponsor is likely to accept in the way of overhead fees and can balance what can be received with what is needed for completion of the study. In our experience, we have almost never failed to agree on a research budget due to an unwillingness of our clinical trials office to negotiate with an industry sponsor.

Another potential form of compensation involves resource materials derived from an industry study. Equipment that is purchased for one study could be used for future research. Laboratory machinery and reagents, computers and software, and other material can often be budgeted into an industry study but used in other research. Institutions and sponsors are at times more willing to purchase these types of resources for investigators than to fund salary support. Such compensation must be acknowledged and disclosed when writing up a paper for publication. Obtaining compensation for research creates an inherent conflict of interest that can be managed, but must be disclosed to the reader in order to determine how much, if any, bias it may have produced.

Publication

The publication of scholarly work resulting from the research should be considered as another form of compensation for performing industry-sponsored research. Many departments within academic medical centers require scholarly work as one of the criteria for academic advancement. Although a researcher could be valued by an academic institution only for bringing in research money, publications arising from their research are important. For this reason, we often seek co-authorship potential as a necessity for participation in clinical trials and industry-sponsored research. Authorship potential should always be clearly discussed before agreeing to participate in the study. We have seen a variety of rules on authorship used by industry for a number of reasons. At times, industry sponsors have sought to have complete decision making capacity over publication of results. This could be important to the sponsor if the result were negative, and has obvious ethical and academic implications. Many investigators who are offered authorship will reserve the right to publish results regardless of the outcome, but at times the industry sponsor will retain the final publication decision. An academically healthy arrangement involves retaining the right of the investigators to publish regardless of the outcome, but allowing the sponsor the option to pre-review (but not edit) the manuscript prior to submission; this allows them to express any concerns, ask for clarification, and make any internal preparations for the dispersal of the results to the public.

Once an industry-sponsored study is approved for publication, determining authorship can also be problematic. The industry sponsor will often coordinate the publications and set the rules of authorship. Sponsors (and the lead author) are often reluctant to include large numbers of authors on a publication; some journals will limit author number as well. It then becomes an issue of who "deserves" to be included as an author. This can be decided in several ways. In smaller industry studies, we have seen the principal investigators of all sites given co-authorship, without regard to subjects enrolled or completed. At these situations, each institution is allowed to have one co-author who is decided upon at the initiation of the study. This method has worked well and is often the most equitable way of including all investigators. Other trials have included only those investigators as authors who enroll a certain number of subjects, or who take part in the conception and implementation of the trial. In either case, investigators should have a clear understanding of authorship prior to taking part in the trial if this is important.

Pitfalls

Some of the pitfalls encountered in industry studies performed in the emergency department are indicated in Box 17.1.

Inadequate funding

The greatest pitfalls in industry-sponsored research that we have encountered involve inadequate funding, overzealous enrollment expectations, and unexpected study changes by the sponsor. Funding difficulties have been described above, and we have realized over the years that underfunding a clinical trial or industry-sponsored study is

Box 17.1 Pitfalls encountered in industry studies performed in the emergency department.

- Underestimate of funds needed to complete the study.
- Difficulty in enrolling subjects.
- Inability to follow up some patient populations.
- Lack of academic recognition for work performed by investigator.
- Pharmacy errors in storage or dosing of study drug.
- Complications on shipping or acquiring study drug or device.
- Errors by study personnel on collecting data.
- Industry cancellation of study prior to completion.
- Lack of institutional support for budget negotiations.
- Prolonged IRB review delaying study initiation.
- Excessive institutional overhead costs.
- Difficulty with informed consent in certain populations.
- Language barriers in certain populations.
- Conflicts of interest with investigators.

worse than not getting approval to be a study site investigator. Younger researchers who are anxious to begin taking part in clinical trials may be willing to take less salary support or do without certain resources in order to be included as an investigator. The usual hope is that participation in the study will improve one's opportunity for industry-sponsored research in the future. To a certain extent this is true, in that many industry sponsors seek investigators with "experience" for their trial. However, we have seen that the complications involved in underfunding a study outweigh the potential benefits from future trials. Again, involving a clinical trials office in industry-sponsored study negotiations can help eliminate some of these problems.

Under-enrollment

Understanding enrollment limitations for one's institution is also important when planning industry studies. We have had several studies in which we met all criteria for enrollment, jumped through all the regulatory hoops, received IRB approval, and then were unable to enroll subjects. This can be frustrating for both the investigator and the sponsor, and potentially lead to adverse considerations of future industry associations. Many times, a failure to enroll subjects is a matter of bad luck. Patients have to present with a certain disorder in order to be enrolled. However, some clinical trials, such one we have done with some antivenoms, require the rare event of an envenomation, thus leaving us at the mercy of both nature and patient's selection of an emergency department for treatment. We have tried in several cases to educate both community and emergency medical service (EMS) agencies with targeted advertising. This advertising at times improves enrollment, but rare disorders are still rare.

When enrollment for studies is low, such as with rare events like envenomations, other pitfalls can occur. To continue employing research assistants, one needs to garner income from study sponsors. If subjects are not enrolled, this income source slows, and many assistants prefer not to work under these uncertain terms. To counter this uncertainty, principal investigators will sometimes also serve as the enrolling research assistant. This can be difficult when the principal investigator has other duties, such as clinical shifts or administrative activity. In the past we have also used a "commission" offered to residents or other clinicians to aid the principal investigator in entering subjects when research assistants are not available. However, IRBs have taken an increasingly negative view of these gifts, citing the potential for conflict of interest.

Training and availability of investigational pharmacists

Another problem with sparse enrollment of industry studies is the interaction with an institution's investigational pharmacy. Investigational pharmacists have become increasingly important to industry studies. While they have historically been subsidized by academic institutions, this is becoming less common, and most large medical institutions now require investigators to add a stipend in their industry-sponsored budget for pharmacy participation. This usually covers drug shipping, storage, preparation, and administration. While most institutions employ one or two pharmacist to fill this role, enrollment of subjects on nights and weekends can be problematic. Our institution actively cross-trains night and weekend pharmacists to aid investigators in obtaining study drug during these off times. However, we have seen many situations where less-experienced pharmacists cover nights or evening shifts and are expected to cover the investigational pharmacy. At times, we have been unable to enroll patients under these situations due to the study complexities of blinding and preparation of study drugs at these hours. In other situations, we have had study drugs inappropriately stored by non-investigational personnel, resulting in loss of all study drug vials.

Market changes

A final pitfall we have encountered is unexpected market changes. Pharmaceutical companies develop drugs or devices based on a perceived need for use. With rising research and development costs, companies are reluctant to devote resources to product development when the expected return may not be profitable. Several years ago we participated in methodology design with a company that was developing an antibody to reverse tricyclic antidepressant poisoning. Animal trials and a few isolated human case reports of compassionate use demonstrated the product's efficacy [13]. Plans were developed to perform a larger Phase 2 trial of the study drug at multiple institutions and investigators spent significant amounts of time with project design. Shortly before full-scale implementation of the project was to occur, the company announced that they were abandoning the effort, citing a lack of marketability of the product. Needless to say, there are multiple potential pitfalls, many unforeseen, when taking part in industry studies.

Conflicts of interest

Investigators face several possible conflicts of interest when taking part in industry studies. Industry sponsors often offer financial incentives to investigators. For example, for Phase 3 trials, investigators and assistants often take part in research planning meetings in preparation for enrollment. The economy of scale in getting investigators from multiple sites together in one location for teaching and information dissemination is obvious. However, as incentive, these meetings have often been held in exotic or resort sites, and include impressive meals and other perks. While many institutions have no regulations over these activities, a growing number do, and administrators are becoming more careful to scrutinize institutional leaders in these activities. Another common industry incentive is speaker's bureaus for lecturing at sponsored events. Significant honoraria are often offered to speakers for these affairs. Industry sponsors market these talks by arguing that there is no one more credible to speak of the virtues of the new drug or device than an investigator. In reality, more academic institutions are examining participation in these sponsored activities as potential conflicts of interest. And more and more publishers and national organizations require speakers and authors to acknowledge participation in any activity that others may deem *could* be considered a conflict of interest.

Institutional pharmacy and therapeutics committees are increasingly looking for conflicts of interest when considering new drug approval. Clinicians who propose new medications for formulary addition at our institution are asked to list financial relationships with the drug or device manufacturer. Clear direction on how to apply these potential conflicts when considering new agents has not been well established but acknowledgement could affect committee decisions.

Finally, IRBs in modern times are giving members a greater awareness and responsibility for identifying potential conflicts of interest in reviewed proposals. This evolving area is discussed in more detail in the next section.

IRB issues

Navigating the IRB at academic institutions has become more challenging. IRBs are now tasked by institutions with more complex goals than just protecting the safety of subjects. In the past decade, our local IRB asked our committee to be "fiscally responsible" when reviewing research proposals. It has become important for the IRB to protect the institution from industry-sponsored "shifting" of costs due to a subject's insurance. In addition, the IRB has increasingly applied conflict of interest criteria to studies. Investigators are asked about financial or other relationships they may have with the industry sponsor. These relationships are somewhat loosely used in the approval process, but are discussed in every review of industry studies.

In the past few years, IRBs have also begun asking for financial compensation for review of industry studies. IRBs members have traditionally spent long hours in careful review of an increasing number of studies. Academic institutions have embraced the idea that industry sponsors should share the cost involved in review of these projects and have begun charging fees for the process. Initially, these fees were small and not applied uniformly. More recently, they have become standard inclusions in investigator budgets, similar to investigational pharmacy fees.

Positive aspects of IRB review of industry-sponsored studies include the committee's assurance that the methodology has undergone several layers of analysis, thus suggesting that statistical design and power analyses of these studies is sound. In addition, Phase 3 industry studies almost always employ a DSMB which assists the IRB in overseeing subject safety.

Recruiting patients

Many young investigators may feel great relief after completing IRB review and site enrollment for industry studies. Unfortunately, the true challenge occurs when recruiting subjects. If the disease or disorder being studied is common and presents predominantly during daytime hours, then recruitment can be easy. But ED patients may present at unconventional times and days, requiring around-the-clock monitoring for enrollment. Most industry studies are not confined to "convenience sampling" and this requires employing multiple research assistants or even co-investigators to cover all times for potential recruitment. Since most IRBs and industry sponsors prefer a limited number of staff in an ED to act as co-investigators for study entry, the burden of entering subjects falls onto the investigator either to be on-call indefinitely or to maintain an active research staff of assistants. Many investigators will end up terminating a project early due to slow or sporadic enrollment of subjects that does not support the research staff.

We have used many types of advertisements to enhance industry study enrollment. Our IRB has now mandated review of all public advertisements and requires each be stamped with an approval authentication. Investigators utilizing unapproved advertisements can be sanctioned. We have posted approved placards for our studies around our campus to recruit volunteers. If our need for industry study volunteers is small, we have often employed our own staff, with co-authorship as an incentive. In some studies where sparse enrollment is anticipated, we have utilized EMS providers to increase study awareness. Our investigators have visited local EMS conferences and meetings to teach about topics related to our research and remind EMS providers about ongoing studies.

Summary

Industry-sponsored research can be both academically and financially rewarding to investigators and institutions. As a source of research dollars, medical companies can lead to support for both present and future studies, and provide seed funding for principal investigators, co-investigators, and multiple research staff. Recent legislation and institutional rules regarding conflict of interest have necessitated caution both from an investigator and institutional perspective, and have caused some shifting in funding expectations. But when experienced research staff is assembled and institutional support generated, industry-sponsored studies continue to emerge as important step in the delivery of medical devices and drugs to the general public, as well as sources of funding for academic departments. After all, fomepizole, the drug of choice for the patient mentioned at the beginning of this chapter, was originally developed in such a manner.

KEY POINTS

- Clinical trials are usually divided into three phases depending on the goals of the study. Phase 1 involves pharmacokinetics and initial safety; Phase 2 studies usually involve e-finding; and Phase 3 studies look for clinical efficacy.
- When designing and proposing industry-sponsored studies, it is important not to underestimate equipment and personnel resources required to complete the trial and obtain meaningful results.
- Most institutions have clinical trials committees or offices that can be helpful in negotiating budgets that include overhead with industry sponsors.
- Investigators should always be aware of potential conflicts of interest when dealing with industry sponsors.

References

1 Brent, J., McMartin, K., Phillips, S, *et al.* (1999) Fomepizole for the treatment of ethylene glycol poisoning. Methylpyrazole for Toxic Alcohols Study Group. *N Engl J Med*, **340**(11):832–838.
2 Dart, R.C., Seifert, S.A., Carroll, L., *et al.* (1997) Affinity-purified, mixed monospecific crotalid antivenom ovine Fab for the treatment of crotalid venom poisoning. *Ann Emerg Med*, **30**(1):33–39.

3 Dart, R.C., Seifert, S.A., Boyer, L.V., *et al.* (2001) A randomized multicenter trial of Crotalinae Polyvalent Immune Fab (Ovine) antivenom for the treatment for Crotaline snakebite in the United States. *Arch Intern Med*, **161**:2030–2036.

4 Sage, T.A., Jones, W.N., and Clark, R.F. (1993) Ondansetron in the treatment of intractable nausea associated with theophylline toxicity. *Ann Pharmacother*, **27**:584–585.

5 Clark, R.F., Chen, R., Williams, S.R., *et al.* (1996) The use of ondansetron in the treatment of nausea and vomiting associated with acetaminophen poisoning. *Clin Toxicol*, **34**(2):163–167.

6 Clark, R.F., Selden, B.S., Curry, S.C. (1991) Digoxin specific fab fragments in the treatment of oleander toxicity in a canine model. *Ann Emerg Med*, **20**(10):1073–1077.

7 Tanen, D.A., Danish, D.C., Clark, R.F. (2003) Crotalidae polyvalent immune fab antivenom limits the decrease in perfusion pressure of the anterior leg compartment in a porcine crotaline envenomation model. *Ann Emerg Med*, **41**(3):384–390.

8 Tanen, D.A., Danish, D.C., Grice, G.A., *et al.* (2004) Fasciotomy worsens the amount of myonecrosis in a porcine model of crotaline envenomation. *Ann Emerg Med*, **44**(2):99–104.

9 Richardson, W.H., Tanen, D.A., Tong, T.C., *et al.* (2005) Crotalidae polyvalent immune fab (ovine) antivenom is effective in the neutralization of South American Viperdae venoms in a murine model. *Ann Emerg Med*, **45**(6):595–602.

10 Richardson, W.H., Tanen, D.A., Tong, T.C., *et al.* (2006) North American coral snake antivenin for the neutralization of non-native elapid venoms in a murine model. *Acad Emerg Med*, **13**(2):121–126.

11 Rangan, C., Nordt, S.P., Hamilton, R., *et al.* (2001) Treatment of acetaminophen ingestion with a superactivated charcoal-cola mixture. *Ann Emerg Med*, **37**(1):55–58.

12 Boyer, L.V., Seifert, S.A., Clark, R.F., *et al.* (1999) Recurrent and persistent coagulopathy following pit viper envenomation. *Arch Int Med*, **159**:706–710.

13 Heard, K., Dart, R.C., Bogdan, G., *et al.* (2006) A preliminary study of tricyclic antidepressant (TCA) ovine FAB for TCA toxicity. *Clin Toxicol*, **44**(3):275–281.

CHAPTER 18

How to design a study that everyone will believe: Prospective studies

Gary Gaddis

St. Luke's Hospital of Kansas City, MO, USA

Introduction

The story of Dr Barry Marshall and Dr Robin Warren and their receipt of the Nobel Prize for Physiology or Medicine in 2005 is the story of how the causative role of *Helicobacter pylori* for gastric and duodenal ulcers (and gastric cancers) came to be broadly understood and believed. However, the story also clearly illustrates important differences between study designs and differences of persuasive power inherent to published observations, case reports, case series, cohort studies, and randomized control trials. In this chapter, Marshall's story serves as the backdrop for an overview of various study designs.

Observational studies

Individual observations represent the lowest level of strength of medical evidence. Observational manuscripts disseminate an observation. Individual observations generally do not permit inference of cause and effect and rarely, if ever, change clinical practice.

Regarding *H. pylori*, observations that bacteria can exist in the stomachs of animals [1] and humans [2, 3] were published as long ago as the late nineteenth and early twentieth centuries. A number of physicians reported the observation of successful treatment of gastritis with various antibiotics in the 1950s and 1960s [4–6]. However, these observations were not followed up by any well-designed clinical trials attempting to convincingly demonstrate cause and effect between these microbes and gastric ulcers. Scientific dogma held that since the stomach was thought to be too acidic to permit bacterial life or growth, any bacteria observed in the stomach must be contaminants. In fact, despite clearly being on the right track, a doctor named John Lykoudis was fined 4000 Greek drachmas in 1968 for prescribing antibiotics for peptic ulcer disease [5]!

Various types of observational studies exist. Published observations, case reports and case series are the simplest forms of observation. In 1981, when Marshall was assigned to a gastroenterology rotation as a young trainee, he was encouraged to collaborate with a pathologist, Robin Warren, who had made some interesting observations of bacteria in human stomachs. At that point, a collaboration was born. Marshall and Warren published their observation of bacteria in stomachs of patients with gastric disease in 1983 [7]. Although Marshall began treating at least one ulcer patient with a two-week course of a tetracycline antibiotic in 1981 [8], the observation of bacteria in human stomachs did not change the widely accepted dogma that excess stomach acid is the principal cause of gastric and duodenal ulcer disease.

A *case report* is a report of a single interesting clinical observation. A *case series* is a group of similar clinical observations that have a common apparent disease cause, or outcome of interest, without any control group for comparison. As stated, case reports and case series cannot demonstrate any evidence of cause and effect, but they can suggest ideas for further research.

Doing Research in Emergency and Acute Care: Making Order Out of Chaos, First Edition. Edited by Michael P. Wilson, Kama Z. Guluma, and Stephen R. Hayden.

Marshall executed a compelling case report when he demonstrated that a volunteer patient (who, it was eventually discerned, was Marshall himself), developed endoscopically-documented gastritis that was induced after ingestion of microbes. Marshall began with histologically normal gastric mucosa, demonstrated by gastroscopy. He developed gastritis after deliberately ingesting a broth, obtained from one of his ulcer patients, containing bacteria we now know as *H. pylori*. The microbe was known to be sensitive to metronidazole. Marshall developed endoscopically-documented gastritis 10 days after ingesting the inoculum, and then used antibiotics to cure himself. He took this extreme measure only after being unsuccessful at causing Helicobacter infection in the stomachs of mice, pigs, and rats. Only later would Marshall learn that Helicobacter could only infect primates [9, 10].

Most case reports are not so dramatic or compelling. Nonetheless, this case report did not change the dogma that excess stomach acid was the primary cause of gastric and duodenal ulcer disease. Neither did a case series from his group, which showed that of 100 consecutive patients presenting for gastroscopy, 77% of the patients with gastric ulcers and 100% of patients presenting with duodenal ulcers had flagellated, gram negative bacilli, then identified as a species of Campylobacter, (and which we now know as *H. pylori*) cultured from their stomachs [11].

Gastroenterologists in the early 1980s remained convinced that excess acidity was the primary cause of ulcers. The histamine receptor blocking drugs cimetidine and ranitidine, which decreased stomach acidity, could be demonstrated to usually bring about improvements in most patients with ulcer disease. Thus, results of histamine-blocker drug therapy reinforced the widely accepted premise that excess acidity was the primary cause of gastric and duodenal ulcers. Perhaps not coincidentally, cimetidine and ranitidine were two of the most profitable drugs at the time, generating sales income of over US$8 billion each year [12]. In the early 1980s, Marshall submitted his case series [11] as an abstract, hoping to present the data at a forum in Australia. However, his abstract was one of only eight not accepted from among the 67 submitted for consideration for presentation at that Australian meeting [13]. (This research was instead presented at an international congress devoted to the topic of Campylobacter, in Brussels, Belgium, and then published in the *Lancet*.) Marshall tried to use his case series data to seek pharmaceutical company funding to further explore his microbial hypothesis, but he was unsuccessful at that point.

Case–control studies are the next level of evidence. Subjects are grouped by outcome. The most usual outcome is the presence or absence of a specific disease. Patients with disease are matched to others without disease for various traits, such as age, gender, or other relevant attributes. The goal of assembling a control group is to assemble a cohort that is highly similar to the case group, except for the presence of disease, and the presence or absence of defined risk factor(s). The diseased and non-diseased groups are then compared for the frequency of presence of the risk factor of interest between the two groups. These studies can be prospective, but are usually retrospective. These studies can support causation, but usually do not.

H. pylori is now known to contain urease, which hydrolyzes urea to ammonia and the bicarbonate ion. The bicarbonate ion buffers stomach pH, contributing to microbial survival, and the ammonia contributes to halitosis associated with gastric ulcer disease due to *H. pylori* infection. If Marshall had executed a case–control series in which he assayed patients' breath for ammonia levels above a normal threshold value, he would have found that "case" patients with the outcome of gastric or duodenal ulcers were more likely to have elevated breath ammonia levels than "control" patients without ulcers. He would have been able to demonstrate an association between ammonia in the breath and ulcers visible upon gastroscopy. However, he would not yet have been able to purport a mechanism by which ammonia was commonly present in patients with ulcers, and he would not have been able to link a specific microbe to ulcer pathogenesis.

Cohort studies

In a *cohort study*, subjects are grouped based upon whether or not they possess a purported risk factor for some specific disease. Subjects are then followed across time to determine who develops disease and who does not. In contrast to case–control studies, the outcome for patients in a cohort study is not known at the time of a subjects' entry into a study. Most cohorts for study are assembled and studied prospectively, but retrospective (also called "non-concurrent") assembly of the patient cohort can occur. By definition, subjects in cohort studies cannot be randomly assigned to study groups.

Marshall *et al.* reported a prospectively assembled cohort study in 1985. The trait possessed by one group, but not the other, was the presence of histologically-demonstrated rod-shaped bacteria on gastric biopsy samples. *H. pylori* could be cultured from 88% of patients with gastric mucosa in which the rod-shaped bacterium could be demonstrated histologically, but in 0% of patients with histologically normal gastric mucosa [14]. This study did not change the dogma that excess stomach acid was the primary cause of gastric and duodenal ulcer disease. Also, this study would not have met Marshall's ultimate objective to demonstrate that antibiotics should be used to cure gastric disease, because it did not attempt to demonstrate the efficacy of antibiotics to cure gastric or duodenal ulcers in this cohort.

Randomized control study designs with a placebo group

Consider a possible study design to determine if antibiotics help decrease the duration or recurrence of ulcer disease, compared to placebo. Before starting such a study, we must consider a number of important factors. The first is *random allocation* of subjects into study groups

Random allocation is the best means to decrease *bias* in study designs. *Bias* means any factor that increases the likelihood of concluding one of the possible outcomes of the study, for a reason other than being due to a treatment's inherent effect. Random allocation ensures factors that affect outcome are balanced between study groups. Think of bias as the equivalent of a head start in a race. Any competitor who has been given a head start is more likely to cross the finish line first, before the other competitors, even though the person given a head start may not be the fastest competitor. Similarly, study groups assembled with a bias toward reaching a specific conclusion can confound a research study's ability to discern the truth, regardless of whether or not one treatment is or is not superior to the other. The best way to minimize bias is for each subject in each population being studied to have an equal chance of being included in any group of the research study. This is accomplished by the process of randomization (outlined in detail in Chapter 12), the random allocation of subjects into the different groups in a study.

"*Blinding*" is another important tool to decrease bias. Blinding means concealing the treatment or group assignment from subjects and/or research team members. Concealment can be done for the patients, the members of the research team who assess outcomes, or, ideally, both. When both the patient and the outcome assessor are "blinded", the study is said to have a "double-blind" design.

Randomized, double-blind designs are important tools to decrease bias. Double-blind research designs help to minimize the likelihood that potential confounding variables are more frequently present in one patient group than in others. For example, patients who subjectively believe their treatment is likely to be effective may be more compliant with treatment than patients who do not believe their treatment will be effective. Blinding is especially important when subjectivity in assessing treatment outcomes is present. When research team members need to adjudicate somewhat subjective outcomes, such as slides of biopsy samples of patients with gastric ulcers, researchers are at risk for classifying an outcome more favorably when they know the patient has received a treatment that they believe will be effective. Researchers are at risk for classifying a subjective outcome less favorably if they know that the patient has received a treatment that they believe will not be effective. In summary, the most ideal situation is for both the subjects and the researchers who are assessing a study's outcomes to be blinded to the treatment condition of the subject.

The researcher must also consider whether or not the condition of *equipoise* is present before beginning to collect data. When equipoise is present, it is plausible that the new treatment being studied might, or might not, be best for the patient, when compared against some alternative treatment. Without equipoise it is unethical to conduct a prospective clinical trial.

When equipoise is present, prospective, blinded, randomized study designs, in which each subject has an equal chance to receive a treatment or a placebo, and in which patients are enrolled before receiving placebo or treatment, minimize bias and can help discern whether the treatment is helpful to decrease the burden of disease. This is why prospective, double-blind, randomized study designs are the benchmark for the study design that can provide the most convincing evidence.

Finally, researchers must also recognize that a *placebo effect* may be responsible for patients obtaining clinical improvement of a disease condition. Human physiology permits medication-free recovery from many illnesses. For example, when researchers have studied the effects of antidepressant medications, depression in some patients will improve if they are given a placebo instead of active medication. (A good rule of thumb is to expect placebo response rates to be of the range 10–20%.)

When any prospective study is executed, the numerical result obtained from one group will rarely, if ever, be identical to the results obtained in other groups. If Marshall and Warren had used an *ineffective* antibiotic to try to cure *H. pylori* in a prospective, randomized, double-blind, placebo-controlled trial, the response rate to the ineffective antibiotic would not have been zero, but would not be likely to have differed markedly from the placebo response rate. If they had used an effective antibiotic, the cure rate with the antibiotic would be expected to numerically and statistically exceed the placebo control and ineffective antibiotic cure rates. Researchers must employ biostatistics to permit inference regarding whether or not any numerical differences observed between groups are unlikely to have occurred due simply to chance.

Randomized clinical trials without a placebo group

As noted above, the most effective means to establish whether a cause and effect relationship exists between some purported risk factor and the development of disease is a prospective, randomized, double-blinded clinical trial. As it stands, being able to do a randomized controlled trial with a placebo group is actually a rarity in medicine, because few diseases or disease states do not already have some sort of proven treatment. Marshall and Warren actually could not have ethically conducted a trial comparing the effect of antibiotic treatment versus placebo upon the subsequent cure rate of patients diagnosed with gastric or duodenal ulcers. When they were delineating the role of microbes in gastric disease, it was already known that H2 blockers such as cimetidine and ranitidine would cause temporary improvements in most patients. Marshall and Warren also knew unequivocally that bismuth helped retard the growth of *H. pylori*. Equipoise would not have been present if a prospective, randomized research design with a placebo group had been employed, because placebo group patients would have been denied the benefits of H2 blocker and/or bismuth treatment.

They knew that instead of having a placebo group, ethical, randomized, prospective, double-blinded clinical trials would need to be designed to compare two or more groups that each receive non-placebo treatments in order to permit equipoise.

They executed at least two such trials. One compared gastric histology in patients given either cimetidine, colloidal bismuth subcitrate (CBS), or CBS plus an antibiotic (amoxicillin or tinidazole) [15]. Cimetidine did not change gastric mucosal histology or decrease bacterial infection, but did bring about temporary symptom resolution. CBS was associated with a reduction in bacterial number and better symptom resolution. Addition of an antibiotic with CBS was associated with a longer term disappearance of microbes than was the case with CBS alone. This trial was ethical because cimetidine and CBS were both known to be efficacious for ulcer treatment.

A follow-up study randomized ulcer patients to receive cimetidine or CBS for eight weeks, while also randomizing subjects to receive either tinidazole or placebo. Thus, there were four treatment groups. Ulcer healing was observed at 10 weeks in 92% of patients in whom *H. pylori* could not be detected, but in only 61% of patients with persistent *H. pylori* [16]. Further convincing evidence was provided by Forbes *et al.*, from Marshall's group, in 1994. This seven year follow-up study demonstrated that an active ulcer was present in 20% of patients in whom *H. pylori* infection could be demonstrated, but in only 3% in whom *H. pylori* assays were negative [17].

Epilogue

Marshall *et al.* built a convincing case that the microbe we now know as *H. pylori* causes most gastric and duodenal ulcers. Marshall's team started with observations. However their research culminated with prospective randomized blinded studies that implicated the role of a microbe in the development and persistence of gastric and duodenal ulcer disease. The research of Marshall *et al.* was critical to eventually overturn prior dogma regarding the most important etiology of gastric and duodenal ulcer disease.

However, it proved difficult to change the medical dogma based strongly upon studies implicating the etiologic role of stomach acidity published in the 1970s. These studies suggested that excess stomach acid was the primary culprit for causing gastric and duodenal ulcers.

It is a given that knowledge translation is never immediate, but it was not until 1994 (which, interestingly, was the year that patent protection ended for ranitidine and cimetidine) that the United States National Institutes of Health convened a consensus development conference, which produced a recommendation that patients with *H. pylori* should be treated with antibiotics [18]. It is unlikely that consensus could have been reached without convincing, prospective, randomized, blinded studies that demonstrated the importance of earlier findings from observational and cohort studies. Also, important contributions of others, who provided data to help develop the three drug cocktail that became widely adopted to cure *H. pylori* disease, have been omitted in the interest of simplicity.

Summary

Various research designs exist to communicate scientific findings. The simplest means to report findings, but least persuasive to influence practice, are isolated observations, case reports and case series. Case–control studies are observational studies that rank above case series in complexity and persuasive power, because they can be used to demonstrate a difference in risk factors for developing an important clinical outcome. However, case–control studies rarely change clinical practice.

Cohort studies are intermediate between observational studies and randomized trials, and can be used to begin to infer cause and effect. These studies can utilize data collected prospectively, but all lack the bias-deceasing effects of randomization of patients into study groups. Also, many cohort studies lack blinding of outcomes by outcome assessors.

The most persuasive medical evidence is obtained from prospective, randomized, double-blinded clinical trials. Placebo groups can be used while maintaining equipoise if no good treatment exists for a disease. However, for most diseases, a non-placebo treatment is available. Therefore, to maintain equipoise, a new treatment regimen must be compared against the current standard of care, which is called an "active control". An ethical research trial regarding such diseases must compare a new, possibly better treatment against the prior standard of care treatment. Even with all of these measures, knowledge translation from bench to bedside may take years to complete.

More details regarding research design concepts can be found elsewhere [19].

KEY POINTS

- Case reports and retrospective studies can report important observations that influence medical opinions and form the basis of prospective study designs. However, case reports and retrospective study designs seldom themselves report findings that change medical practice.
- Various retrospective and prospective study designs have strengths and weaknesses that influence the goals and design of prospective, randomized trials.
- Prospective, randomized, double-blinded study designs are the least biased and most persuasive study designs. It is unusual for major changes of medical dogma or widely-held belief to become widely accepted as true without data from such a trial.

References

1 Bizzozero, G. (1893) Ueber die schlauchförmigen drusen des magendarmkanals und die beziehunger ihres epithels zu dem oberflächenepithel der schleimhaut dritte mitteilung. *Archiv Mikroskopische Anat*, **43**:82–152.
2 Krienitz, W. (1906) Ueber das auftreten von mageninhalt ei carcinoma ventriculi *Dtsch Med Wochenschr*, **22**:872.
3 Luger, A. (1917) Ueber spirochaeten und fusiforme bazillen im darm, mit einer beitrag zur frage der lamblien-enteritis. *Wien Klin Wochensch*, **52**:1643–1647.
4 Mozorov, I.A. (2005) *Helicobacter pylori* was discovered in Russia in 1974. In: B. Marshall (ed.) *Helicobacter pioneers: firsthand accounts from the scientists who discovered helicobacters, 1892–1982*. Blackwell, Oxford, pp. 105–118.
5 Rigas, B. and Papavassiliou, E.D. (2005) John Lykoudis: The general practitioner in Greece who in 1958 discovered etiology of, and a treatment for, peptic ulcer disease. In: B. Marshall (ed.) *Helicobacter pioneers: firsthand accounts from the scientists who discovered helicobacters, 1892–1982*. Blackwell, Oxford, pp. 75–84.
6 Lieber, C.S. (2005) How it was discovered in Belgium and the USA (1955–1976) that gastric urease was caused by a bacterial infection. In: B. Marshall (ed.) *Helicobacter pioneers: firsthand accounts from the scientists who discovered helicobacters, 1892–1982*. Blackwell, Oxford, pp. 39–52.
7 Warren, J.R. and Marshall, B.J. (1983) Unidentified curved bacilli on gastric epithelium in active chronic gastritis. *Lancet*, **1983**;1273–1275.
8 Thagard, P. (1997) Discovery 3: Peptic ulcers can be treated with antibiotics. In: *Ulcers and Bacteria I: Discovery and Acceptance*. http://cogsci.uwaterloo.ca/Articles/Pages/Ulcers.one.html (last accessed 9 May 2015).
9 Marshall, B.J., Armstrong, J.A., McGechie, D.B., Glancy, R.J. (1985) Attempt to fulfil Koch's postulates for Pyloric Camphylobacter. *Med J Aust*, **142**:436–439.
10 Warren, J.R. (2005) The discovery of *Helicobacter pylori* in Perth, Western Australia. In: B. Marshall (ed.) *Helicobacter pioneers: firsthand accounts from the scientists who discovered helicobacters, 1892–1982*. Blackwell, Oxford, pp. 151–164.
11 Marshall, B.J. and Warren, J.R. (1984) Unidentified curved bacilli in the stomach of patients with gastritis and peptic ulceration. *Lancet*, **1**(8390):1311–1315.
12 Larsen, H.R. (nd) *The Great Ulcer Drug Rip-off*. http://www.yourhealthbase.com/ulcer_drugs.htm (last accessed 9 May 2015).
13 Thagard, P. (1997) *Discovery 2: The hypothesis that H. pylori cause ulcers*. In: *Ulcers and Bacteria I: Discovery and Acceptance*. http://cogsci.uwaterloo.ca/Articles/Pages/Ulcers.one.html (last accessed 9 May 2015).
14 Marshall, B.J., McGechie, D.B., Rogers, P.A., and Glancy, R.J. (1985) Pyloric Camphylobacter infection and gastroduodenal disease. *Med J Aust*, **142**:439–444.

15 Marshall, B.J., Armstrong, J.A., Francis, G.J., *et al.* (1987) Antibacterial action of bismuth in relation to Camphylobacter pyloridis colonization and gastritis. *Digestion*, **37**(Suppl 2):16–30.

16 Marshall, B.J., Goodwin, C.S., Warren, J.R., *et al.* (1988) Prospective, double-blind trial of duodenal ulcer relapse after eradication of *camphylobacter pylori*. *Lancet*, **2**(8626/8627), 1437–1441.

17 Forbes, G.M., Glaser, M.E., Cullen, D.J.E., *et al.* (1994) Duodenal ulcer treated with *Helicobacter pylori* eradication: Seven year follow-up. *Lancet*, **342**:258–260.

18 Thagard, P. (1997) Causation and Cure. In: *Ulcers and Bacteria I: Discovery and Acceptance*. http://cogsci.uwaterloo.ca/Articles/Pages/Ulcers.one.html (last accessed 9 May 2015).

19 Mayer, D. (2010) *Essential Evidence-Based Medicine*, 2nd edn. Cambridge University Press, Cambridge.

CHAPTER 19

How to design a study that everyone will believe: Effectiveness, safety, and the intention to treat

Ashleigh Campillo[1], Christopher J. Coyne[2], and Juan A. Luna[3]

[1] UCSD Department of Emergency Medicine Behavioral Emergencies Research (DEMBER) laboratory, University of California, San Diego, CA, USA
[2] UCSD Department of Emergency Medicine, UC San Diego Health System, San Diego, CA, USA
[3] California State University San Marcos, CA, USA

Real world issues that occur in clinical research

- Patients do not adhere to the protocol (e.g., do not take prescribed study medication, do not follow study schedules).
- Patients withdraw from the study or are lost to follow-up.
- Patients are erroneously included in the study that may not have been eligible to participate.
- An adverse event occurs and a patient must be removed from the trial.
- A patient receives treatment in the arm they were not originally randomized to (crossover).

All of these "oops" moments will lead to missing or inaccurate data. Sometimes, even if the researchers did nothing wrong, it will still prove difficult to measure a patient if they move, die for a reason unrelated to the study, or simply do not want to participate.

In other words, no matter how well designed the protocol is or how conscientious the researcher and staff are, missing data points will occur. Any time you throw a human subject into the mix (at least as far as research goes), things can get pretty complicated. Luckily, there are a few techniques to address and analyze these incomplete data sets. At the end of this chapter, you will know how to deal with missing data (the bane of many researchers' existence) that can result from conducting efficacy and effectiveness studies. Just remember, these skills do not absolve you from being a conscientious researcher with well-designed protocols mentioned before. You will just be better equipped to address the common problem of missing data. (Sloppy collection of data cannot be fixed so easily; Chapters 10, 11, and 12 give an overview).

Which came first: The efficacy or the effectiveness study and what is the difference anyway?

Efficacy and effectiveness trials are two important types of studies in clinical research that are often misunderstood. So, let us start with a couple of definitions so you do not fall into the quagmire of confusion.

Efficacy: In pharmacology, for example, efficacy is the measure used to determine a drug's ability to produce its indicated effect *under ideal and controlled circumstances*.

Efficacy studies (also referred to as experimental or explanatory studies) often have very strict inclusion and exclusion criteria, which generate a homogeneous patient population. They also use detailed protocols, employ protocol-trained physicians and research staff, and may have extensive associated patient interventions including patient education, appointment reminders, medication reminders, and so on [1, 2].

Doing Research in Emergency and Acute Care: Making Order Out of Chaos, First Edition. Edited by Michael P. Wilson, Kama Z. Guluma, and Stephen R. Hayden.
© 2016 John Wiley & Sons, Ltd. Published 2016 by John Wiley & Sons, Ltd.

- Efficacy studies aim to answer the question, "Does this treatment work?"

Effectiveness: Effectiveness is an all-encompassing term that measures a drugs ability to produce its indicated effect *under usual or real world circumstances.* It measures an overall treatment strategy more than a pure effect of treatment.

Effectiveness studies (or pragmatic studies) have less restrictive inclusion and exclusion criteria, and therefore generate a heterogeneous patient population. They typically use less specific protocols, occur in a standard practice environment, do not require highly trained research staff, and may not be associated with extensive patient interventions [1, 2].

- Effectiveness studies aim to answer the question, "Does this treatment strategy work in the real world?"
  These study types do, however, have some similarities:
- They usually follow general Randomized Control Trial design schema (Chapter 18).
- They are both prone to patient withdrawal and protocol deviations.
- They use Intention-to-Treat analysis to address missing data issues.

So your patient is a no-show for the rest of the study. Now what? Intention-to-Treat Analysis

According to The International Conference on Harmonisation of Technical Requirement for Registration of Pharmaceuticals for Human Use (ICH) the Intention-to-Treat (ITT) is defined as follows:

> "The principle that asserts that the effect of a treatment policy can be best assessed by evaluating on the basis of the intention to treat a subject (i.e., the planned treatment regimen) rather than the actual treatment given. It has the consequence that subjects allocated to a treatment group should be followed up, assessed and analysed as members of that group irrespective of their compliance to the planned course of treatment."
>
> ICH E9 Statistical Principles for Clinical Trials [3]

We have found an easier way of defining ITT that we hope you appreciate. Intention-to-treat analysis can be described as, "once randomized, always analyzed." Unfortunately we cannot take credit for making that up, although we would like to because it is pretty catchy [4]. Despite having a memorable catch phrase, intention-to-treat analysis is sadly misunderstood, misrepresented, and applied inconsistently in primary literature. Many researchers throw caution to the wind, excluding large subsets of their randomized patient populations from analysis without adequately describing their reasoning. Randomization is important because it ensures that factors affecting outcome are evenly balanced between groups [5]. This goes for both factors known to affect the outcome of interest as well as unknown factors. If you do not analyze patients according to the groups they were originally allocated to, you run the risk of unbalancing those factors (especially the unknown factors) that affect outcome and introducing bias. ITT is a means of preserving the benefit of randomization. With ITT, there are a few very specific instances where you can exclude randomized patients from analysis; otherwise it is no longer an ITT analysis [6]. Reading this section provides more information on this handy technique, including the pros and cons and the rules that go along with its use. You do not want to be one of those researchers who forgets the slogan of intention-to-treat.

Intention-to-treat: Who's included?
- All patients post-randomization are ideally to be included in analysis.

Intention-to-treat: Who can be excluded?
- Per ICH Guidelines and expert suggestions there are two circumstances in which randomized patients could be excluded from analysis:
  (i) A critical error was made in which an ineligible patient was enrolled and randomized to a research arm (eligibility violation).
  (ii) A major protocol violation occurred in which no trial medication was taken/given to/received by the patient (methodological error).

(Caveat A to condition (ii): No data exist on the patient post-randomization.

Caveat B to condition (ii): Trial design must be appropriate, For example, if a trial has an arm in which patients receive a pain medication upon request, patients cannot be excluded for not requesting the target medication [3].)

Any plans to exclude patients from analysis should be planned for prospectively (e.g., in your study protocol) when possible [7]. Planning ahead for protocol deviations, data that are really extreme on your scale (i.e., outliers) and early withdrawal offers you the opportunity to design the best overall data analysis strategy. The importance of stringent documentation on all research protocol related events, especially with regard to excluding patients from data analysis, cannot be stressed enough [8, 9]. Having records on these events will come in very handy when preparing a manuscript. Reviewers do not appreciate when patients conveniently disappear from analysis without any offered explanation.

The good the bad and the ugly: Pros and cons of intention-to-treat analysis

We must be critical thinkers when we approach ITT analysis; this is a book on research after all.

Pros:
- Maintains sample size and statistical power of study.
- Maintains integrity of random sample by eliminating selection bias for compliant participants.

If we were to consistently exclude non-compliant patients from analysis and not report data on the complete data set, we would be introducing bias. There may be some characteristics that are different between the group complying with treatment and the group not complying.
- Prevents overestimation of effectiveness and efficacy of treatment.
- Prevents Type I error (Chapter 27).
- Prevents splitting patients into arbitrary subgroups for analysis.

Cons:
- May underestimate the risk of adverse side effects.
  - Patients experiencing side effects drop out without reporting any of these effects.
- Dilutes efficacy data of the treatment being evaluated.
  - Non-compliant and compliant patient endpoints are analyzed as all compliant.
- It is an overly cautious means of analyzing patient treatment data that does not provide useful information on the efficacy of treatment (remember the difference between efficacy and effectiveness).
- Susceptible to Type II error (Chapter 27) [10–12].

Filling in the blanks: Types of missing data and techniques for replacing missing data points

Some of you may have been reading along and have asked yourself, "This ITT analysis is all fine and dandy, but is not getting to the point of the actual missing data. You cannot analyze missing data." Well you get a gold star. You are absolutely right; you cannot analyze data that does not exist. This next section will introduce the types of missing data and a few standard techniques used for imputation, or substituting missing data values.

Types of missing data
Missing completely at random
When data are said to be missing completely at random (MCAR), it means that there is no observed or unobserved relationship between the missing variable and any characteristic of treatment population or any other study related variables. This is to say that the reason for missing data is unsystematic. For example, you are missing data for a participant on a given follow-up visit because they could not come due to a scheduling error. Another example could be that a blood sample was lost due to a study coordinator dropping the laboratory draw tube. This is a discrete instance where you would not have information for this subject that exists for the rest of your data set [13, 14].

Missing at random

When data are missing at random (MAR) there is a relationship between the missing variable and some observed characteristic of the treatment population/other study related variables. Try not to get caught up on the "randomness" of this phrase because, in fact, the missing data may not be missing randomly at all. For instance, you are collecting survey information on young adults who present to the emergency department with suicidal ideation for a study that focuses on gender-specific psychological interventions. After finishing data collection, you find that 60% of young men fail to answer whether they had a history of depression. Both men and women have equal likelihood to not answer the question, but there is an observable relationship between failure to answer the question and gender [15].

Missing not at random

When data are missing not at random (MNAR) there is a relationship between the missing variable and some unobserved variable or hypothetical outcome. The easiest way to conceptualize MNAR is to think about patients who drop out of a trial or who are lost to follow-up. For instance, consider a clinical trial examining the efficacy of a new acne medication taken orally. One of the potential side effects of this drug is hormone-related migraines. Over time, the trial experiences a huge dropout rate of women of child bearing age for what can be assumed to be incidences of side effects. We now have to infer a hypothetical outcome for the remainder of the missing data points [16, 17].

One size does not fit all: Choosing the appropriate technique to fill in missing data

Now that you are familiar with the different types of missing data that can arise during a clinical research study, we will move on to the different ways of substituting missing data points.

Complete case analysis

When you chose to analyze only the cases in which you have complete data sets you are performing a complete case analysis. In order to do this, you "delete" all cases in which there is any missing data. The glaring issue with this method is that you are ignoring the number one rule of intention-to-treat analysis, which is that all patients are to be analyzed once they are randomized. Methodologically speaking, you also decrease the power of your study by decreasing your sample size with every case that you remove from your data set. In the worst case scenario, you would whittle your sample down to an n of 1 which would be pitifully insignificant and unreportable.

- When to apply: Complete case analysis can be appropriately applied to data MCAR. Remember, however, when excluding participants due to lack of compliance or missing data you run the risk of decreasing your sample size and the power of your study. You may want to consider using a different method of analysis.

Single imputation techniques

Although no current stringent recommendations exist on the best practices for data imputation, single imputation is often the least favorable method of replacing missing data. Why? Well, this method often introduces the greatest bias to a study's outcome, produces unrealistic p-values, and underestimates variability, which can result in misleading confidence intervals. Despite these obvious issues, single imputation is still employed in many clinical research studies, including pharmaceutical trials [16]. Tread carefully if you plan on using single imputation and make sure you provide adequate justification in your methods section as to why it is the appropriate statistical technique for dealing with missing data. You may want to consult a statistician.

Baseline observation carried forward

As the name implies, baseline observation is used for the missing data points for a participant. Any increase or decrease in performance status is disregarded and the value in question is simply put back at square one. On one hand this can be a conservative model of imputation. On the other, it can be an overly optimistic method of imputation. If a patient fared worse on treatment, then were we to impute their baseline data it would appear that the treatment was more efficacious than it really was.

- When to apply: Because of the obvious issue of biasing your outcome data, it is not recommended to use BOCF in any circumstance.

Worst case scenario

In the worst case scenario model, we assume that all patients who withdrew from the treatment arm fared worse after they dropped out of the study while all patients who withdrew from the control arm did better. This model is appropriate for studies in which the final endpoint is measured as a discrete, dichotomous outcome (e.g., dead/alive, no evidence of disease/disease progression, etc.). This method is the most conservative approach to imputation, which may have some benefit when reporting results of analysis. If your treatment is successful, it implies the results are not due to faulty imputation or lack of reporting of patient drop outs [14–17]. On the other hand, this conservative approach has obvious risks. If after analysis, results show treatment was unsuccessful, there would be no definitive way to discern if it was due to the treatment itself or due to the imputation technique chosen and, thus, a consequence of the number of total dropouts.

Last observation carried forward

Last observation carried forward, or LOCF, is when the last recorded observation for a withdrawn participant is used for all subsequent missed visits for the duration of the trial. This method allows for analysis of data over the duration of the trial, removing focus on simple endpoint data. It preserves the number of total analyzable participants in the trial while still maintaining a conservative estimate of patient performance after dropout.

LOCF is not without flaws. It is an unrealistic model of patient performance, especially those with advanced stage cancers and cardiac disease. It does not plot progression or regression of disease or take into account disease processes [16].

- When to apply: LOCF is commonly applied in a wide array of trial designs for all missing data types. If you decide to use LOCF, use with caution.

Hot deck imputation

Hot deck imputation is the process of replacing missing data points from one subject with data points from another similar subject within the same treatment group. The same issues arise with hot deck imputation, namely a lack of variability between subjects.

Mean imputation

In mean imputation the missing data point is replaced by the mean (or average) value for the variable in question. This, of course, assumes that the missing value is numerical [18].

- When to apply: Mean imputation can appropriately estimate treatment outcomes in data MCAR but not in data MAR.

Imputation with Variance

Maximum-likelihood estimation

Another technique recommended by methodologists is maximum-likelihood estimation. In this scenario, a population parameter is identified as being the most probable to generate the missing sample data. Using a log-likelihood function, the mean between observed data points and the variables of interest is calculated [17]. Think back to algebra and think of it like a least squares calculation. Now we understand some of that algebra class may have sounded like Greek, but the main point of maximum-likelihood estimation is to introduce artificial variability to imputed data. However, do not worry, most statistical software packages have maximum-likelihood estimation functions so you would never need to do this by hand.

- When to apply: This technique can be applied appropriately to MAR, MCAR, and MNAR depending on sensitivity analysis.

Multiple imputation

A more sophisticated, and by that we mean complicated, technique of imputing data has emerged known as multiple imputation. Using hierarchical linear modeling or HLM[1] variation is introduced into missing data variables in a way that simple imputation techniques cannot. Without getting into too much depth, HLM imputes data from patients who have withdrawn from a longitudinal study after receiving, or participating in, at least three treatment cycles. What happens next offers the key difference between single imputation and multiple imputation [13, 17]. Through complex computerized linear regression modeling, each unique data point is generated with introduced variation. This process is repeated until you have a number of complete data sets with imputed data generated the same way. After the imputed data sets have been generated, they are then analyzed and pooled together. The pooling process entails estimating variances between the within-imputation group and between-imputation group caused by the first steps of the MI process.

---

[1] Also known as growth curve analysis, empirical Bayes models, random effects regression, and a number of other names that most statisticians understand but make our eyes glaze over. HLM is also an advanced technique in itself used to handle missing data [13, 19].

Multiple imputation has some obvious advantages over previous methods of data imputation, in that it can offer the most realistic substitution for missing variables. This is imperative for pharmaceutical trials that test chemotherapy or cardiac interventions as their patient populations are expected to have widely variable outcomes overtime. In such cases, single imputation for all missing data is unrealistic and has the potential to bias outcome analyses [13, 17].

- When to apply: Applicable to MCAR, MAR, MNAR depending on sensitivity analysis.

Summary

In this chapter you have learned:

- The difference between efficacy and effectiveness studies
- All about Intention-to-treat analysis
- How to handle missing data like a pro

Now the next time you are working on a study and a participant drops out because they feel like the trial medication leads them to compulsively over-eat pizza, you will not need to dive face-first yourself into a deep-dish pizza in a fit of stress-eating despair. No, you now have a good overview of intention-to-treat analysis and data imputation techniques.

KEY POINTS

- Efficacy studies aim to answer the question, "Does this treatment work?", while Effectiveness studies aim to answer the question, "Does this treatment strategy work in the real world?"
- Intention-to-treat analysis maintains sample size and statistical power, and prevents Type I error, but may underestimate the risk of adverse side effects and dilute the efficacy data of the treatment being evaluated.
- Missing data are not all the same and should be treated differently according to whether they are missing completely at random (MCAR), missing at random (MAR), and missing not at random (MNAT).
- Missing data can be handled in many ways, including the complete case technique, single imputations techniques and imputation with variance techniques.
- All techniques for handling missing data have their unique pros and cons, and should be chosen based on the type of study and missing data encountered.

References

1 Signal, A., Higgins, P., and Waljee, A. (2014) A primer on effectiveness and efficacy trials. *Clin Transl Gastroenterol*, **5**:e45.
2 Revicki, D. and Frank, L. (1999) Pharmacoeconomic evaluation in the real world effectiveness versus efficacy studies. *Pharmacoeconomics*, **15**(5):423–434.
3 ICH Expert Working Group (1998) ICH Harmonised Tripartite Guideline, Statistical Principles for Clinical Trials E9, Current Step 4 version dated 5 February 1998. http://www.ich.org/fileadmin/Public_Web_Site/ICH_Products/Guidelines/Efficacy/E9/Step4/E9_Guideline.pdf (last accessed 10 May 2015).
4 Gupta, S. (2011) Intention-to-treat concept: A review. *Perspect Clin Res*, **2**(3):109–112.
5 Kruse, R.L., Alper, B.S., Reust, C., *et al.* (2002) Intention-to-treat analysis: who is in? Who is out? *J Fam Pract*, **51**(11):969–971.
6 Fergusson, D., Aaron, S., Guyatt, G., and Herbert, P. (2002) Post-randomisation exclusions: the intention to treat principle and excluding patients from analysis. *BMJ*, **325**(7365):652–654.
7 Roland, M. and Torgerson, D. (1998) Understanding controlled trials: What are pragmatic trials? *BMJ*, **316**(7127):285.
8 Hollis, S. and Campbell, F. (1999) What is meant by intention to treat analysis? Survey of published randomised controlled trials. *BMJ*, **319**(7211):670–674.
9 Schulz, K., Altman, D., and Moher, D. (2011) Consort 2010 statement: Updated guidelines for reporting parallel group randomized trials. *Int J Surg*, **9**(8):672–677.
10 Ellenberg, J. (2005) Intention to treat analysis. In: P. Armitage and T. Colton (eds) *Encyclopedia of Biostatistics*, Vol. **4**. John Wiley & Sons, Inc., pp. 1–5.
11 Sommer, A. and Zeger, S. (1991) On estimating efficacy from clinical trials. *Stat Med*, **10**(1):45–52.
12 Streiner, D. and Geddes, J. (2001) Intention to treat analysis in clinical trials when there are missing data. *Evid Based Ment Health.*, **4**:70–71.

13 Norman, G. and Streiner, D. (2008) Analysis of longitudinal data: Hierarchical linear modeling. In: G.R. Norman and D.L. Streiner, *Biostatistics: The Bare Essentials*. BC Decker Inc., Hamilton, ON, pp. 186–193.

14 Dziura, J., Post, L., Zhao, Q., *et al.* (2013) Strategies for dealing with missing data in clinical trials: From design to analysis. *Yale J Biol Med*, **86**(3):343–358.

15 Baraldi, A. and Enders, C. (2010) An introduction to modern missing data analyses. *J Sch Psychol*, **48**(1):5–37.

16 Schafer, J. (2005) Missing data in longitudinal studies: A review. Presented to The American Association of Pharmaceutical Scientists, Nashville, TN, 9 November 2005.

17 Woltman, H., Feldstein, A., MacKay, C., and Rocchi, M. (2012) An introduction to hierarchical linear modeling. *Tutor Quant Methods Psychol*, **8**(1):52–69.

18 Andridge, R. and Little, R. (2010) A review of hot deck imputation for survey non-response. *Int Stat Rev*, **78**(1):40–64.

19 Raudenbush, S. and Bryk, S.W. (2002) *Hierarchical Linear Models: Applications and Data Analysis Methods (Advanced Quantitative Techniques in the Social Sciences)*, 2nd edn. Sage Publications Inc.

CHAPTER 20

How to design a study that everyone will believe: Emergency department operations and systems

Vaishal Tolia

Department of Emergency Medicine, University of California, San Diego Health System, San Diego, CA, USA

Studying operations and flow in an acute care setting

So how do you study the processes of an acute care setting, such as the emergency department (ED)? Well, as has been mentioned previously in other chapters (e.g., Chapter 3), the first step in carrying out research is asking a thoughtful and important question. This continues to hold true even if the focus of research is based on operations and systems of an emergency department. In industry, as well as in medicine, operations-based research helps in solving problems that need timely decisions. Data-driven analytic techniques help manage the ability to make challenging decisions in dynamic environments, and there are, indeed, none more dynamic or complicated than the emergency department.

Medical directors often have to find unique solutions to each problem specific to their institution and geography, as well as keep a very diverse faculty and resident group happy and feeling that they have the tools to effectively and efficiently do their jobs. If that is not hard enough, managing relationships with nursing and hospital administration is another major operational area. All of these problems and innovative solutions require lots and lots of evaluation (in other words, research!), and there are multiple questions that can be asked. The most common problems (er, opportunities for research) that you will encounter in your emergency department include:

- Evaluation of flow and throughput (i.e., how quickly patients are seen and discharged).
- Performance improvement.
- Staffing optimization.
- Patient experience.
- Finances.
- Marketing.

Common goals of medical directors and department operation leaders include improved patient care, enhanced patient experience, fewer patients who leave the ED without being seen by a provider (LWBS), decreased length of stay (LOS) for all patients, fewer "diversion hours" where ambulances go to other emergency departments, and meeting state and national benchmarks for excellence [1]. Outside of the interesting research questions involved with all of these, measuring success and failure is important for medical directors, so that they can both appropriately recognize high performers as well as help lesser performers improve areas that are below par. This is important to realize, because unlike data collected purely for research purposes in other types of studies (Chapter 11), data collected for operations research in the emergency department is collected solely to help the department improve. Thus, the type (and even the quality) of the data is based solely on the needs of particular department. This, of course, may make it difficult to generalize a study in this area to other areas of the country (or even in the same hospital!). Other areas of the hospital, such as the intensive care unit, operating room, and so on have their own set of challenges and metrics that require focused research. Many of the same concepts are applicable here as well.

Doing Research in Emergency and Acute Care: Making Order Out of Chaos, First Edition. Edited by Michael P. Wilson, Kama Z. Guluma, and Stephen R. Hayden.
© 2016 John Wiley & Sons, Ltd. Published 2016 by John Wiley & Sons, Ltd.

Benchmarking

If every department collected data differently, of course, it would be difficult, if not impossible, to carry out impactful research in this area. However, there are areas of notable agreement. Welch *et al.* described a consensus on operational metrics in 2010 at the second summit of convened experts in emergency department operations. These experts concluded that in order to improve performance in all areas of ED care and processes, terminology and metrics needed to be standardized, so as to more easily compare between departments [2]. There has been an increased emphasis on standardization due to the regulatory burdens that every emergency department are facing and because outside organizations are analyzing flow in performance in comparing it to national "standards" in order to set goals for accreditation [3, 4].

The consensus group convened by Welch *et al.* also helped develop a set of metrics by which emergency department operations are characterized. "Timestamps" such as census (number of patients in a given time period), admission rate (admitted patients as compared to the total census), case-mix index (complexity of patients), transfer rate (patients transferred as compared to the census), arrival to provider time (time from arrival to patient being seen by the provider), length of stay (total time in the ED), and availability of data, are key features (among many others) of operation-based research (Figure 20.1).

Emergency departments (naturally!) try to reduce many of these times to optimize flow. Medical directors often look at these metrics on a monthly basis (if not more frequently) to evaluate trends and focus on areas of improvement. One notable change in ED flow patterns at several institutions that was an outcome of this data set was the creation of "pods." These are care-specific areas in the ED with the staff divided into smaller teams with improved communication and reduction in commonly cited delays. Several institutions (including our own) have shown a reduction in many of these benchmarked metrics, such as overall length of stay for discharge patients.

This benchmarking allows easy comparison between emergency departments and allows any ED to target particular areas where performance is lacking. Obtaining this data is also useful for operation leaders and medical directors to

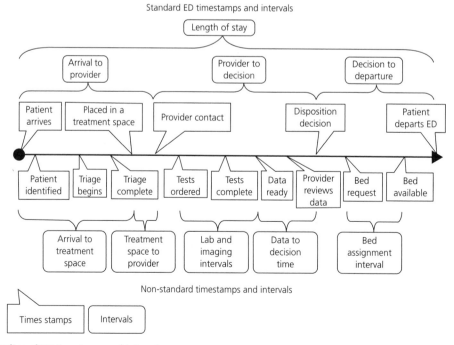

Figure 20.1 Timeline of ED timestamps and intervals.

create improvement, since systems and processes impact these metric measurements. In many situations, internal funding, external funding, and reimbursement are directly tied to performance. Thus, having a standardized set of data to present to both hospital administration and other regulatory bodies is essential to optimal functioning and support. Again, all of this data means that you can ask questions about how a particular factor impacts the day-to-day operations of your ED.

Informatics

If a question about benchmarking does not interest you, there are other interesting questions about how all of this benchmarking data are stored and utilized. The field of informatics is concerned with exactly that. Informatics in medicine generally is an important topic, since not only is the meaningful use of electronic health records a major issue, but the ability to perform high quality research is based upon the ease of access to accurate and interpretable patient data. In addition, mobile technologies, web-based technologies, and simulation are important tools. Most emergency department charting systems are being replaced by electronic health records, and most modern physicians rely on electronic sources of information instead of upon printed textbooks. In other industries, such as the airlines, simulation-based education and training have been mainstays, but are now becoming ever more popular in emergency medicine.

The conversion from print to electronic methods of storing and delivering information raises a whole host of questions for researchers in this area: How and what information should be stored? What is the optimum way to provide needed information so that clinicians do not have to "hunt" through various parts of the chart? How can patient information be utilized in order to make a simulation more realistic? From a regulatory standpoint, how can patient privacy and maintenance of records be protected, yet easily available to providers who need it? Informatics research has spawned fellowships and many research opportunities that involve a wide variety of topics, some of which include: ease of health record access, meaningful use of the EMR and data it produces, and identification of at risk situations in patient care (among many others).

Improving operations-based research

As noted previously, studies in this area often cannot be generalized to other departments (i.e., lack external validity). Still, you have probably had the experience (like many people) of returning from a great conference where you discussed innovative solutions with amazing physicians and administrators from other departments. If it works well somewhere else, why can you not replicate it immediately at your home institution with similar or better results?

Wise administrators know that the most important questions in a busy department do not necessarily involve the specific intervention of interest, but rather how the intervention is going to affect the current environment and processes already in place. For example, one of our emergency departments suffers from a common problem, that of holding inpatient admissions for an extended period (often days), which may pull valuable resources such as nursing away from other patients. This is a unique challenge to this particular clinical site and comes with it its own set of solutions. This clinical site is also the only one that has a dedicated emergency department base observation unit, which has had a positive impact on this boarding problem by creating alterative care pathways that are more efficient. Focusing on solutions often involves the medical director further highlighting the problem to hospital leadership, so that specific areas (operating room scheduling, inpatient discharge, nurse staffing, etc.) can be addressed, as they all impact (and can help disimpact!) the flow. Our other clinical site, on the other hand, is our level I trauma centre and primary teaching facility and we deal with the challenges of a very vulnerable population as well as a high proportion of psychiatric patient's that require significant time and resources.

One process improvement strategy recommended by the American Heart Association & American Stroke Association is an attempt to reduce the time to fibrinolytic therapy for patients arriving by ambulance with concern for acute ischemic stroke. Unloading stable stroke patients directly from the paramedic gurney onto the CT scanner has significantly decreased time to neuroimaging as well as that of initiation of fibrinolytic therapy.

One of the process improvement measures that we employed was to send patients who are stable directly to the CT scan and have them unloaded onto the scanner directly from the paramedic gurney. We had a large volume of data prior to this singular intervention, which we employed at both of our clinical sites, and we were able to show a significant reduction in time to lytic therapy, which improved the care for the patient as well as our measured metrics related to the care of the acute stroke patient. Having a strong study design is fundamental to provide both internal and external validity, particularly when the impact of the study may require resources, finances, and oversight from those outside of the department of emergency medicine. Having a dedicated research network and staff that can focus on operational issues is important for not only study design but also implementation of findings as well as multicenter application of the study and ultimately the expansion of better process methods. Randomization is also easier with multiple sites, as department-specific measured confounding variables are less likely to have an impact. Though it goes without saying, patient-based research and outcome measures are generally the focus of emergency department operations studies. Developing partnerships with funding agencies, specialty colleges in emergency medicine, and industry, especially with a focus on improving healthcare delivery efficiency and cost, is an important first step to dealing with emergency department-based operational challenges.

Asplin and Yealy, in their February 2011 article in *Annals of Emergency Medicine*, describe other key requirements for operations-based research in the emergency department [5]. The following are necessary to conduct operations-based research: proper infrastructure; ability to perform multicenter analysis; study design focusing on patient centered outcomes, especially those that go along with benchmarked metrics (mentioned previously); and projects that have the opportunity for impact and propagation. In addition, the institution has to have a focus and an interest in operation-based research, as well as the ability to act upon findings that improve health care delivery and patient outcomes.

Conclusion

Although many physicians may not like the fact that data about their performance with patients is being collected and compared in multiple ways, collecting and analyzing data about the processes and flows of a typical emergency department are essential for efficiency. Research on this data, or operations-based research, allows for the comparison of this data across different systems. Like it or not, modern emergency departments operate in the current era of benchmarking data, evolving informatics, increasing regulatory burdens, and demands from society to become more patient-oriented. Medical directors will continue to need high quality data to inform these decisions. The area of operations-based research has tremendous need for skilled researchers, especially ones who can use rigorous methodology and high-quality study designs.

KEY POINTS

- Collecting and analyzing data about ED flow is important to improving efficiency.
- There are multiple questions that can be asked about ED flow, including evaluation of flow and throughput, staffing optimization, and patient experience.
- Research on ED flow has defined generally agreed-upon timestamps

References

1 Rathlev, N.K., Chessare, J., Olshaker, J., et al. (2007) Time series analysis of variables associated with daily mean emergency department length of stay. *Ann Emerg Med*, **49**:265–271.
2 Welch, S.J., Stone-Griffith, S., Asplin, B., et al. (2011) Emergency department operations dictionary: results of the second performance measures and benchmarking summit. *Acad Emerg Med*, **18**:539–544.
3 The Joint Commission (2005) *A Comprehensive Review of Development and Testing for National Implementation of Hospital Core Measures.* http://www.jointcommission.org/assets/1/18/A_Comprehensive_Review_of_Development_for_Core_Measures.pdf (last accessed 10 May 2015).
4 Glickman, S.W., Schulman, K.A., Peterson, E.D., et al. (2008) Evidence-based perspectives on pay for performance and quality of patient care and outcomes in emergency medicine. *Ann Emerg Med*, **51**:622–631.
5 Asplin, B.R. and Yealy, D.M. (2011) Key requirements for a new era of emergency department operations research. *Ann Emerg Med*, **57**(2):101–103.

How to design a study that everyone will believe: The challenges of doing international research

Vicken Y. Totten

Department of Emergency Medicine, Kaweah Delta Health Care District, CA, USA

Quality work

The most important part of designing a study that everyone will believe is, of course, performing quality work. It is even more important for international work than it is for national work. Quality work means doing a study with an interesting question, a strong design, enough data so that the results are believable with a relatively narrow confidence interval, a good analysis demonstrating where the results are applicable, and an interesting discussion.

So, in this chapter, let us assume that you already have an interesting question, you have carried out quality work and your statistical analysis is appropriate. Let us also assume that you are making no claims about your work that are not supported by the data. This chapter covers only issues that pertain when more than one country is involved, that is, "international" research (not about research which compares countries! That would be "comparative" research.)

"Inter-nation-al" means between and among nations

How is international research different from research at home, you ask? Well, very different, yet much the same. "International research" could mean that your coresearchers are from and in another country or that you are gathering data in one other country or in more than one country. Perhaps your work is intended for readers outside your own country. If you want to be taken seriously and if you want to be believed, you will have to take into account differences in culture, ethics, applicability, language, and presentation.

> *"The man ain't got no culture."*
>
> Paul Simon, a *Simple Desultory Philippic*

Are you working with researchers from another culture? They may have different expectations than you do. Better make sure you have addressed all expectations first, before you start to gather data! Such as? Expectations about time-frames, about payment; and what will happen to the data, who collects it and who owns it, who will be an author, and in what order. Other things, you will have to ask if there are other things.

Before you start gathering any data, discuss your plans and set your expectations. "Soon" can mean so many different durations. Set firm expectations of time, and do it very early. Otherwise you may be frustrated by "we-do-it-tomorrow" attitude – or you may frustrate others with your potentially more efficient sense of time. Decide who will be authors, and in what order, in advance. In many cultures, the highest ranking person takes the first author's

---

Doing Research in Emergency and Acute Care: Making Order Out of Chaos, First Edition. Edited by Michael P. Wilson, Kama Z. Guluma, and Stephen R. Hayden.

place regardless of the amount of work done by that person. The chairman's name is on everything carried out in his shop. The professor will be first author, even when the trainee did all the work. It used to be that way here too, not so many decades ago [1, 2].

Ethics

When you have designed your study, before you collect one single datum, ask yourself about the ethics of what you want to do. It IS ethical, isn't it? Of course it is. You would not do anything else, would you? Then tell yourself that you are biased and go to seek approval from the appropriate ethics board for the country where you plan to gather your data. In the USA it is an Institutional Review Board (IRB); without IRB approval, you will not get published. And you do want this published, don't you? Why else would you do all this hard work? It cannot be to get rich! No one ever got rich writing academic research.

IRB? We don't need an IRB!

Ah, but you do. If you are a researcher based in the USA, your home institution will probably demand that your research be inspected and accepted by *its* Institutional Review Board first (Chapters 8 and 16). They will also likely demand that your work be approved by an ethics board in the other country(ies). No significant journal will publish your work without a statement that the work was reviewed by an IRB *or its equivalent.*

Equivalent? What is an IRB equivalent?

If you are going to carry out research in a developing country, that country might not have as well developed an IRB system as in the USA. So, what to do? Most universities anywhere in the world have an ethics board of some kind. Usually one of these can be affiliated with your site and provide ethical oversight. If that will not work, you can go to the Ministry of Health. Every country has one. Getting access may be a problem. That is why it is very helpful to have a collaborator who is from the country(ies) in which you will be working. Remember, even when payola (bribery) is the expectation in that country, it is not considered a legitimate business expense in the USA (so do not try to deduct it from your taxes!), and it is illegal for any US government employee to pay a bribe.

Is it ever ethical to do abroad what you would not do at home?

Yes and No. This is a question often debated in "international medicine." Although the same general ethical principles guide all the signatories to the Declaration of Helsinki, the relative weights given to each principle may differ. (The Declaration is periodically revised. Search the web for the most recent version if you need details [3]. In addition, see Chapter 8, which is all about ethics in research.) In some cultures, the individual's choices are more important than the good of the group. In others, just the opposite: the tribe/group is more important than the individual. And so on.

The US government's Belmont Report more succinctly cites three ethical principles as "respect for persons," "beneficence," and "justice" [4] Respect the people who sacrifice for your research. Yes, they do sacrifice. At a minimum, they have sacrificed their time, their outcomes, their data, and their privacy. Your research must not take advantage of people. Beneficence implies that the populace that made the sacrifice for your research must also be the populace that benefits from your work. Your work should leave no one worse off than they were before.

One perennially debated issue is: "Isn't something better than nothing at all?" The answer is not always as obvious as you might suspect.

> Should we trial new HIV drugs in sub-Saharan Africa? The drug will benefit those who get it – at least as long as they get it. What will they do when the trial is over? Will the populace be better off when you leave, or will your (temporary) benefit of offering medicines and some health care drive out the local practitioners, leaving the people in this area worse off when you leave than they were before you came with your medicines?

Sometimes there does not even seem to be an upside. Take this real-life example involving an antibiotic for meningitis as an example: In a devastating 1996 meningitis outbreak in Kano, Nigeria, the pharmaceutical company Pfizer tested a new meningitis antibiotic called Trovan. The clinical trial, reportedly called a "philanthropic" venture by the company, involved children. It was eventually fraught with controversy (and panel inquiries) regarding whether or not study patients – typically illiterate and distraught parents – were appropriately consented for the trial, whether there was adequate oversight of the trial, or even whether the trial had undergone an adequate ethics review before being instituted. The problem seemed to center around the actions of the local in-country investigator for the trial. Use of the drug was later severely restricted by the US Food and Drug Administration (in 1999) due to reports of liver damage and deaths; European regulators eventually banned the drug [5].

This real-life case highlights issues involving (i) ethical concerns in testing a new drug in a patient population that will likely not be able to afford the drug (and benefit from it) once it is out and (ii) doing so with a local (in-country) partner with whom there may be miscommunication or misunderstanding as to what constitutes good clinical practice.

Sometimes, though, there are questions that cannot be investigated in your home area. Under those circumstances, yes, there are things you might do abroad that you cannot do at home. Perhaps the disease of interest is not present. Perhaps, the physical or medical environment is different. Some questions require a particular venue in order to find an answer. It would be tough to study malaria in Iceland!

> Some of my own work in postpartum hemorrhage could not be done in a resource-rich venue, because withholding better care is never ethical. For example, we have reason to believe that an abdominal tourniquet using a swathe of cloth, twisted tight with a stick, might decrease mortality from postpartum hemorrhage among women *who have no access to surgical care or medications*. It would be unethical to study this device in the USA because the USA has plenty of access to surgery and medications. We could ethically ONLY perform this study where there is no other alternative or when the device was used only to "buy time" to get the woman to more definitive care.

Be respectful

If you are going to work outside your home country, be respectful. That means that you must treat the people – both your collaborators and your patients – in a way that benefits them as well as you. When you leave, your in-country co-investigators should be pleased with the relationship. They should not feel that you were trying to "use" them, impose your values on them, or disrespected them. The next researcher should be welcomed.

> There is a maternity hospital in Africa that works with many tiny remote maternity clinics where our abdominal tourniquet might offer life-saving benefits. The chief obstetrician at the maternity hospital is reluctant to partner with us because a few years ago he partnered with a major American university. When the researchers left, they took all the data with them. Neither he nor his hospital benefited. He has not been named on any of the papers. He is now understandably reluctant to trust another American.

Applicability

Research is a systematic method to answer a question. Ideally, you want your results to apply everywhere. Unfortunately, since you can never really measure the whole universe at once, both your question and your results will only apply to similar populations. That is why you have to collect demographics and describe your setting well enough that your readers can tell if your research applies to their population.

Any study of humans is applicable at least to some other humans. And sometimes what we do not think would be applicable turns out to actually be applicable. For example, IVs are very rare in developing countries, but diarrhea and dehydration are not. The World Health Organization (WHO) developed cheap, easily-made rehydration electrolyte formulations to be given by a parent to a dehydrated child, one sip every 30 seconds, for hours. It works so well, that in the USA we have had to rethink our automatic use of IVs for administering fluids. Many small children would be grateful for skipping the IV!

Readers? What readers?

You want to publish. Research, by definition, is "investigation with the purpose of developing generalizable knowledge." So of course you want to publish. But where? And how are you going to get your results to the readers who can best make use of your results? Fortunately, there are lots and lots of medical journals. You already know to whom your work is applicable. Think now: Which journals serve those readers? How can you best get your message across? It is possible that a journal may not be the best way. Yes, paper-based journals are traditional, but in many developing countries mail is either not reliable, or simply not available. Besides, a subscription to a major journal may cost about a year's pay. The Internet, on the other hand, has good penetration. If you want your work to reach readers in less developed areas, make sure that the journal you aim for has an on-line presence and perhaps even open access.

You might consider a regional journal, local to the area where your data were gathered. There is a new *African Journal for Emergency Medicine* (http://www.afjem.org/), which might be a good venue if your work involved Africa. Likewise, the *European Journal of Emergency Medicine* (http://www.eusem.org/journal/) looks favorably on work carried out in and between European countries.

Even though you may be writing for Asia, the current international language for medicine is English. If you want your research to be read by many people, write it in good, technical English, and in the journal's favorite format. Fortunately, most journals give you a fair amount of guidance: section headings, word counts for each section, even some standard language. Write your article in the style the journal asks for; you are more likely to get published.

KISS, KISS!

Keep it short and simple. Do not use a $10 word when a $1 will do. Convoluted turns of phrase may turn off readers of indifferent ability in English. See examples below.

Example of simplification

Maybe you wrote: "2132 patients were enrolled, but due to lack of basic information and exclusion criteria, 1970 cases of chest pain were analyzed."

The copy editor changed it to: "2132 patients were enrolled, but due to missing data and exclusion criteria which were met, only 1970 cases could be analyzed."

Or:

Perhaps you wrote: "The medications of the patient that was taken before the arrival of the patient to the emergency room were …"

And it was changed to: "The medications that the patient took before ED arrival were …"

Summary

International research has its own challenges. To design a study that everyone will respect, it first has to be good research. A study is "international" when the researchers are working in or with countries that are not their own, or if the data are being gathered in a country not their own. Every country has its own history, pride of place, and people in power. All those people deserve your respect. Research – no matter who you are or who your patients are – has to everywhere adhere to the same ethical principles. The way those ethical principles are weighted is determined by the cultural context.

Two good ways to make sure that you have taken the local context into account are, firstly, to make sure that at least one researcher in your study is from, lives in, and understands the country where the data are being collected and, secondly, to get ethical oversight from a local IRB or its equivalent.

Finally, the most ethical research is research that brings benefit. That includes publication. Ethicists claim that being a research patient is one way to contribute to generalizable knowledge. The ethical researcher, being respectful of the patients' sacrifice, should not waste the patient's efforts by failing to publish the data they helped to create.

Finally, do not be afraid to share your ideas and ask for help. A wise man once said, "The best way to seem smart is to surround yourself with even smarter people, then help them do more than they ever dreamed they could."

KEY POINTS

- Quality work is the most important part of being believed.
- International research is when …
  - Data is gathered outside your own country … or …
  - Your coworkers are outside your own country… or …
  - Your results are intended for an audience outside your own country
- Ethically, do not waste the patient's efforts by failing to publish the data.
- Do not be afraid to share your ideas and ask for help.

References

1 Calvello, E.J., Broccoli, M., Risko, N., *et al.* (2013) Emergency care and health systems: consensus-based recommendations and future research priorities. *Acad Emerg Med,* **20**(12):1278–1288. doi: 10.1111/acem.12266.

2 Weiner, S.G., Totten, V.Y., Jacquet, G.A., *et al.* (2013) Effective teaching and feedback skills for international emergency medicine "train the trainers" programs. *J Emerg Med,* **45**(5):718–725. doi: 10.1016/j.jemermed.2013.04.040.

3 World Health Organization (2001) World Medical Association Declaration of Helsinki. Ethical Principles for Medical Research Involving Human Subjects. *Bull World Health Organ,* **79**(4):373–374. http://www.who.int/bulletin/archives/79(4)373.pdf (last accessed 10 May 2015).

4 US DHSS (1979) *The Belmont Report. Ethical Principles and Guidelines for the Protection of Human Subjects of Research.* http://www.hhs.gov/ohrp/humansubjects/guidance/belmont.html (last accessed 10 May 2015).

5 Stephens, J. (2006) Panel Faults Pfizer in '96 Clinical Trial In Nigeria. *The Washington Post.* http://www.washingtonpost.com/wp-dyn/content/article/2006/05/06/AR2006050601338.html (last accessed 10 May 2015).

CHAPTER 22

The development of clinical prediction rules

Benton R. Hunter[1] and Christopher R. Carpenter[2]

[1] Department of Emergency Medicine, Indiana University School of Medicine, Indianapolis, IN, USA
[2] Department of Emergency Medicine, School of Medicine, Washington University in St Louis, St. Louis, MO, USA

Your scenario

You are 11 hours into a 12-hour shift. The eager 4th year student walks up to present another chest pain patient (which you estimate to be roughly the 84th such patient today). He tells you about the 46-year-old male who has had intermittent sharp chest pain for about two days, and shows you an EKG, which appears normal, along with a set of laboratory test results that are most notable for a troponin of 0. You go to see the patient, who looks well and describes sharp pain that is very short-lived but that seems to come on with exertion. As you walk out of the room and meet back up with the student, you decide that you are done thinking about this and tell him: "Let's just get him admitted to rule out unstable angina." The student looks a bit perplexed, and, clearly trying not to offend you, inquires why the faculty in this one department seems to have such different opinions about which patients to admit for chest pain. He is even more confused, he sheepishly admits, because he does not understand what makes this patient different to the one he presented with YOU yesterday with a nearly identical presentation, that you sent home on the spot. As you start to wax poetic about the medico-legal environment, the voice in your head starts laughing at yourself as you consciously recognize that these decisions are often based as much on your mood, fatigue level, and desire to wrap up your patients prior to sign out as they are by the objective criteria from the patient's presentation. If only there was a widely accepted method to easily, reliably, and accurately determine who is safe to go home without further workup! Those thoughts of a chest pain utopia start you thinking about what it would take to make such a dream become reality.

What is a clinical decision instrument?

In the emergency department (ED), medical decision making often occurs in a chaotic climate by over-tasked clinicians operating with an evolving information stream. Clinical decision instruments (CDIs), also known as clinical decision rules, attempt to bring order from chaos via original research-derived constellations of history or physical examination findings, and occasionally laboratory test results. The objective of a CDI is to significantly alter the post-test probability of a disease process (diagnostic CDI) or anticipated outcome (prognostic CDI) [1–3]. These algorithmic tools assist healthcare providers to predict clinical outcomes with known sensitivity and specificity. Examples of CDIs abound in contemporary emergency medicine and include diagnostic CDIs such as the Well's criteria for pulmonary embolism [4, 5] and deep venous thrombosis [6, 7], the Canadian cervical spine rule for blunt neck injury imaging [8, 9] and prognostic CDIs like the TIMI score [10].

Validated and reliable CDIs serve several purposes for clinicians. Some provide estimates of pretest probability to help guide the need for, or interpretation of, further testing. Imagine you are seeing a child with right lower quadrant pain. You do not want to miss appendicitis, so you might be inclined to order a CT scan to dictate your management. However, if you had a validated CDI by which this child's estimated risk of appendicitis is less than 1%, you could feel safe documenting in your chart that a CT is not necessary to rule out appendicitis. Alternatively, if the estimated probability of appendicitis was 90%, then even a negative CT would not accurately eliminate the possibility of appendicitis, and further observation would be necessary. CDIs provide quantitative structure to Bayesian analysis. CDIs provide a quantitative estimate (sensitivity and specificity) for several of these diagnostic components.

Doing Research in Emergency and Acute Care: Making Order Out of Chaos, First Edition. Edited by Michael P. Wilson, Kama Z. Guluma, and Stephen R. Hayden.

© 2016 John Wiley & Sons, Ltd. Published 2016 by John Wiley & Sons, Ltd.

Box 22.1 Checklist of standards for developing a clinical decision instrument.

1 Is there a need for the decision instrument?
Prevalent clinical condition
Potential overuse of diagnostic resources
Practice variation
Healthcare provider (physician, physician extender, nurse) attitude
Clinical accuracy of healthcare provider (baseline gestalt)
2 Were reproducible and acceptable methods used to derive the CDI?
Explicit definitions (outcome, predictor variables)
Reliability of predictor variables
Representative subject selection
Sample size
Mathematical techniques
Sensibility of the CDI
Ability of the CDI to significantly alter post-test probability
3 Has the CDI been prospectively validated and adapted/refined?
Prospective validation in real-world setting
Representative subject selection
Accurate and reliable application of the rule by intended users
Outcomes
Ability of the CDI to significantly alter post-test probability
Healthcare providers' interpretation of the CDI
Refinement or adaptation of the CDI
Potential effects (time or resource consumption)
4 Has the CDI been successfully and meaningfully implemented into clinical practice?
Clinical trial
Effect on use
Ability of the CDI to significantly alter post-test probability
Acceptability
5 Would use of the CDI be cost effective?
6 How will the CDI be disseminated and implemented?

Source: Stiell and Wells 1999 [1]. Reproduced with permission of Elsevier.

What is Bayesian analysis? Quite simply, it is one means of assessing uncertainty. In clinical settings, diagnostic uncertainty ensues when a patient presents with a symptom (chest pain, abdominal pain, headache, fever, etc.) and a list of possible etiologies. Each possible cause of the symptom has a pretest probability (likelihood of being the true etiology) ranging from 0 to 100% and the sum of all potential causes should equal 100%. Using Bayes' Theorem clinicians can modify the pretest probability for each diagnosis based upon the presence or absence of individual diagnostic "tests", including history, physical examination, laboratory tests, and imaging. This modified estimate of disease likelihood is called "post-test probability".

While some evidence-based medicine opponents suggest that unstructured human estimation of pretest probability is a fatal flaw of evidence-based diagnostic reasoning [11], validated CDIs provide accurate and reproducible estimates of disease prevalence or anticipated incidence. CDIs can also reduce practice heterogeneity and reduce testing rates without missing diagnoses [12, 13]. Although CDIs sound appealing in response to the growing problem of "over-diagnosis" [14, 15], researchers face multiple challenges in developing, validating, and disseminating these instruments [16, 17]. This chapter summarizes the research approach to CDI development, which occurs in phases that can take over a decade to complete (Box 22.1) [2].

Choosing a CDI focus

Not every problem that we face in medicine needs a CDI. There is a reason that so many researchers have tried to validate different CDIs to rule out acute coronary syndrome [16, 18–24] or syncope [25–29], but no one has yet tried to develop a rule for finger dislocation or pheochromocytoma. Understanding this reality ensures that researchers will pursue potentially worthwhile CDIs. Useful CDIs meet the following criteria:

- Testing for the condition is common (a CDI for diagnosing pheochromocytoma is unlikely to spare millions of people from urine metanephrine testing).
- The CDI can supplant more advanced testing that is costly (i.e., stress testing for CAD) [30], inaccurate (stress testing for CAD) [30], difficult to obtain (stress testing anyone?), or potentially harmful.
- Significant diagnostic and therapeutic practice variability exists. Variability is a threat to patient safety and increases malpractice risk [31]. For example, in women with abdominal complaints, one ED clinician might diagnose and treat pelvic inflammatory disease (PID), while another clinician evaluating the same patient might send a culture and wait to treat, and yet another interprets the same findings as inconsistent with PID and neither tests nor treats [32]. A uniform and accurate approach could minimize both overtreatment and undertreatment.

The perceived need or desire for a CDI in a clinical scenario depends upon careful analysis of these criteria. A more direct approach is to survey clinicians' desires for and acceptability of decision aides [33, 34]. Failure to assess these perspectives can yield an accurate and reliable CDI that clinicians do not incorporate into practice [35, 36].

Developing a CDI: Research methods

Derivation
In order to optimize your odds of deriving a pragmatic and effective CDI, balance several factors before proceeding, including:

- **Is there a need?** Assessing and quantifying the likely acceptance of the CDI. Can you prove that testing for the disease process is prevalent, highly variable, and that developing this particular CDI is a priority for the clinicians who would ultimately use this tool?
- **Which candidate variables to include?** "Candidate variable" refers to a historical, physical examination, or laboratory finding to potentially be used as part of the CDI. For example, fever, vomiting, or right-sided pain might all be candidate variables in a CDI to rule out appendicitis. Remember that the overall effectiveness of a CDI to reduce resource consumption requires that non-ED physicians understand and accept the validity of the CDI, so these professionals should be included in the derivation phase. For example, the Canadian Head CT Rule was derived after obtaining consensus of clinically significant head injury from 129 neurosurgeons, neuro-radiologists, and ED physicians [37].
- **Complexity:** Incorporating more variables into your CDI usually improves overall accuracy at the expense of overly cumbersome bedside application (e.g., the Pneumonia Severity Index [38]).
- **End-product:** Decide whether it is better to derive a nomogram (an often complex system for mathematically defining an unknown variable based on the interaction between two or more known variables) or scoring system. A scoring system (e.g., ABCD to predict stroke after transient ischemic attack [39] or Wells score to predict DVT/PE [deep vein thrombosis/pulmonary embolism] [40]) is often easier to use at the expense of less precise estimates for the outcome of interest.

Here is a personal example of a CDI dream that failed to meet these prederivation criteria and was therefore never derived. Geriatric abdominal pain is a prevalent ED chief complaint with significant and recognized practice variability [41, 42]. Emergency physicians have also identified an abdominal pain CDI as a high-priority research product [33]. However, a readily available diagnostic test (CT) for geriatric abdominal pain already exists [43, 44] and the long-term radiation risks of CT are of less concern for older adults. In addition, the differential diagnosis for abdominal pain is far more complex than a single diagnosis (ankle fracture, pulmonary embolism) encompassing dozens of intra-abdominal and extra-abdominal culprits. A geriatric abdominal pain CDI would either have to focus on one diagnostic possibility (cholecystitis) or risk lack of acceptance from end-users. In fact, after two years of trying to bring general surgeons, emergency physicians, geriatricians, and radiologists together to identify the candidate predictor variables, funding evaporated and no CDI was developed. The initial problem was simply too complex and CT offered an easily available, well-accepted alternative to the unknown of a geriatric abdominal pain CDI.

The methodology for developing a CDI is explicit [2]. Subjective variables and outcomes need to be clearly defined so that any future clinician or researcher understands how each of these was measured, using what equipment, by whom, at what stage in the ED evaluation. The individual assessing the presence or absence of candidate variables at the bedside should be unaware of the outcome(s) of interest and vice versa. This reduces the risk of various forms of diagnostic bias [45]. Patient selection should reflect the target population (site, age, stage and severity of illness) in whom the CDI will be used. A rule-of-thumb sample size calculation is to estimate ten outcomes (not ten subjects, but ten individuals with the outcome of interest) for each variable included in the CDI. However, the most important sample-size consideration is usually whether the precision around the point estimate of sensitivity will be sufficient to inform medical practice [1, 2]. In most cases, a CDI is used to "rule out" a disease process.

Statistical analysis of candidate variables assesses their association with the outcome(s) of interest. In other words, how likely is it that the observed association between this predictor variable and the outcome(s) are by chance alone? Prespecified inclusion criteria (for example, associations with p<0.10 and with kappa >0.60, signifying good inter-observer agreement) are then used to select significant variables for inclusion in the statistical model that will form the CDI (see Recursive Partitioning later). CDI researchers need to report sensitivity, specificity, positive and negative likelihood ratios, and receiver operating characteristic area under the curve. In addition to the overall diagnostic accuracy of the model, it is essential to assess the reliability (reproducibility) of each predictor variable because a CDI element that yields differing interpretations by various clinicians will not be useful.

> Imagine that a CDI is derived to rule out cervical spine injury in patients after blunt trauma. The rule is 100% sensitive when "validated" among 200 patients, six of whom had an injury. Despite the CDI catching all six injuries in this small group, one could imagine it very possible that, in a group of 20 000 patients with 600 injuries, it might miss many injuries. In fact, in this example, assuming a specificity of 50% for the CDI, the 95% confidence interval (precision) around the sensitivity goes as low as 55%. This illustrates why it was necessary for the NEXUS group [46] to enroll over 34 000 patients (with more than 800 injured patients) to ensure that the confidence intervals around their sensitivity for cervical spine injury were sufficiently narrow.

Internal validation

Internal validation refers to the ability of the CDI to accurately distinguish patients with and without disease (or outcomes in prognostic situations). Most CDIs are initially validated in the same populations and institution(s) in which they were derived, either retrospectively from a registry of patients or prospectively. Common statistical approaches to cross-validate a CDI on the same population include the "jackknife" and "bootstrap" methods [1]. Retrospectively validated CDIs are prone to overestimating accuracy by overfitting the statistical model and are, therefore, a lesser quality of evidence than prospectively validated CDIs [2]. One significant disadvantage of prospective validation is that data collection is expensive, time consuming, and often inconvenient for patients and clinicians. The major disadvantage of retrospective validation is that researchers cannot assess candidate variables not documented in the data source or the inter-rater reliability of candidate variables. Validation trials can yield refined CDIs that are easier to use or more accurate, but refined CDIs need to again go through the validation process, since they are essentially a newly derived CDI.

External validation

CDI accuracy should be quantified in multiple settings and patient populations that differ from the one in which it was derived (external validation) to ensure that the instrument works in disparate settings. CDIs that perform well in derivation trials, but are significantly less accurate in external validation studies are common [47, 48]. A few basic tenets are essential in external validation studies:

1 **Ensure that definitions, application, and interpretation of the rule are the same as in the derivation/ internal validation of the rule.** CDIs often rely heavily on physical examination or history features, so failure to explicitly replicate the technique and timing of history or examination can alter findings from one study to another [49]. For example, if the derivation study asked patients to report chest pain on a 1-to-10 Likert scale before receiving any nitroglycerin or morphine, whereas the validation study asked a simple yes/no chest pain question at the end of the emergency department evaluation, two different symptoms are being ascertained. The questions must be asked in the same way every time across settings.

2 **Be wary of applying the rule to populations with very different disease prevalence.** If the pretest probability (or prevalence in a study) is substantially higher in the validation study than it was in the original, then the post-test probability of disease will also be higher. For example, in the USA, the Pulmonary Embolism Rule-out

Criteria (PERC) instrument is able to reproducibly demonstrate a prevalence of PE<2% in low risk patients with a "negative" PERC [50, 51]. However, attempts to validate PERC in Europe led to a much higher post-test probability of PE after a "negative" PERC due to the 21% prevalence of PE in the European study, compared to 7–8% in the US trials [52]. The effect is also true for outcome rates in prognostic trials [53].

3 **Avoid trying to apply the CDI too broadly in patients or diseases that are dissimilar to those studied during development of the CDI.** While it would be nice to have a CDI that works anywhere, at any time, on anyone, it is usually necessary to define a reasonably narrow disease process and patient population. A CDI to rule out meningitis that performs well in developed countries is unlikely to perform similarly in less developed nations, where vaccination is underutilized, health care is less accessible, and the spectrum of organisms that cause meningitis differ. In addition to geographic differences in disease or patients, there may be temporal changes, such that a CDI performs differently today than it may 10 years from now. A decision instrument designed today to rule out abdominal injury after blunt trauma might have performed very differently in 1970, when bedside ultrasound and computed tomography were not available, and when many cars lacked seat belts or airbags and traffic laws were more variable.

Impact analysis – "The next painful step"

Accurate and reliable CDIs need widespread acceptance, which necessitates real-time assessment in the hands of clinicians at the bedside. If one objective of the CDI is decreased resource use (testing or admissions), then impact analysis researchers should assess whether this decrease manifests. You will also want to show that the decrease in testing or admissions does not result in missed diagnoses or bad outcomes. Few decision aids progress to this level of evidence [12, 13, 54, 55]. CDIs face numerous barriers to meaningful implementation, including malpractice concerns, workflow constraints, overestimated personal diagnostic aptitude, or misunderstanding the design or intent of the CDI [16, 17, 33, 34].

The ideal impact analysis trial randomizes patients to CDI or "standard care" without the CDI, a design that is difficult to organize and often prohibitively expensive. Usually, researchers use a cluster-randomized trial, in which clinicians at some sites use the CDI and "control" clinicians at other sites do not. Another option is to study clinician behavior at a single site both before and after teaching and implementation of the CDI [56]. Regardless of the methods, the goal of impact analysis is to verify and quantify patient-centric or societal effectiveness and safety in real-world clinical practice.

Advanced topics

Recursive partitioning versus logistic regression

Univariate analysis alone does not explore the relationship of predictor variables with other variables and the outcome. Logistic regression analysis and χ^2 recursive partitioning do evaluate these intervariable relationships with the outcome, but these two methods have important differences (Chapter 32 provides more explanation of these tests). Logistic regression analysis is technically appropriate to predict binary outcomes, but yields the highest overall accuracy for a model at the expense of decreased sensitivity [8, 57, 58]. However, emergency medicine CDIs often seek to identify a lower-risk subset of patients in order to safely defer ED testing to outpatient settings, so clinically acceptable CDIs preferentially maximize sensitivity at the expense of specificity. In contrast, recursive partitioning analysis (Figure 22.1) progressively subdivides the population into groups of patients with a particular outcome and can preferentially optimize sensitivity at the expense of specificity [2]. Recursive partitioning is a non-parametric modeling technique that is capable of assessing a large number of predictor variables with complex interactions. One form of recursive partitioning is the classification and regression tree (CART) analysis [59], but other forms such as Random Forests™ exist [60]. The basic concept is sequential splitting of data to lump groups that share a predictor variable and the primary outcome. Bivariate association models are run for each predictor variable with each step to identify the one with the strongest association with the outcome. The study population is then split into two or more subgroups based on the optimal cut point of the strongest predictor variable. Partitioning continues until a stopping condition is met. Figure 22.1 shows an example of recursive partitioning and stopping conditions [61].

Incorporation of clinician gestalt into CDIs

Experienced physician clinical instinct is often an independently-predictive tool to estimate the probability of a disease or outcome [62]. Since a CDI works alongside clinician's judgment, why not incorporate that judgment into the tool formally?

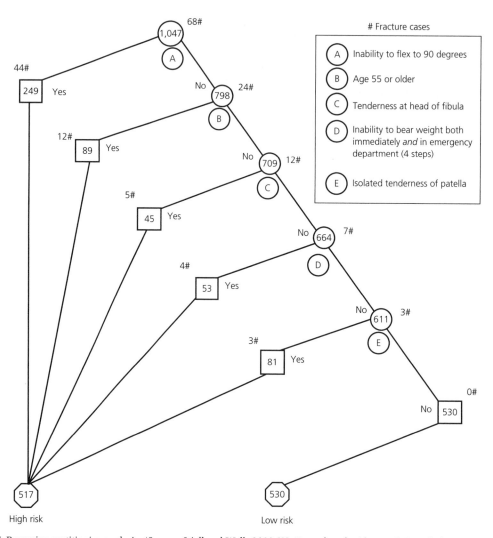

Figure 22.1 Recursive partitioning analysis. (Source: Stiell and Wells 1999 [1]. Reproduced with permission of Elsevier.)

One challenge is that by incorporating gestalt into a CDI it can open the clinician to medico-legal scrutiny. A series of objective "yes or no" facts about the patient is easy to document accurately and defend if the instrument "fails." When a clinician "fails" or is wrong, it is said to represent cognitive error, and a lawyer can argue that the next clinician would have made a "better" decision [63]. In addition, incorporating gestalt into CDIs introduces subjectivity due to variability in the level of experience and accuracy of different clinicians' gestalt or instincts [64].

The benefit of incorporating gestalt is that it incorporates many measurable and unmeasured variables that may be more powerful than any "yes or no" historical or examination features. The Wells criteria for PE/DVT incorporates gestalt indirectly by asking, "Is another diagnosis more likely?" [40] The PERC rule does not directly incorporate gestalt, but indirectly incorporates gestalt because it was designed to be used only in low-risk populations (<15% probability of PE) [65]. Although either clinician gestalt or another PE CDI can be used to define "low risk" patients in whom the PERC rule is appropriately applied, early evidence indicates that gestalt may be superior to some CDIs in defining the low risk subset [66]. Incorporating gestalt into a decision rule may have substantial upsides and downsides. These must be weighed against each other and carefully considered before deciding whether clinician judgment or gestalt should be included as a potential part of your CDI.

The future of CDI research

Valid CDIs are often unrecognized and underused by clinicians [36, 67, 68]. Efficient dissemination and implementation of well-developed, valid, and clinically effective CDIs sometimes requires over a decade from the derivation phase until widespread uptake of the tool [69]. In the future, quicker knowledge translation will require disruptive innovation by embedding valid and reliable CDIs into clinical decision support systems (i.e., computerized physician order entry) in a manner that does not disrupt department flow [70]. CDI researchers should contemplate how to disseminate and integrate the rule during the initial derivation phase in order to minimize the risk that clinicians subsequently ignore, misuse, or misinterpret valid, reliable, and impactful CDIs.

KEY POINTS

- CDIs can provide valid and reliable estimates of disease or outcome probability.
- The methods of deriving, validating, refining, and disseminating CDIs are complex and time-consuming, often requiring over a decade to complete and requiring input from multiple emergency medicine (EM) and non-EM stakeholders.
- The optimal statistical modeling approach to derive CDIs is recursive partitioning.
- CDIs should be evaluated and validated in multiple different emergency department or other clinical settings, and on a variety of patient populations before they can be widely applied.
- The role of clinician gestalt, either as part of the CDI or in addition to the CDI, should be evaluated during the derivation phase.

References

1 Wasson, J.H., Sox, H.C., Neff, R.K., and Goldman, L. (1985) Clinical prediction rules. Applications and methodological standards. *N Engl J Med*, **313**(13):793–799.

2 Stiell, I.G. and Wells, G.A. (1999) Methodologic standards for the development of clinical decision rules in emergency medicine. *Ann Emerg Med*, **33**(4):437–447.

3 Pines, J.M., Carpenter, C.R., Raja, A.S., and Schuur, J.D. (2013) Clinical decision rules. In: J.M. Pines, C.R. Carpenter, A.S. Raja, and J.D. Schuur *Evidence-Based Emergency Care: Diagnostic Testing and Clinical Decision Rules*, 2nd edn. John Wiley & Sons Ltd, pp. 36–43.

4 Wells, P.S., Anderson, D.R., Rodger, M., *et al.* (2000) Derivation of a simple clinical model to categorize patients probability of pulmonary embolism: increasing the models utility with the SimpliRED D-dimer. *Thromb Haemost*, **83**(3):416–420.

5 Chunilal, S.D., Eikelboom, J.W., Attia, J., *et al.* (2009) Does this patient have pulmonary embolism? In: D.L. Simel and D. Rennie (eds) *The Rational Clinical Examination: Evidence-Based Clinical Diagnosis*. McGraw-Hill; New York, pp. 561–575.

6 Anand, S., Wells, P.S., Hunt, D., *et al.* (2009) Does this patient have deep vein thrombosis? In: D.L. Simel and D. Rennie (eds) *The Rational Clinical Examination: Evidence-Based Clinical Diagnosis*. McGraw-Hill; New York, pp. 227–234.

7 Wells, P.S., Owen, C., Doucette, S., *et al.* (2009) Does this patient have deep vein thrombosis? In: D.L. Simel and D. Rennie (eds) *The Rational Clinical Examination: Evidence-Based Clinical Diagnosis*. McGraw-Hill; New York, pp. 235–246.

8 Stiell, I.G., Wells, G.A., Vandemheen, K.L., *et al.* (2001) The Canadian C-spine rule for radiography in alert and stable trauma patients. *JAMA*, **286**(15):1841–1848.

9 Stiell, I.G., Clement, C.M., McKnight, R.D., *et al.* (2003) The Canadian C-spine rule versus the NEXUS low-risk criteria in patients with trauma. *N Engl J Med*, **349**(26):2510–2518.

10 Chase, M, Robey, J.L., Zogby, K.E., *et al.* (2006) Prospective validation of the Thrombolysis in Myocardial Infarction Risk Score in the emergency department chest pain population. *Ann Emerg Med*, **48**(3):252–259.

11 Phelps, M.A. and Levitt, M.A. (2004) Pretest probability estimates: a pitfall to the clinical utility of evidence-based medicine? *Acad Emerg Med*, **11**(6):692–694.

12 Perry, J.J. and Stiell, I.G. (2009) Impact of clinical decision rules on clinical care of traumatic injuries to the foot and ankle, knee, cervical spine, and head. *Injury*, **37**(12):1157–1165.

13 Stiell, I.G., Clement, C.M., Grimshaw, J., *et al.* (2009) Implementation of the Canadian C-Spine Rule: prospective 12 centre cluster randomised trial. *BMJ*, **339**:b4146.

14 Welch, H.G. (2011) *Overdiagnosed: Making People Sick in the Pursuit of Health*. Beacon Press, Boston MA.

15 Hoffman, J.R. and Cooper, R.J. (2012) Overdiagnosis of disease: a modern epidemic. *Arch Intern Med*, **172**(15):1123–1124.

16 Reilly, B.M., Evans, A.T., Schaider, J.J., *et al.* (2002) Impact of a clinical decision rule on hospital triage of patients with suspected acute cardiac ischemia in the emergency department. *JAMA*, **288**(3):342–350.

17 Green, S.M. (2013) When do clinical decision rules improve patient care? *Ann Emerg Med*, **62**(2):132–135.

18 Christenson, J., Innes, G., McKnight, D., *et al.* (2006) A clinical prediction rule for early discharge of patients with chest pain. *Ann Emerg Med*, **47**(1):1–10.

19 Fesmire, F.M., Hughes, A.D., Fody, E.P., *et al.* (2002) The Erlanger chest pain evaluation protocol: a one-year experience with serial 12-lead ECG monitoring, two-hour delta serum marker measurements, and selective nuclear stress testing to identify and exclude acute coronary syndromes. *Ann Emerg Med*, **40**(6):584–594.

20 George, T, Ashover, S, Cullen, L, *et al.* (2013) Introduction of an accelerated diagnostic protocol in the assessment of emergency department patients with possible acute coronary syndrome: The Nambour Short Low-Intermediate Chest pain project. *Emerg Med Australas.*, **25**(4):340–344.

21 Goldman, L, Cook, EF, Johnson, PA, *et al.* (1996) Prediction of the need for intensive care in patients who come to the emergency departments with acute chest pain. *N Engl J Med*, **334**(23):1498–1504.

22 Jalili, M, Hejripour, Z, Honarmand, AR, and Pourtabatabaei, N. (2012) Validation of the Vancouver Chest Pain Rule: a prospective cohort study. *Acad Emerg Med*, **19**(7):837–842.

23 Xavier-Scheuermeyer, F, Wong, H, Yu, E, *et al.* (2014) Development and validation of a prediction rule for early discharge of low-risk emergency department patients with potential ischemic chest pain. *CJEM*, **16**(2):106–119.

24 Xavier Scheuermeyer, F, Wong, H, Yu, E, *et al.* (2013) Development and validation of a prediction rule for early discharge of low-risk emergency department patients with potential ischemic chest pain. *CJEM*, **15**(0):1–14.

25 Grossman, SA, Bar, J, Fischer, C, *et al.* (2012) Reducing admissions utilizing the Boston Syncope Criteria. *J Emerg Med*, **42**(3):345–352.

26 Grossman, S.A., Fischer, C., Lipsitz, L.A., *et al.* (2007) Predicting adverse outcomes in syncope. *J Emerg Med.*, **33**(3):233–239.

27 Reed, M.J., Newby, D.E., Coull, A.J., *et al.* (2010) The ROSE (risk stratification of syncope in the emergency department) study. *J Am Coll Cardiol*, **55**(8):713–721.

28 Saccilotto, R.T., Nickel, C.H., Bucher, H.C., *et al.* (2011) San Francisco Syncope Rule to predict short-term serious outcomes: a systematic review. *CMAJ*, **183**(15):E1116–E1126.

29 Serrano, L.A., Hess, E.P., Bellolio, M.F., *et al.* (2010) Accuracy and quality of clinical decision rules for syncope in the emergency department: a systematic review and meta-analysis. *Ann Emerg Med*, **56**(4):362–373 e361.

30 Health Quality Ontario (2010) Stress echocardiography for the diagnosis of coronary artery disease: an evidence-based analysis. *Ont Health Technol Assess Ser*, **10**(9):1–61.

31 Williamson, J.A.H. and Runciman, W. (2009) Thinking in a crisis: Use of algorithms. In: P. Croskerry, K.S. Cosby, S.M. Schenkel, and R.L. Wears (eds) *Patient Safety in Emergency Medicine*. Lippincott, Williams, & Wilkins, Philadelphia, PA, pp. 228–234.

32 Kane, B.G., Degutis, L.C., Sayward, H.K., and D'Onofrio, G. (2004) Compliance with the Centers for Disease Control and Prevention recommendations for the diagnosis and treatment of sexually transmitted diseases. *Acad Emerg Med*, **11**(4):371–377.

33 Eagles, D., Stiell, I.G., Clement, C.M., *et al.* (2008) International survey of emergency physicians' priorities for clinical decision rules. *Acad Emerg Med*, **15**(2):177–182.

34 Brehaut, J.C.., Graham, ID., Wood, T.J., *et al.* (2010) Measuring acceptability of clinical decision rules: validation of the Ottawa acceptability of decision rules instrument (OADRI) in four countries. *Med Decis Making.*, **30**(3):398–408.

35 Arkes, H.R., Shaffer, V.A., and Medow, M.A. (2007) Patients derogate physicians who use a computer-assisted diagnostic aid. *Med Decis Making*, **27**(2):189–202.

36 Smith, C., Mensah, A., Mal, S., and Worster, A. (2008) Is pretest probability assessment on emergency department patients with suspected venous thromboembolism documented before SimpliRED D-dimer testing? *CJEM*, **10**(6):519–523.

37 Stiell, I.G., Wells, G.A., Vandemheen, K.L., *et al.* (2001) The Canadian CT Head Rule for patients with minor head injury. *Lancet*, **357**(9266):1391–1396.

38 Fine, M.J., Auble, T.E., Yealy, D.M., *et al.* (1997) (1985) A prediction rule to identify low-risk patients with community-acquired pneumonia. *N Engl J Med*, **336**(4):243–250.

39 Rothwell, P.M., Giles, M.F., Flossmann, E., *et al.* (2005) A simple score (ABCD) to identify individuals at high early risk of stroke after transient ischaemic attack. *Lancet.*, **366**(9479):29–36.

40 Wells, P.S., Anderson, D.R., Rodger, M., *et al.* (2001) Excluding pulmonary embolism at the bedside without diagnostic imaging: management of patients with suspected pulmonary embolism presenting to the emergency department by using a simple clinical model and d-dimer. *Ann Intern Med*, **135**(2):98–107.

41 Pines, J.M., Mullins, P.M., Cooper, J.K., *et al.* (2013) National trends in emergency department use, care patterns, and quality of care of older adults in the United States. *J Am Geriatr Soc*, **61**(1):12–17.

42 McNamara, R.M., Rousseau, E., and Sanders, A.B. (1992) Geriatric emergency medicine: A survey of practicing emergency physicians. *Ann Emerg Med*, **21**(7):796–801.

43 Esses, D., Birnbaum, A., Bijur, P., *et al.* (2004) Ability of CT to alter decision making in elderly patients with acute abdominal pain. *Am J Emerg Med*, **22**:270–272.

44 Hustey, F.M., Meldon, S.W., Banet, G.A., *et al.* (2005) The use of abdominal computed tomography in older ED Patients with acute abdominal pain. *Am J Emerg Med*, **23**:259–265.

45 Kohn, M.A., Carpenter, C.R., and Newman, T.B. (2013) Understanding the direction of bias in studies of diagnostic test accuracy. *Acad Emerg Med*, **20**(11):1194–1206.

46 Hoffman, J.R., Mower, W.R., Wolfson, A.B., *et al.* (2000) Validity of a set of clinical criteria to rule out injury to the cervical spine in patients with blunt trauma. National Emergency X-Radiography Utilization Study Group. *N Engl J Med*, **343**(2):94–99.

47 Carpenter, C.R. (2009) The San Francisco Syncope Rule did not accurately predict serious short-term outcome in patients with syncope. *Evid Based Med*, **14**(1):25.

48 Perry, J.J., Sharma, M., Sivilotti, M.L, *et al.* (2011) Prospective validation of the ABCD2 score for patients in the emergency department with transient ischemic attack. *CMAJ*, **183**(10):1137–1145.

49 McDermott, D. and Quinn, J. (2009) Response to "failure to validate the San Francisco Syncope Rule in an independent emergency department population". *Ann Emerg Med*, **53**(3):693.

50 Kline, J.A., Courtney, D.M., Kabrhel, C., *et al.* (2008) Prospective multicenter evaluation of the pulmonary embolism rule-out criteria. *J Thromb Haemost*, **6**(5):772–780.

51 Kline, J.A., Mitchell, A.M., Kabrhel, C., *et al.* (2004) Clinical criteria to prevent unnecessary diagnostic testing in emergency department patients with suspected pulmonary embolism. *J Thromb Haemost*, **2**(8):1247–1255.

52 Hugli, O., Righini, M., Le Gal, G., *et al.* (2011) The pulmonary embolism rule-out criteria (PERC) rule does not safely exclude pulmonary embolism. *J Thromb Haemost*, **9**(2):300–304.

53 Charlson, M.E., Ales, K.L., Simon, R., and MacKenzie, C.R. (1987) Why predictive indexes perform less well in validation studies. Is it magic or methods? *Arch Intern Med*, **147**(12):2155–2161.

54 Marrie, T.J., Lau, C.Y., Wheeler, S.L., *et al.* (2000) A controlled trial of a critical pathway for treatment of community-acquired pneumonia. CAPITAL Study Investigators. Community-Acquired Pneumonia Intervention Trial Assessing Levofloxacin. *JAMA*, **283**(6):749–755.

55 Renaud, B., Coma, E., Labarere, J., *et al.* (2007) Routine use of the Pneumonia Severity Index for guiding the site-of-treatment decision of patients with pneumonia in the emergency department: a multicenter, prospective, observational, controlled cohort study. *Clin Infect Dis*, **44**(1):41–49.

56 Atlas, S.J, Benzer, T.I., Borowsky, L.H., *et al.* (1998) Safely increasing the proportion of patients with community-acquired pneumonia treated as outpatients: an interventional trial. *Arch Intern Med.*, **158**(12):1350–1356.

57 Heckerling, P.S., Tape, T.G., Wigton, R.S., *et al.* (1990) Clinical prediction rule for pulmonary infiltrates. *Ann Intern Med*, **113**(9):664–670.

58 Kharbanda, A.B., Taylor, G.A., Fishman, S.J., Bachur, R.G. (2005) A clinical decision rule to identify children at low risk for appendicitis. *Pediatrics*, **116**(3):709–716.

59 Breiman, L., Friedman, J., Stone, C.J., and Olshen, R.A. (1984) *Classification and Regression Trees.* Chapman & Hall/CRC, Washington DC.

60 Breiman, L. (2001) Random forests. *Mach Learn*, **45**(1):5–32.

61 Garge, N.R., Bobashev, G., Eggleston, B. (2013) Random forest methodology for model-based recursive partitioning: the mobForest package for R. *BMC Bioinformatics*, **14**:125.

62 Penaloza, A., Verschuren, F., Meyer, G., *et al.* (2013) Comparison of the unstructured clinician gestalt, the Wells score, and the revised Geneva score to estimate pretest probability for suspected pulmonary embolism. *Ann Emerg Med*, **62**(2):117–124.

63 Kachalia, A., Gandhi, T.K., Puopolo, A.L., *et al.* (2007) Missed and delayed diagnoses in the emergency department: a study of closed malpractice claims from 4 liability insurers. *Ann Emerg Med*, **49**(2):196–205.

64 Nordenholz, K.E., Naviaux, N.W., Stegelmeier, K., *et al.* (2007) Pulmonary embolism risk assessment screening tools: the interrater reliability of their criteria. *Am J Emerg Med*, **25**(3):285–290.

65 Carpenter, C.R., Keim, S.M., Seupaul, R.A., and Pines, J.M. (2009) Differentiating low-risk and no-risk PE patients: the PERC score. *J Emerg Med*, **36**(3):317–322.

66 Penaloza, A., Verschuren, F., Dambrine, S., *et al.* (2012) Performance of the Pulmonary Embolism Rule-out Criteria (the PERC rule) combined with low clinical probability in high prevalence population. *Thromb Res*, **129**(5):e189–193.

67 Runyon, M.S., Richman, P.B., and Kline, J.A. (2007) Emergency medicine practitioner knowledge and use of decision rules for the evaluation of patients with suspected pulmonary embolism: variations by practice setting and training level. *Acad Emerg Med*, **14**(1):53–57.

68 Corwin, M.T., Donohoo, J.H., Partridge, R., *et al.* (2009) Do emergency physicians use serum D-dimer effectively to determine the need for CT when evaluating patients for pulmonary embolism? Review of 5,344 consecutive patients. *AJR Am J Roentgenol*, **192**(5):1319–1323.

69 Stiell, I.G. and Bennett, C. (2007) Implementation of clinical decision rules in the emergency department. *Acad Emerg Med*, **14**(11):955–959.

70 Zimlichman, E. and Levin-Scherz, J. (2013) The coming golden age of disruptive innovation in health care. *J Gen Intern Med*, **28**(7):865–867.

CHAPTER 23

Testing the safety and efficacy of devices: Device safety, as well as obtaining an IDE (investigational device exemption) from the FDA

Sean-Xavier Neath

Department of Emergency Medicine, University of California, San Diego, CA, USA

Medical device safety and regulation is a constantly changing field. The concepts and pathways in place at the time of this chapter's writing may well have changed by the time you are prepared to launch your medical innovation. The reader is advised to consult the most current versions of regulatory guidance for the countries in which you might be working. These are usually available directly on-line through governmental web sites.

Creative people (clinicians included!) frequently come up with brilliant innovations to solve common problems by inventing a device that can make something faster, or safer, or better. Without medical devices, acute medical care cannot happen. Often we think of pharmaceuticals as the backbone of modern medicine. This is perhaps true. But without an IV cannula to deliver the medications, *in vitro* diagnostics to monitor a drug's effect on critical patient biomarkers, the occasional high-charge zap from a defibrillator, or the misting from a correctly-placed ET tube, our medications really cannot do much for our patients.

In the medical industry "medical devices" refers to a large range of innovations from implantable devices to *in vitro* diagnostics. Almost everything that is not a pharmaceutical or a biologic is considered a "device" for regulatory purposes.

The following maps out the steps for creation of new devices from start to finish. As a researcher you may find yourself inserted at various stages in the process depending on what degree of product development has already taken place.

Step one: Protect your invention

This is frequently called "getting IP (intellectual property) around" your innovation. Depending upon the nature of your innovation, you may benefit from various patents and trademarks for elements and concepts of your device. Not surprisingly, these protections will vary from country to country. The extensive world of patents and intellectual property is beyond the scope of this chapter. However, that said, if you are testing the safety and efficacy of a device that YOU have invented, you are probably going to be spending a lot of your (and other peoples') cash on this project. And you (as well as your other investors) are going to be somewhat aggrieved if some *other* company starts selling a knock-off (imitation) of your invention just days before the formal launch of your product. If you are reading this chapter because of your interest in testing *other* people's devices for safety and efficacy, intellectual property rights will not necessarily be a major concern for you. However, try to learn a bit about the fascinating process of intellectual property and medical device development ... at the very least you will come away with an understanding of why it often costs millions of dollars to bring a medical device to market. Prototype manufacturing can be really expensive, especially for

Doing Research in Emergency and Acute Care: Making Order Out of Chaos, First Edition. Edited by Michael P. Wilson, Kama Z. Guluma, and Stephen R. Hayden.
© 2016 John Wiley & Sons, Ltd. Published 2016 by John Wiley & Sons, Ltd.

more complex devices. Clinical trials are increasingly more costly to perform; this is related to more exacting regulatory requirements from an increasing number of regulatory bodies.

Step two: Innovate

Find a clinical issue for which an innovative solution is lacking. Map out the design process; develop prototypes and pilots as needed.

Step three

Manufacture and sell the device worldwide, making huge profits while curing legions of sick.

Step four

Recognize that step three, unfortunately, is not really that simple!

One of the most difficult aspects of getting a medical device to market is the having the knowledge required to navigate a device through the regulatory process necessary for approval. In the United States, medical devices are subject to the regulations spelled out in the Federal Food Drug and Cosmetic (FD&C) Act ,which is a part of the Title 21 Code of Federal Regulations, an enormous body of laws administered mostly by the US Food and Drug Administration (FDA). These controls are the baseline requirements that apply to all medical devices necessary for marketing, proper labelling, and monitoring of performance once the device is on the market.

The information given here details the process of device clearance in the United States, but be forewarned that each country has it is own specific requirements. Movements towards harmonization have made some headway in Europe, where the members of the European Union (EU) have agreed on some general requirements. Nevertheless, some country-specific regulations remain even in the EU. Unfortunately; global harmonization of medical device approval pathways is still a long way from realization.

Most of the time if you are testing a novel medical device, you will probably be working with some type of manufacturer or established medical-device maker. However, since the world of medical devices is a smaller and less robustly-funded than the giant pharmaceutical industry, the "medical device manufacturer" might actually be a small local start-up company, perhaps lacking staff for a comprehensive regulatory and reimbursement division. Therefore, an understanding of the process is very important for clinicians participating in the device development process, as partnerships are often formed between small device start-up companies and their clinician investigators.

The FDA unit that serves the regulatory role for medical devices has the somewhat unusual name of the "Center for Devices and Radiological Health" (CDRH). The CDRH describes three stages for obtaining marketing clearance in the United States. It is recommended that the most up-to-date version of this information is viewed on-line at the CDRH section of the FDA web site [1].

Stage one in the marketing process is to make absolutely sure that the product you wish to market is actually a *medical device,* as opposed to a drug or some unusual hybrid device/drug that is submitted to a different agency [2]. True medical devices meet the definition of a medical device as listed in section 201(h) of the FD&C Act. For example, the product may be a drug or biological product that is regulated by a division of the FDA other than the CDRH or for which there are different provisions in the FD&C Act.

The second stage is to determine how the FDA may classify your device – which one of the three classes of perceived risk the device may fall into. However, unless the device is "exempt" the FDA will actually classify your device. Classification identifies the level of regulatory control that is necessary to assure the safety and effectiveness of a medical device. Most importantly, the classification of the device will identify, unless exempt, the type of regulatory submission pathway the "sponsor" (manufacturer) must complete in order to obtain FDA clearance/approval for marketing. There are currently two major pathways in the United States for devices: premarket notification (also known as the "510(k)" pathway) and premarket approval (also known as "PMA" pathway). Generally, the 510(k) pathway is preferred by device developers as it is typically less burdensome. Semantically, a device whose marketing has been permitted by the FDA using data from the 510(k) pathway is called "FDA cleared" and a device permitted after successfully navigating the PMA pathway is called "FDA approved". This carries some implications with respect to wording in advertisements, but essentially a device authorized by either pathway can now be marketed in the United States.

FDA clearance or approval also frequently carries important status for marketing in other countries, as FDA clearance frequently serves as a proxy for clearance or partial clearance in many countries.

The third stage of FDA clearance involves the development of data necessary to submit a marketing application and to obtain FDA clearance to market. For some 510(k) submissions and almost all PMA applications, clinical performance data are required to obtain clearance to market. In these cases, conduct of the trial must be done in accord with the FDA's Investigational Device Exemption (IDE) regulation [3]. Investigations covered under the IDE regulation are subject to differing levels of regulatory control and scrutiny depending on the perceived level of risk of the new device. The IDE regulation distinguishes between significant and non-significant risk device studies and the procedures for obtaining approval to begin the study differ accordingly. Also, some types of studies are actually completely exempt from the IDE regulations. The IDE exemption process is discussed in a later section of this chapter.

The design of your trial is absolutely critical. This point cannot be emphasized enough. Many theoretically solid medical devices have been shelved due to failure to satisfy the FDAs endpoints for *both* safety and efficacy. This comes at great cost to the sponsors and to the clinical investigators. In the process of rejecting a submission, the FDA can provide feedback that would theoretically allow a sponsor to repeat a trial in a more successful fashion. However, in reality, by this point most clinical trial budgets have been completely exhausted and the device is permanently shelved. The memoir "Innovation Breakdown: How the FDA and Wall Street Cripple Medical Advances" is primarily focused on the battle to obtain approval for a device that detects melanoma, but also includes interesting stories of other devices which were temporarily or permanently shelved due to complications in the approval pathway [4].

Trial design should be thoroughly vetted internally and externally to predict any potential downstream problems that will reduce the device's chance of approval. This begins from the very first sentences of the application where the "intended use" statement is constructed. The FDA approves a medical device for the "intended use" (or indication) based on successful demonstration of safety and efficacy in the data set. After clearance, any other use of the device will be considered "off-label "unless the sponsor re-applies to the FDA with new data for a new indication or "claim extension".

Interestingly, because the FDA mission statement clearly states it is not in the business of *practicing* medicine, the limitation of the device's intended use label does not necessarily prevent physicians from actually *using* an already-approved device for an off-label purpose. For example, tongue depressors can be used for splinting fingers and Foley catheters have been used to remove nasal foreign bodies in children, and wrapped layers of surgical suture are frequently employed to help remove stuck finger rings. The important nuance here is that the *manufacturers* and *distributors* of the devices cannot *promote* the use of these devices for purposes for which they are not cleared. Therefore, defining the intended use of the device is critical from the very beginning.

The FDA also points out that there are other requirements beyond matter-of-fact data supporting safety and efficacy. The device developer must be aware of FDA requirements on product labelling, quality control, and postmarketing surveillance of the device.

Lest the above discussion of regulatory issues suck the wind out of your sail of enthusiasm for bringing your invention to market, keep in mind that, on average, the FDA clears about 3000 new devices each year under the 510(k) pathway as well as an additional number under the less-frequently used PMA pathway [5]. Once "cleared" or "approved," a device approved by either pathway can be sold in the United States.

Step five: Obtain reimbursement for your device

You have got your device to market. Now you have to sell it to recover costs associated with its development. In theory, you can price your product at whatever amount you want, and sell it, as long as the marketing and sales team that offers your product adheres to the various regulations that require the presentation of the product be related to its "on-label" features. Remember that the FDA cleared the device based on the indications supported in your data, and indications not supported in the FDA-reviewed data are viewed as "off-label". So while the FDA is not in the business of practicing medicine and physicians can actually legally use your product however they see fit for direct non-clinical trial patient care, advertising for non-FDA approved indications is illegal.

In reality, to obtain proper reimbursement for your invention involves pursuing the three elements outlined here. A complete discussion of medical device reimbursement is beyond the scope of this chapter, but the essential features are:

- *Coverage*: "Obtaining coverage" requires convincing the major paying entities, such as the Centers for Medicare and Medicaid Services (CMS), and insurers, such as Blue Cross and Aetna, that your device is proven and medically necessary. FDA approval is only the first step in this process. Your experiment design portfolio should include other studies that are designed to convince payers that this device does something new, important, and should be on their list of "covered" services.

- *Coding*: In the United States, "obtaining a code" refers to the process of obtaining a desired CP T® (Current Procedural Terminology) code from an American Medical Association (AMA) organization called CPT-HCPAC. This can be an iterative process. That is, when your device is first approved the supporting evidence available may only supports its association with a generic (and often low paying) CPT code. As more evidence of the uniqueness of your device is demonstrated, you can argue for a better code by "cross-walking" to existing codes for comparable technology. Some ability also exists to apply for a novel CPT code. Up-to-date information on CPT coding is generally best found on the web site of the American Medical Association [6].
- *Payment*: Payment is determined by contractual terms between healthcare providers and payers. This is an area where industry frequently must assist because the cost of the technologies may exceed the expectation of the payer's perception of the benefit. This is also where "cost effectiveness" studies can play a key role in the adoption of new technology.

When a groundbreaking device is substantially more expensive than devices that are already on the market, medical device manufacturers can seek a new code to receive appropriate reimbursement by applying for an "add-on payment," which is a temporary provision for new technologies.

Obtaining an IDE (Investigational Device Exemption) from the FDA

In the process of investigating medical devices, the clinician may encounter an element of the Institutional Review Board (IRB) application that they have not had to address before when doing chart-based studies or surveys. You will see a question similar to this on your IRB application:

"If this study involves a device that is not FDA approved, has the Investigational Device Exemption (IDE) or 510(k) reference been provided?"

The purpose of an IDE is to allow an investigational device to be used in a clinical study to collect safety and effectiveness data for a marketing application. An IDE also permits a device to be shipped lawfully so that it can be studied in a clinical investigation.

IDE is a process that involves the clinical investigators, their IRBs, and the industry sponsors of the trial with the FDA to determine if the study for the device being considered is low enough risk that a more stringent set of proof/requirements can be "waived."

The FDA was not initially set up to relinquish its authority at any stage in product development. However, the concept of IDE was developed "To encourage discovery and development of useful medical devices for human use, to the extent consistent with the protection of the public health and safety and with ethical standards, while maintaining optimum freedom for scientific investigators in their pursuit of that purpose" [7].

That freedom therefore allows you a way to test devices, with certain conditions attached and as long as you follow certain procedures along with your IRB. The broader issue of the IRB application and process has been discussed in greater detail in Chapter 7 of this book.

An important step is to determine whether an IDE is even required for your device. This is based on the level of risk associated with the device; if low-risk, an IDE may sometimes not be required. Other times, if the device is deemed to be a "non-significant risk," very abbreviated requirements from the FDA need to be met. If a device is considered to be "significant risk" then the complete IRB process needs to be completed. It is your IRB who actually makes the determination of what level of risk a device may pose. If your IRB is uncertain, the FDA will make the decision.

Examples of *Exempt devices* that do not typically require an IDE would be: 510(k)-cleared or PMA-approved devices (if used in accordance with approved labelling), most *in vitro* diagnostic devices (unless being used to assign patients for a therapeutic purpose or involving an invasive sampling regimen), consumer-preference testing, combinations of legally-marketed devices, and devices to be used solely on animals.

Non-significant risk devices are devices that do not pose a significant risk to human subjects. Examples include most daily-wear contact lenses, contact lens solutions, and Foley catheters. A non-significant risk device study requires only IRB approval prior to initiation of a clinical study. Sponsors of studies involving non-significant risk devices are not required to submit an IDE application to the FDA for approval.

Significant risk devices present the potential for serious risk to the health or safety of a subject. Significant risk devices may include implants, devices that support or sustain human life, and devices that are substantially important in diagnosing, curing, mitigating or treating disease, and devices important in preventing impairment to human health. Examples include sutures, cardiac pacemakers, hydrocephalus shunts, and orthopedic implants. Extended-wear contact lenses are considered "significant risk" (whereas daily-wear contact lenses are considered "non-significant" risk).

The reader is advised to consult the FDA web site for examples of device risk categories [8]. If your proposed device is similar to any of the ones on the list, it is likely that an IDE will be required.

The sponsor of the study is ultimately responsible for submitting the IDE application to the FDA. The FDA encourages sponsors to work consultatively prior to the submission of the IDE in a process called "pre-IDE". After these consultative meetings, the IDE application is submitted [9]. The FDA then either approves, conditionally approves, or rejects the IDE. After obtaining either approval or conditional approval, the sponsor can typically move forward with the IRB process of the institution(s) involved in the study. FDA and IRB approval is a process that may take some time, perhaps in the order of months. One approach that may be taken to optimize efficiency of review and shorten the time to initiation of a trial is to submit a contemporaneous IRB application that includes a statement to the effect that (i) an IDE application has been/will be submitted, (ii) FDA approval will be forwarded to the IRB once received, and (iii) no trial procedures will be initiated without both FDA and IRB approval (and IRB review of FDA communications).

Summary

Medical device investigation continues to play an increasing role in acute care research. While the regulatory elements of medical device approval might appear daunting, a suitable understanding of the pathways makes navigating the process more manageable for the clinician-researcher. Local assistance can often be obtained from the investigator's own IRB staff. Additional resources are available directly from the regulatory bodies themselves, such as the FDA and AMA. Consulting firms exist to assist with the development and FDA submission process; many offer start-to-finish suites of services to the individual investigator, institution, or small company to bring their innovation to market. Larger companies will have in-house professional staff that provide many of these same services. If you are involved in testing a device for a larger company, they will usually provide the institutional investigator with templates and step-by-step guidance through the process. There can be a great deal of personal and professional satisfaction for researchers who bring new technologies to market. Novel technologies in medicine tend to endure for years, sometimes decades, and can make far-reaching changes in the practice of medicine. Best of luck on your venture in developing your medical device!

KEY POINTS

- The development of new medical devices is critical in the evolution of acute care medicine.
- Regulatory pathways for marketing novel devices vary by region, as well as by perceived risk of the new device.
- Protection of intellectual property is important early in the development of new products.
- Up-front work planning and executing clinical trials (with an eye towards regulatory approval) will prevent needless delays in getting your device to clinicians.

References

1 US Food and Drug Administration (2015) *Medical Devices*. http://www.fda.gov/MedicalDevices (last accessed 11 May 2015).
2 US Food and Drug Administration (2014) *Is the Product a Medical Device?* http://www.fda.gov/MedicalDevices/DeviceRegulationandGuidance/Overview/ClassifyYourDevice/ucm051512.htm (last accessed 11 May 2015).
3 U.S. Food and Drug Administration (2014) *Device Advice: Investigational Device Exemption (IDE)*. http://www.fda.gov/MedicalDevices/DeviceRegulationandGuidance/HowtoMarketYourDevice/InvestigationalDeviceExemptionIDE/default.htm (last accessed 11 May 2015).
4 Gulfo, J.V. (2014) *Innovation Breakdown: How the FDA and Wall Street Cripple Medical Advances*. Post Hill Press.
5 Emergo Group (2013) *How Long it Takes the FDA to "Approve" a 510(k) Submission*. http://www.emergogroup.com/research/download-fda-510k-review-times-research (last accessed 11 May 2015).
6 American Medical Association (nd) *CPT – Current Procedural Terminology*. http://www.ama-assn.org/ama/pub/physician-resources/solutions-managing-your-practice/coding-billing-insurance/cpt.page (last accessed 11 May 2015).
7 US Food and Drug Administration (2014) *US Code of Federal Regulations Section 520(g) 21CFR*. http://www.accessdata.fda.gov/scripts/cdrh/cfdocs/cfcfr/CFRSearch.cfm?fr=812 (last accessed 21 May 2015).
8 US Food and Drug Administration (2015) *IDE Approval Process*. http://www.fda.gov/medicaldevices/deviceregulationandguidance/howtomarketyourdevice/investigationaldeviceexemptionide/ucm046164.htm (last accessed 11 May 2015).
9 US Food and Drug Administration (2015) *IDE Application*. http://www.fda.gov/MedicalDevices/DeviceRegulationandGuidance/HowtoMarketYourDevice/InvestigationalDeviceExemptionIDE/ucm046706.htm (last accessed 11 May 2015).

CHAPTER 24

Privacy in research: How to collect data safely and confidentially

Gary M. Vilke and Edward M. Castillo

Department of Emergency Medicine, University of California San Diego, San Diego, CA, USA

Overview

So you are embarking on a research project; to be successful you will need data. This is true whether you are carrying out a retrospective review of hospital records (Chapter 14), prospectively collecting data for a clinical trial (Chapters 11 and 18), or carrying out an interventional study (Chapter 19). When the data come from patients, as opposed to mice or gel runs in a bench research laboratory, there are issues of privacy. This chapter addresses some of the challenges and how you can work to navigate the treacherous Institutional Review Board (IRB) waters (Chapters 8 and 16) and remain in compliance with The Health Insurance Portability and Accountability Act (HIPAA) of 1996.

Prior to HIPAA, research was much easier in terms of collecting patient data. A researcher had to submit a proposal to the IRB requesting to collect patient data and create a plan to keep the material safe and secure. Relative to today, proposals did not have to be very specific and it was not very difficult to get a proposal through a standard IRB, even at conservative university settings. Then, the implementation of HIPAA changed all of that. The pendulum swung so far in the other direction, that research and data collection was often delayed for months trying to get IRB approval, as IRB committees tried to understand the best way to maintain compliance with HIPAA.

> *"Every time I submit a new IRB application the requirements for patient privacy and maintaining data confidentiality change – it is an unpredictable moving target."*
>
> Senior researcher

What is HIPPA?

To understand what HIPAA means to you as a researcher, we need to better understand what HIPAA was intended to do and who and what are affected by this privacy rule. The HIPAA Privacy Rule was intended to address potential concerns for patient privacy posed by the development and national adoption of electronic medical records and the associated patient information databases. HIPAA was designed to provide a new floor level of federal protection for health information that would span across all 50 states. Compliance with the Privacy Rule was required as of April 2003, but there was considerable confusion about interpreting the Privacy Rule and the specific changes it requires in the way healthcare providers, hospital systems, health plans and others use, maintain, and disclose health information. This was good news if you were a patient, but not so good news if you were a researcher.

So what does this HIPAA Privacy Rule actually do? Basically, in simplistic terms, it sets forth detailed regulations regarding the types of uses and disclosures of an individuals' personally-identifiable health information, called "protected health information" (PHI), which is permitted by "covered entities." These covered entities include health plans, healthcare clearinghouses, and healthcare providers who transmit information via an electronic format. A major goal of the HIPAA Privacy Rule was to ensure that individuals' health information was properly protected while allowing the flow

Doing Research in Emergency and Acute Care: Making Order Out of Chaos, First Edition. Edited by Michael P. Wilson, Kama Z. Guluma, and Stephen R. Hayden.

of information needed to maintain and promote high-quality health care. If a patient's information is safe and protected but not available to a physician who is actively caring for a patient, then this would obviously be a disservice to the patient specifically and the entire healthcare team in general.

For researchers, the HIPAA Privacy Rule also set out requirements for the conduct of health research. The Institute of Medicine Committee on Health Research and the Privacy of Health Information was charged with two principal tasks: (i) to assess whether the HIPAA Privacy Rule is having an impact on the conduct of health research, defined broadly as "a systematic investigation, including research development, testing and evaluation, designed to develop or contribute to generalizable knowledge"; and (ii) to propose recommendations to facilitate the efficient and effective conduct of important health research while maintaining or strengthening the privacy protections of personally identifiable health information. (More information about this can be found in the references for further reading at the end of this chapter.)

Beyond the challenges of day-to-day maintenance of health-related information for real-time patient care, researchers were concerned that HIPAA could hinder their access to health information needed to conduct research. Gunn and colleagues studied this in 2004 and concluded that the Privacy Rule is indeed fundamentally changing the way that healthcare providers, health plans, and others use, maintain, and disclose health information and the steps that researchers must take to obtain health data. In their paper, they go on to say that the Privacy Rule requires researchers who seek access to identifiable health information to obtain written authorization from patients, or, alternatively, to demonstrate that their research protocols meet certain Privacy Rule requirements that permit access without written authorization. To ensure continued access to data, researchers will need to work more closely than before with healthcare providers, health plans, and other institutions that generate and maintain health information.

Informed consent and impact on privacy

Informed consent is an ethical and legal requirement for research involving human participants; it is discussed in more detail in Chapter 16. However, some discussion as to how it impacts you, the researcher, and the privacy issues of your patients is needed here. Informed consent is the process where a study participant is informed about all aspects of the research project so the participant can make an informed and educated decision regarding their participation. After studying all aspects of the proposed study and having the opportunity to ask questions, the participant voluntarily confirms his or her willingness to participate in a particular study – he or she gives you their consent. The concept of informed consent is embedded in the principles of The Nuremberg Code, The Declaration of Helsinki and The Belmont Report (Chapter 8).

Informed consent is an inevitable requirement that you must address prior to every research project you want to embark on involving human beings as participants. However, under some circumstances, informed consent can be waived by the IRB. Despite this, the protection of PHI is still mandatory. This is common in retrospective studies, including medical record reviews. In these types of studies, the patient is typically not available for you to obtain an informed consent, either written or verbal, and a waiver of informed consent is generally appropriate. If a waiver of individual HIPAA authorization is requested for research uses of PHI, the HIPAA Privacy Rule requires that eight conditions must be satisfied in order to grant that waiver. These eight conditions must be clearly addressed in the IRB proposals:

1 Demonstrating that the use of disclosure of PHI involves no more than minimal risk to the patient.
2 Describing how granting the waiver will not adversely affect privacy rights and the welfare of the individuals whose records will be used.
3 Describing how the project could not practicably be conducted without a waiver of informed consent.
4 Describing how the project could not practicably be conducted without the use of PHI.
5 Describing an adequate plan to protect identifiers from improper use and that a disclosure plan is included in the research proposal.
6 Describing an adequate plan to destroy the patient identifiers at the earliest opportunity, or offering a justification for retaining the patient identifiers and describing how the information will be protected.
7 Providing a project plan that includes written assurances that PHI will not be re-used or disclosed for other purposes.
8 Providing, whenever appropriate, additional pertinent information to subjects about the research project after participation.

Protected health information and anonymity

If you are embarking on a prospective research project in which you will be collecting data in real-time, the IRB will generally require you to obtain informed consent both for the study and the use of PHI prior to enrolling the patient into the study. To protect patient privacy, the PHI needs either to be collected with no patient identifiers, or in such a manner that patient confidentiality is strictly maintained. The method of collecting PHI is the difference between anonymity and confidentiality. *Anonymity* is the collecting of data that do not have any patient identifiers. Additionally, there is no link between response or information and a specific study participant. This differs from *confidentiality*, in which information collected from patients has patient-identifying information or contains a link between response or information and a specific study participant. You, the researcher, must make every effort to prevent anyone outside of the study from having access to the information linking the individual patients with their information. Examples of PHI or identifying information are shown in Box 24.1.

Box 24.1 Examples of patient identifying information.

Name
Address
Phone number
Fax number
Social security number
Account numbers
Medical record number
Relatives' names
Relatives' addresses
Relatives' phone numbers
Employer name
Employer address
Date of birth
Date of death
Other dates specific to the individual
Voiceprints
Fingerprints
Full face photos
Other identifying images (tattoos, scars)

Protecting and storing the data

If data include PHI, they need to be protected for privacy issues. These data can come in different forms, such as data collection tools, on-line or computerized surveys, other questionnaires, video or audio tapes, and field notes. In addition, unless identifying information is removed, aggregated data sets and spreadsheets must also be accounted for by you and your research team.

If it is essential that you collect patient identifying information as part of the study, for example, a medical record number so that you can gather additional data at a future date or have access to a patient's name or phone number for follow-up information, then you must provide confidentiality for the patient's data. You may need to be creative in order to accomplish this. There are number of strategies that can be implemented, depending on the type of study you are embarking on, and a number of practices that can be utilized to increase the level of confidentiality.

Common strategies include using study codes on documents containing data, such as a completed survey tool or questionnaire, which help keep the data separate from identifying information. You can keep the study code along with identifying information locked in a separate location with restricted access to this document. By limiting who has access to the code sheet, such as only the principle investigator or study coordinator, you also minimize the risk of information being compromised.

If not needed for future follow up or further analysis, removing cover sheets or face sheets from data collection tools after the information has been acquired from the study participant will separate PHI from the data. If the data are computerized, assigning security codes or passwords to these records will limit access while adding an increased level of security. Once records are no longer needed, having a plan to properly destroy paper files or delete computerized records is also a technique to reassure the IRB that you are protecting the information of your study patients. If data are not destroyed, they should be encrypted on password-protected computers. Lastly, the plan for limiting who has access to any of the study records should be spelled out in the study plan.

In this electronic age, there are host of high-tech ways to maintain and store data using on-line data entry and storage. Most industry-based research utilizes some form of on-line case report forms (CRFs) that are vetted with appropriate log-in security, access limitations and firewall protection. A low cost, but high-tech way of collecting and storing data can be through Research Electronic Data Capture, also known as REDCap. The REDCap Consortium is composed of over a thousand active institutional partners spanning over eighty countries. The consortium supports a secure web application designed specifically to support protected data capture for research studies. The REDCap application allows researchers to build and manage online surveys and databases quickly and securely, and is currently in production use or development build-status for more than 120,000 projects with over 156,000 users spanning numerous research focus areas across the consortium.

At the other end of the technology spectrum, though it may seem basic, use of a locked filing cabinet or desk drawer also counts toward protecting the PHI of study patients. These filing cabinets should be kept in a locked office or secured room, and this practice should be specifically referred to in the IRB application. Okay, now that you are an educated expert in privacy issues, here is a real-world example of a prospective study. This is sample language that was used in an IRB application on a clinical trial in which patients who met study inclusion criteria were to have certain demographic and PHI documented and then blood drawn at specific time intervals. There were no medications being administered as part of this trial.

> All research data will be stored in a password-protected computer database. The access to this database is restricted to those involved in the data management and data analysis activities. To minimize the potential loss of confidentiality, patients will be assigned a unique number as their subject identifier code. No personal health identifiers will be used. The unique subject code will be used to label all study documents. The blood specimens will be assigned unique specimen codes different from the subject codes. A separate paper and electronic document will link the subjects with their subject codes and the specimen codes. This document will be kept in a secure location in a locked cabinet or on a password-protected computer. Only the principal investigator and study coordinator will have the key to the secure location as well as the password to the computer containing the document linking the subjects with the subject and specimen codes. All other electronic documents will be labeled only with subject codes and will not contain patient identifiers. These electronic documents will only be stored on specified research only computers. If any study documents are transferred to the sponsor, the forms will only contain subject codes and no patient identifiers will be included on the forms.

Obviously, as a researcher, you should modify and tailor this type of language to suit your needs and the expectations of your particular IRB. This example merely highlights the issues of protecting patient privacy in a real world, tangible example. Now go forth and research, and when dealing with subject privacy, remember the language on many police cars, "To protect and serve."

KEY POINTS

- If you are performing research using patients, you must be familiar with HIPPA.
- Informed consent is a requirement that you must address prior to every research project involving human beings as participants.
- The method of collecting PHI is the difference between anonymity and confidentiality.
- If collected data include PHI, these data need to be protected for privacy issues.
- There are many different acceptable techniques to protect data.

Futher reading

1 Gunn, P.P., Fremont, A.M., Bottrell, M., *et al.* (2004) The Health Insurance Portability and Accountability Act Privacy Rule: a practical guide for researchers. *Med Care,* **42**(4):321–327.
2 McRae, A. and Weijer, C. (2008) US Federal Regulations for emergency research: a practical guide and commentary. *Acad Emerg Med,* **15**(1):88–97.
3 Nass, .SJ., Levit, L.A., Gostin, L.O. (eds) (2009) *Beyond the HIPAA Privacy Rule: Enhancing Privacy, Improving Health Through Research. Institute of Medicine (US) Committee on Health Research and the Privacy of Health Information: The HIPAA Privacy Rule.* National Academies Press, Washington, DC.
4 Offerman, S.R., Nishijima, D.K., Ballard, D.W., *et al.* (2013) The use of delayed telephone informed consent for observational emergency medicine research is ethical and effective. *Acad Emerg Med,* **20**(4):403–407.
5 Petrini, C. (2013) Clinical trials with subjects unable to give consent: some ethical-legal paradoxes. *Med Leg J,* **81**(Pt 3):128–131.

CHAPTER 25

How do I establish a research assistant program?

Judd E. Hollander

Department of Emergency Medicine, Thomas Jefferson University, Philadelphia, PA, USA

> "I want to do research but everyone is too busy to help me collect data."
>
> Most emergency medicine researchers

What is an research assistant program and why do I need one?

Presumably, if you are reading this chapter, you have already either decided that you want to do your own research or you are interested in developing a robust research program. In both cases you have figured out you need a research infrastructure [1–3]. This chapter will help you get that going.

Axiom 1. It's not the about the project. It's about the program.

You cannot run a successful research program unless you are are passionate about doing it. This author is unaware of any program that has survived when a chair assigned someone who does not love research to initiate the program. It is just too much work and not enough reward. If that is what happened to you, go get a new job, because this one will make you miserable. The rest of the chapter assumes you actually want to do a lot of research and are willing to lay the groundwork for a successful research career. If that is the case, it is more important to grow the program and develop the infrastructure than to complete your next project.

Axiom 2. Funding begets more funding.

You are not going to get funding until you prove you can perform. Let us use the venture capital analogy. Where do you think venture capitalists put their money? It goes to companies with the highest likelihood of providing a return on investment. If you were a pharmaceutical company with a new product, would you pay yourself to do the research? A six-month delay in getting to market might mean your company loses millions of dollars or you lose your job. They want to have studies conducted by sites that have proven ability to meet timelines and deliver the highest quality research. They are not in the business of "giving you a shot at it."

Axiom 3. It takes time and money to make money and save time.

If you are developing a robust research program, you need to invest your time and your department's money upfront. You cannot wait for your first funded study to hire staff to conduct a study. You either need to hire people first or you need to volunteer your time and find others to do the same. You need to live and breathe the first study.

> "If you build it, they will come"
>
> Field of Dreams

Doing Research in Emergency and Acute Care: Making Order Out of Chaos, First Edition. Edited by Michael P. Wilson, Kama Z. Guluma, and Stephen R. Hayden.

Remember if you do not perform well on this study, you decrease the likelihood of getting funding next time.

Developing a research assistant program (or as it is called at several places including Thomas Jefferson University, an academic associate program) is one way to rapidly develop a robust research infrastructure with relatively little financial commitment. In fact, you can even get external funding for your program from your university (more on that later).

The term "academic associate" rather than "research assistant" is preferable because it is an academic position; the students are being taught, they have classes and they are not the same as paid research assistants. The title, Academic Associate, allows them to introduce themselves to the patient without the patient believing he or she is being approached to be a "guinea pig" in a clinical trial. Unfortunately, patients sometimes think that when they hear the word "research." The term "academic associate" will, therefore, be used throughout the remainder of the chapter.

Why do you need an academic associate program?

This is easy – you need help with data collection, your colleagues do not help while they are seeing patients, you do not have money, and you have not yet figured out how to make research thrive in your department.

What does an academic associate program cost my department?

This author has started two of them with *no* financial contributions from the department. However, it works better if you get time to oversee the program (it does take 20–30 hours a month) and if you have a small kitty to buy pizza or something nice during the classroom sessions. Within a short period of time, all this can be funded off clinical trial revenue, if budgeted appropriately.

Axiom 4. You – the faculty member – need to run the show.
That is just reality. Students come to the program to interact with faculty. They do not come to meet your research coordinator or nurse. If you are not heavily involved, it will not run well. Do not try to pass the buck.

What do other research faculty get out of it?

Data collectors in the emergency department (ED) 17 hours per day, 7 days per week. Is there a need to say more?

What do research faculty have to do in return for use of the academic associates?

Axiom 5. It is not fair to the students to be free labor without something in return.
It is the belief of this author that faculty who use the program should contribute to the program and the author has had a policy of requiring faculty with ongoing studies to attend four academic associate meetings per semester and lecture one or two times per year. Seems fair to ask in return for 17 hours a day, 7 days per week of data collection. Although hard to believe, some people have thought that this was an unreasonable request. Guess what? They cannot use the academic associates.

What do non-research faculty get out of it?

They will never again be asked to enroll patients in clinical studies. The academic associates basically conduct research without interfering with the clinical operations of the department. They will, however, periodically ask faculty to help fill out clinical data forms (since academic associates cannot do physical examinations), but they will not have to consent patients for studies ever again.

Sounds great. How do I establish an academic associates program?

Before your program begins, you need to decide what model you want to use. There are three main options:

- Official course credit through a university.
- Volunteer.
- Paid positions.

Obviously the course credit option takes a little more work. You need to figure out how to create a new course at the university, write a proposal with a syllabus, demonstrate need, show how it will help students, and then wait for university approval. This author achieved this twice in just a couple months – once it was tapped into a pre-established elective program; the other time a new course was created within the undergraduate university.

> "Where do we send the money?"
>
> Director of the Post-Baccalaureate Program

This was the best question – in the experience of this author - that was ever asked about the academic associate program. It turns out that universities pay their biology professors a baseline salary and then a per course stipend. When the course was set up at one university, they expected to pay for teaching the course. All of sudden there was money available to pay for this author's effort (translation: reduce clinical load). It was also possible to get a stipend for a teaching assistant , which compensated the research nurse and research fellow for their extra effort.

Axiom 6. Work with, rather than against your hospital, so they embrace the program.
You will also need to work out other logistics within your hospital or university, such as patient orientation research training, Health Insurance Portability and Accountability Act (HIPAA) compliance training and inform your Institutional Review Board (IRB) of the program. IRB approval of the data collection methods using the academic associates was received, with an agreement on a monitoring program for student compliance with all regulatory concerns. Although it took time to work this out, it was much better than revisiting the use of academic associates every time a new study proposal was submitted to a new primary reviewer. As an aside, the Food and Drug Administration audited one study performed in the program and no issues were raised.

How many students do you take?

In this authors program, associates double-cover the ED from 7 AM to midnight, 7 days a week in 4–6 hour prespecified blocks. If students do not fit into two blocks (8–12 hours) a week, we do not take them. Our experience suggests that students who come only once a week tend to perform poorly.

What exactly is the curriculum?

The basic curriculum in our program is 8–12 hours per week of hands-on time in the ED where students screen every patient who comes into the ED for enrollment in the ongoing clinical studies. For the first two weeks of each semester (first four shifts), they have either a research coordinator or a second semester academic associate mentor them continuously in the ED. After that, there are research coordinators on site to assist academic associate should questions arise. Before the advent of such robust coordinator coverage, academic associates would call the principal investigator of the study that gave rise to the question and discuss it with the physician (any time of day or night).

We have the following mandatory sessions for the academic associates:

- Mini-orientation – a two-hour small group (5–8 student) session before the first shift to review all the studies in detail.

- Major orientation – a 4–5 hour orientation for the whole class after students have done three or four shifts, so they have some clinical experience already. This session includes introductions, policy and procedures, and review of all study details. It is designed to help crystalize information learned thus far.
- Three other mandatory classes are coupled with full faculty project updates during the semester. They are:
  - Data collection methods.
  - Research design.
  - Putting it all together.
- Three optional classes, designed to be fun for the students, are also offered. They include things like ultrasound laboratory, suture laboratory, airway laboratory or lectures on chest pain, trauma or other topics we may be studying. They vary semester to semester depending upon which studies are ongoing.
- Asynchronous learning is accomplished through a series of internally produced training videos as well as reading materials providing scientific background on the studies.

  Academic associates are required to take the following examinations:
- Mid-term on the scientific literature.
- Mid-term on ED operations, data collection and study implementation and conduct.
- Final examination focusing on research design.

  We also conduct in shift observations and peer evaluations.

Are you really crazy enough to have classes and examinations for volunteers?

Yes. When we have run the program without course credit, we have the same curriculum and same requirements. It just works better. See Axiom 7 below.

How do students sign up, get trained and supervised?

We require students to complete patient-oriented research modules (CITI modules) before attending an informational session and signing up for the program. That makes sure people who sign up have appropriate training before they ever walk into the ED, and that they are committed to the program.

We hold a series of small group meetings that students must attend *in person*, in order to sign up. We explain the program, the mandatory attendance requirements (miss two shifts/classes and you fail; miss one, down a full letter grade) and make students sign a pledge that they will not drop the class. They then pick shifts and are enrolled.

After enrollment, the hospital will enable access to HIPAA training and academic associates must complete HIPAA training before their mini-orientation.

Axiom 7. There are plenty of students who want to do this. You set the rules and be unbending. It works better.

It is really hard to publish a paper that says, "We enrolled patients from 7 AM to midnight 7 days per week except when Wendy missed her shift Tuesday morning." As researchers we do not have the luxury to tolerate absences and non-compliance. Your studies might change practice and it needs to be conducted rigorously. Our students and their advisors know this.

Once created, where do you find students?

Do not worry about this – it will not be an issue. You can probably just tap into your local premed club or postbaccalaureate program and within days find more students than you need. If you do not have a university affiliation, I know several colleagues who have approached non-affiliated local universities and set up collaborative referral sources. It works quite well.

How many clinical studies can you conduct at the same time?

The optimal number is 5–8. Less than that and students get bored. More results in missing eligible patients. Obviously it varies on the intensity of the studies. We usually have at least one biomarker study with serial samples and at least one survey that enrolls up to 30 patients per day in the group.

Can the academic associates do more than just collect data in the ED?

Of course they can. Once trained to conduct research, a few of the more experienced students get involved in monitoring compliance, completing case report forms for sponsors and helping with IRB approvals, contracts, and so on. Obviously, increased responsibility can only go to the students with the highest performance. We tend to not allow academic associates to be the last person to touch or review anything. The success of the research program is dependent upon maintaining the highest regulatory standards and having too many hands in the brew is never a good idea. We do not allow academic associates to enter data in the clinical databases. Academic associates do consent patients for observational studies but when a study is interventional and requires more medical knowledge than they can reasonably possess, they are not allowed to conduct the informed consent.

Academic associates are encouraged to develop ideas for secondary manuscripts and we have had many present at our national meetings and author papers. The academic associates who have completed two semesters in our program, and are considered the best in the group, tend to be hired as research coordinators. This is a tremendous pipeline for well-trained employees.

What do the students get out of it?

They obviously feel like they get a lot out of it, since we always have a waiting list. Sometimes it has been as many as 40 students long!

Student benefits include:

- Learning clinical research skills.
- Opportunity to do more than just volunteer in the ED.
- Learning to interact with patients and physicians.
- Developing mentee–mentor relationships with faculty and residents.
- Finding people to write letters of recommendation.
- Developing a skill set that leads to clinical research jobs during the gap year.
- Having clinical anecdotes to speak about on medical school interviews.
- We have even had two pairs of academic associates get married.

KEY POINTS

- A research assistant program is not just free labor.
- Give a lot to the students and you will get a lot in return.
- Research careers grow faster by investing in infrastructure than by worrying about one project at a time.
- Run the program like it is a privilege for the students to be able to participate, they will treat it like a privilege and then it will actually be one.
- Academic associates are a tremendous help with patient screening and enrollment. You do not want them involved in preparation of your IRB documents, protocol development and regulatory monitoring. They do not have training, generally want to please and will try to do more than they should, creating more work for you.

References

1 Hollander, J.E., Valentine, S.M., and Brogan, G.X. (1997) The Academic Associate Program: Integrating clinical emergency medicine research with undergraduate education. *Acad Emerg Med*, **4**(3):225–230.

2 Hollander, J.E. and Singer, A.J. (2002) An innovative strategy for conducting clinical research: The Academic Associate Program. *Acad Emerg Med*, **9**(2):134–137.

3 Sparano, D.S., Shofer, F.S., and Hollander, J.E. (2004) Participation in the Academic Associate Program: Effect on medical school admission rate. *Acad Emerg Med*, **11**:695–698.

CHAPTER 26

How to complete a research study well and in a minimum of time: The importance of collaboration

Austin Hopper[1] and Michael P. Wilson[2]

[1] Department of Emergency Medicine Behavioral Emergencies Research laboratory (DEMBER), UC San Diego Health System, San Diego, CA, USA
[2] Department of Emergency Medicine, UC San Diego Health Systems, Department of Emergency Medicine Behavioral Emergencies Research Lab, CA, USA

Collaboration is a key force in the world and "is founded on the premise that individuals have special areas of expertise or capability that can be shared with other partners to enhance their overall capacity for mutual benefit, to increase effectiveness and to optimally align resources" [1]. Collaboration gave us Tango and Cash, Butch Cassidy and the Sundance Kid, and Maverick and Goose. Collaboration is also something that should be managed carefully and attentively, or your productive team can turn from Van Halen in to Van Hagar.

Collaboration can take many forms. It generally involves a Principal Investigator (PI) with an MD, PhD or MD/PhD working together with postdoctoral fellows, research staff, graduate students and/or undergraduate students, among others. Collaboration can be as simple as members of the same department working together to something as complex as multiple universities working in conjunction with federal and industry interests. Often, collaboration is the primary avenue for mentoring graduate students and postdoctoral fellows and a driving factor for many senior researchers to collaborate [2].

Collaboration allows the joining of researchers with complementary skills. Medicine, science and technology are becoming increasingly specialized. As research projects attempt to tackle questions that require a wide range of skills to assess, collaboration allows individuals to use their specific talents to benefit the group as a whole. Through this mechanism the individual production of each researcher can be enhanced. Martin-Sempere *et al.* found that researchers participating in established collaborative groups had higher scientific productivity [3]. They also found that participating in these groups encouraged participation in funded projects and increased opportunities for publication. Funding sources, particularly funding from the federal government, advocate for, and often require, collaboration. The NIH's roadmap plans for further investment in interdisciplinary research as well as collaboration with industry. The National Science Foundation in the USA and the Framework Programmes in the European Union have also increased funding for collaboration between diverse fields and organizations.

Lee and Bozeman found that the number of collaborating researchers is the strongest predictor of productivity [4]. In a sample survey of researchers from American universities, the authors determined a positive correlation between collaboration and scientific productivity. Loucks-Horsley *et al.* found that stimulation of new ideas, insights and perspectives may happen at a faster rate in collaborative research teams than with individuals working on their own [5]. This phenomenon may increase as experts from diverse backgrounds work together. Collaboration can also develop enhanced networks for future collaborations. As researchers interact they can take advantage of each other's contacts to initiate future collaborative endeavors. Often being invited to collaborate can be seen as an acknowledgement of respect and confidence and, in itself, can foster future collaboration and increased job satisfaction [4]. Now that we have established why you want to collaborate with others, let us go over the details of how it is done.

Doing Research in Emergency and Acute Care: Making Order Out of Chaos, First Edition. Edited by Michael P. Wilson, Kama Z. Guluma, and Stephen R. Hayden.
© 2016 John Wiley & Sons, Ltd. Published 2016 by John Wiley & Sons, Ltd.

Working with your team

The primary goal you should keep in mind as you seek out collaborators is the focus of your research. This will dictate who you want to collaborate with for the project based on what objectives you have and the skills and tasks necessary to fulfill them. It is also essential to choose team members who can work together harmoniously as well as be dependable. As you recruit you should make these objectives, and the expectations you have for each member of your group, as clear as possible. Do not be afraid to go over everything multiple times as the project progresses; redundancy is your friend. If you have worked successfully with specific people in the past, that is fantastic. If you have not, key things to look for are experience, dependability, and, most importantly, interest in the topic. You can train someone on how to do almost anything but you cannot force them to be passionate about something. (Playing the cello in elementary school orchestra taught the first author that!)

Communication is essential to maintaining the effectiveness of your group once you have assembled it. Technology makes staying in contact superficially easy, but meetings are still key. E-mails get lost behind other e-mails and can frequently be misunderstood. Whether face to face or over a conference call/video, make sure you have regularly scheduled interaction with your collaborators. Be as flexible as possible to allow maximum attendance, though in the interest of efficiency submeetings can be effective as well. If three members of your team are working on adjusting the patient recruitment protocol, the statistician does not necessarily need to be there.

Meetings also allow progress updates to be immediately assessed and responses to be formulated. This is an opportunity to take advantage of the different backgrounds, experiences and outlooks of your collaborators. Listen to alternative opinions about improving the study design or responding to challenges; this variety of viewpoints is one of the reasons you are collaborating in the first place. Allowing others to input also makes the group stronger and more cohesive. Use each meeting as a time to set new goals as well, as goals create expectations which result in outcomes.

As PI it is your responsibility to ensure that all of your collaborators are adhering to the guidelines approved by the Institutional Review Board (IRB). When interacting with collaborators at other institutions you must ensure that any data sharing is approved by both IRBs. Any participants, including undergraduate assistants, must go through the appropriate training programs for clinical research methodology and ethics as well. Though not unique to collaboration, keep everything you can in writing, from training documentation to study protocols to progress updates; this becomes more of an issue the more people you have involved.

The collaborator standing next to you

Patients arriving at an emergency department can expect to be met by teams that include emergency physicians, nurses, allied health workers and other specialists. This team-based approach has been shown to provide improved service to the patient, but it can also improve the ability to conduct research [6]. Nurses and physicians regularly work together to help patients, it only makes sense for them to combine their broad range of perspectives and experiences to further clinical research. Many organizations offer specific funding opportunities focused on nurse/physician collaboration, such as the Emergency Nurses Association Foundation (ENAF) and the Emergency Medicine Foundation (EMF) Team Grant, which annually funds a nurse/physician team in research [7].

Nursing and research have long gone hand in hand. Florence Nightingale was not just a nice lady with a lamp; through describing her nursing experiences she was a pioneer in the graphical representation of statistics and the first female member of the Royal Statistical Society. Nurses can play a vital role as the fulcrum between behind the scene research design, disseminating study information and recruiting patients [8]. Being a member of the research team allows nurses insight into the rationale behind research projects and gives a sense of purpose behind the activities they engage in that are associated with the project. A commonly perceived barrier to nurse participation in research is time constraints, both for active participation and learning new skills. When collaborating with nurses this must be taken into account and addressed, potentially through time allowance for education and research activities [9].

Being a participant in a multidisciplinary research group can also improve a nurse's ability to translate research findings into better patient care [10]. The Emergency Nurses Association Position Statement advocates that "exposure to a broad range of perspectives through collaboration may strengthen the application of research to practice by the emergency nurse while improving the nurse's research skills." [7] Additionally, Short *et al.* reported that those seeking advancement to senior clinical leadership positions often required research experience [6]. Many nurse researchers have high profile leadership roles not only in research, but also in policy development [11]. In addition to improving clinical abilities, establishing a research and publication "track record" allows opportunities for academic career advancement [12].

The collaborator down the hall

Prevailing wisdom dictates that physicians in different specialties only come together on Saturdays to golf, but often it is essential to work with other departments to conduct research. Collaborating with other departments and specialties is a necessity for studies requiring any follow-up after a patient leaves the emergency department [13]. The emergency department is also frequently the initial point of contact for patients of interest to other specialties. Successes in collaborative research include the epidemiology of injury, early diagnosis of myocardial infarction, hemorrhagic shock and post-traumatic or asphyxial brain injury [13]. Whether it is identifying and recruiting patients for someone else's project or interacting with another department to have them collect data for one of yours, any opportunity to work with other specialties enhances collegiality and improves relationships with experienced researchers in other fields, which benefits all involved. Forming a multidisciplinary research committee has been identified as a key component for identifying research protocols that can take advantage of collaboration between departments and pooling of resources [13]. To keep things running smoothly remember that relative level of participation and investment in the completion of the research project should be mirrored in any subsequent recognition or publication, a topic expanded on below.

Dirty jobs: Assigning authorship

Being an author on a manuscript is the academic equivalent of charting a hit single or starring in a movie but without all the annoying fans and millions of dollars. In all seriousness, authorship is often used as a marker of success and experience, so this is an important issue. A by-product of collaboration is a long list of people who have contributed to your research project and, as such, expect to be listed as an author. Since YOU want to share credit and foster continued relationships, this is great. Unfortunately, assigning authorship is not a problem-free process. Who exactly gets to be an author? How should you order the authors? What can you do to resolve any disputes that arise? Sometimes this can be like high-school gym class. In other words, when you are picking the teams everyone wants to be on board and thinks it is obvious they should be picked first. Luckily, there are some guidelines to help you avoid any gym class-like headaches (although you are on your own if it comes to rope climbing).

Firstly, let us tackle who you should include as an author. The International Committee of Medical Journal Editors (ICMJE) recommends that authorship be based on the following four criteria [14]:

1 Substantial contributions to the conception or design of the work; or the acquisition, analysis, or interpretation of data for the work; AND
2 Drafting the work or revising it critically for important intellectual content; AND
3 Final approval of the version to be published; AND
4 Agreement to be accountable for all aspects of the work in ensuring that questions related to the accuracy or integrity of any part of the work are appropriately investigated and resolved.

To be listed as an author, all four criteria put forward by the ICMJE should ideally be met. In turn, anyone who contributes to all four of these aspects should also be recognized as an author. These expectations should be directly communicated to all members and made abundantly clear before working on a project in order to avoid any potential conflicts about authorship after the fact. Additionally, the ICMJE recommends that every author should be able to identify which aspects of the project their co-authors have worked on, as well as have confidence in the integrity of the contributions that these co-authors have made. This should not present a problem, as we have already gone over selecting collaborators you can trust ("Working with your team"). These criteria are not meant to be exclusionary. In other words, if someone has participated in the first step, you should give them the opportunity to participate in all following steps if they are willing to contribute productively. Do not be a bully.

In a 2008 article, Feeser and Simon highlight several instances where authorship might be bestowed on those who do not fit ICMJE guidelines and who have not contributed significantly to the project [15]. This may be done for a variety of reasons, including:

• Honorary authorship: Generally given to someone senior to the authors of the project as an expression of gratitude or with the intention of fostering future collaboration; more negatively, this can be done in an attempt to ensure publication by including a "big name" author.
• Coercion authorship: This form of authorship inclusion comes as a result of pressure from a senior member of a laboratory or a department to be included on a project that he or she has not contributed to.

- Ghost authorship: The reverse of the first two, ghost authorship is an instance where significant contributions were made by one or more individuals who are not listed as authors on the project. This may be a result of team members leaving, exclusion of junior members, or from draft preparation of industry-sponsored articles by industry employees.

These three problematic aspects of authorship are more than hypothetical. Honorary and coercion authorships can result in the contribution of members who actually did work being devalued by including inappropriate authors who did not contribute. Ghost authorship potentially introduces bias to the research project.

So now that you have determined who your authors are, here comes the fun part: ordering them. Sounds easy right? Unfortunately, not so much. To quote a wise, two foot tall green guy from Star Wars "Ready, are you? What do you know of ready?" Authorship is the hallmark of research productivity and can be a contentious issue. The first author bears most of the responsibility for design and content of the manuscript, as well as for making the final decisions on authorship order. After *numero uno* the authors are traditionally listed in order of level of contribution, with the last author frequently being a supervisor of the research project [16]. When in doubt of who exactly goes where, Ahmed *et al.* have developed an objective scoring system for ordering your authors [17]. By associating number values to author contribution levels of none (0), minimal (1), some (3), or significant (5), the author's individual contribution to different categories can be calculated. Authors are then ranked in order of descending score. An example of this format can be seen in Table 26.1.

For colleagues that have contributed to the project, but not at a level significant enough to be considered a co-author, credit should still be given. The ICMJE recommends acknowledging as contributors those who have acquired funding, contributed administrative support, or given writing, editing, and investigative assistance. These individuals can be acknowledged individually or as a group and the exact contributions should be specified (e.g., "served as scientific advisors," "critically reviewed the study proposal," "collected data," etc.).

Feeser and Simon also recommend several different tactics for resolving disputes concerning authorship [15]. As mentioned earlier, open and direct communication is necessary to make expectations for authorship clear to all parties involved. This topic should be touched on repeatedly as the project evolves and as contributions change in order to maintain clarity on possibly changing author lists and orders. Secondly, pay attention to the ICMJE guidelines. If someone meets all four requirements they should be listed as an author. While you may want to include an author who has contributed extensively in one or more of the four areas but not as much in another, anyone who covers all four bases is without a doubt on your team of authors. Thirdly, in the absence of clear consensus on author order, you should make use of objective tools such as the scoring system developed by Ahmed *et al.* Following these techniques from beginning to end of the project should allow most problems and disagreements that assigning authorship entails to be avoided [15, 17].

Table 26.1 An example of assigning authorship according to the ranking system developed by Ahmed *et al.* [17]. Authors are given scores of 0, 1, 3 or 5 in each category. Points are totaled for each author with credit given in descending order of points.

	Initial idea	Study design	Data collection and oversight	Data analysis	Preparation of the manuscript	Editing and proofing the manuscript	Corresponding author and public interactions	Total Score
Author A	5	5	1	1	1	5	3	21 2nd Author
Author B	5	1	3	5	5	1	5	25 1st Author
Author C	3	3	5	3	0	1	0	15 3rd Author

Source: adapted from Feeser and Simon [15] and Ahmed *et al.* [17].

KEY POINTS

- Collaboration can enhance the productivity of all involved, though care must be taken to foster respectful relationships within the group.
- Communication and cooperation are essential and the PI must take care to balance the goals of the project with those of each member of the team.
- By delineating clear goals, boundaries and roles for each member and being responsive and considerate of their differing backgrounds and perspectives, each member's unique skill set can be utilized to accomplish goals not possible for any single member alone.

References

1 VanWormer, A., Lindquist, R., Robiner, W., and Finkelstein S. (2012) Interdisciplinary collaboration applied to clinical research: an example of remote monitoring in lung transplantation. *Dimens Crit Care Nurs*, **31**(3):202–210.
2 Bozeman, B. and Corley, E. (2004) Scientists collaboration strategies: implications for scientific and technical human capital. *Res Policy*, **33**(4):599–616.
3 Martin-Sempere, M.J., Rey-Rocha, J., and Garzon-Garcia, B. (2002) The effect of team consolidation on research collaboration and performance of scientists: Case study of Spanish university researchers in geology. *Scientometrics*, **55**(3):377–394.
4 Lee, S. and Bozeman, B. (2005) The impact of research collaboration on scientific productivity. *Soc Stud Sci*, **35**(5):673–702.
5 Loucks-Horsley, S., Hewson, P.W., Love, N., and Stiles, K.E. (1998) *Designing Professional Development for Teachers of Science and Mathematics*. Corwin Press, Thousand Oaks, CA.
6 Short, A., Holdgate, A., Ahern, N., and Morris, J. (2009) Enhancing research interest and collaboration in the interdisciplinary context of emergency care. *J Interprof Care*, **23**(2):156–168.
7 Emergency Nurses Association (2006) Emeregency nurses association position statement: collaborative and interdisciplinary research. *J Emerg Nurs*, **32**(5):385–387.
8 Fawcett, T.J. and McCulloch, C. (2014) Pursuing a career in nursing research. *Nurs Stand*, **28**(28):54–58.
9 Chapman, R. and Combs, S. (2005) Collaboration in the emergency department: an innovative approach. *Accid Emerg Nurs*, **13**(1):63–69.
10 Institute of Medicine (2006) Emergency Medical Services: At the Crossroads. The National Academies Press, Washington, DC.
11 Messmer, P.R., Zalon, M.L., and Phillips, C. (2014) ANF schollars (1955–2012): stepping stones to a nursing research career. *Appl Nurs Res*, **27**(1):2–24.
12 Emden, C. (1998) Establishing a 'track record': research productivity and nursing academe. *Aust J Adv Nurs*, **16**(1):29–33.
13 Lewis, L.M., Callaham, M.L., Kellermann, A.L., *et al.* (1998) Collaboration in emergency medicine research: a consensus statement. *Ann Emerg Med*, **31**(2):160–165.
14 International Committee of Medical Journal Editors (2014) Recommendations for the Conduct, Reporting, Editing and Publication of Scholarly Work in Medical Journals: Roles and Responsibilities of Authors, Contributors, Reviewers, Editors, Publishers and Owners: Defining the Role of Authors and Contributors. http://www.icmje.org/icmje-recommendations.pdf (last accessed 12 May 2015).
15 Feeser, V.R. and Simon, J.R. (2008) The ethical assignment of authorship in scientific publications: issues and guidelines. *Acad Emerg Med*, **15**:963–969.
16 Marco, C.A. and Schmidt, T.A. (2004) Who wrote this paper? Basics of authorship and ethical issues. *Acad Emerg Med*, **11**(1):76–77.
17 Ahmed, S.M., Maurana, C.A., Engle, J.A., *et al.* (1997) A method for assigning authorship in multiauthored publications. *Fam Med*, **29**(1):42–44.

PART 3
Getting it out there: Analyzing and publishing your study

Eliminating common misconceptions to enable intelligent use of biostatistics: How can a novice use statistics more intelligently?

Gary Gaddis

St. Luke's Hospital of Kansas City, MO, USA

Would you use a chisel to drive a screw? Would you use a hammer to smooth a wooden surface? Hopefully, you would not. Just as a good carpenter would not use tools inappropriately, an experienced researcher would not use the wrong biostatistical tool to categorize or analyze research data.

Biostatistics is a difficult topic to master. However, for a researcher, statistical tests and techniques are tools in their research "toolbox." Like a good carpenter, no researcher learns the appropriate use of all of their tools overnight. However, with time and mentoring, both the carpenter and the biomedical researcher can become expert at use of the tools of their trade.

You can gain expertise at analyzing, presenting, and discussing research data by applying the lessons about statistical tools that are presented in this book. Data are the raw materials to which the tools of biostatistics are applied.

This chapter will teach you to distinguish different types of data, so you can use the correct tools to analyze and present that data, instead of committing statistical errors.

Recognizing types of data [1]

Medical researchers almost always collect or tally numbers. Three types of numeric (quantitative) data exist. Each of these types of data is described and analyzed by different statistical tools. Researchers *must* be able to distinguish types of data, in order to be able to select the proper statistical tools to describe and analyze that data without committing a statistical error. Types of data include:

- *Nominal data*: Rates, proportions, or frequencies of observations classed into named categories. (The names of the categories are chosen by the researcher.)
- *Ordinal data*: Numeric data collected using a rank-ordered scale.
- *Interval or ratio data*, which is also called *"parametric data"*: Data that can be expected to fit the Gaussian, or "normal" distribution. Ratio data have a minimum value of zero (such as age or degrees Kelvin), while interval data can have a negative value (such as degrees Celsius). Otherwise, they are essentially identical.

(Qualitative data, by which subjects provide the words to answer research questions, are seldom studied in medical research, and will not be further described in this chapter.)

A landmark study that strongly influenced clinical practice and contains all three types of quantitative data is that of Sullivan *et al.* [2]. This manuscript, "Early Treatment with Prednisolone or Acyclovir in Bell's Palsy", was produced by a group in Scotland and was published in the *New England Journal of Medicine*. This manuscript delivered strong and clear evidence that full recovery from Bell's Palsy is enhanced by prednisolone, but not by acyclovir [2]. The manuscript also provides examples of the statistical concepts discussed in this chapter.

Doing Research in Emergency and Acute Care: Making Order Out of Chaos, First Edition. Edited by Michael P. Wilson, Kama Z. Guluma, and Stephen R. Hayden.

© 2016 John Wiley & Sons, Ltd. Published 2016 by John Wiley & Sons, Ltd.

Table 27.1 Proportions of patients manifesting a Grade 1 House–Brackmann scale (complete recovery from Bell's palsy).

Characteristic	Prednisolone	No Prednisolone	p-value	Acyclovir	No Acyclovir	p-value
Time	(n = 251)	(n = 245)		(n = 247)	(n = 249)	
At 3 months	205/247 (83.0%)	152/239 (63.6%)	<0.001	173/243 (71.2%)	184/243 (75.7%)	0.50
At 9 months	237/251 (94.4%)	200/245 (81.6%)	<0.001	211/247 (85.4%)	226/249 (90.8%)	0.10

Source: Adapted from Sullivan *et al.* 2007 [2].

Nominal data

Nominal data consist of numeric rates, proportions, or frequencies. The primary outcomes Sullivan *et al.* studied were frequencies of full facial motor recovery observed three months and nine months after initiation of treatment for Bell's Palsy.

The four treatment conditions were prednisolone without acyclovir, acyclovir without prednisolone, prednisolone plus acyclovir, and no active medication. The two primary outcomes reported were whether or not full recovery of facial nerve function ("Grade 1 on House–Brackman Scale") was achieved at three months and at nine months after onset of Bell's Palsy. Table 27.1 shows the data regarding the frequency of full facial nerve recovery that appeared in Table 2 of the Sullivan *et al.* manuscript. Although patients were randomized into one of four groups as noted above, the results were tallied as frequency data, as noted here in Table 27.1.

Ordinal data

Ordinal data are data grouped into rankings, from low to high or from high to low. Sullivan *et al.* used the ordinal "House–Brackman" score [3] for judging the degree of facial palsy, which can be scored from 1 (no paralysis) to 6 (total paralysis).

A critical feature of any ordinal data is that an incremental difference of one rating point does not have a consistent meaning. The amount of difference between House–Brackman scores of 1 versus 2 is not equivalent to the difference between scores of 5 versus 6. CHADS2 scores for risk of stroke with atrial fibrillation [4] and Glasgow Coma Scale scores [5] are other examples of ordinal data that are probably more familiar to many clinicians. Notice that these ordinal data are dimensionless; there are no units of measure that can be applied to ordinal data.

For all of these scoring systems, *there is no consistent level of difference between scores on an ordinal data scale*. A consequence of this distinction is that it is inappropriate to attempt to calculate a mean or standard deviation for ordinal data.

Interval or ratio (parametric) data

Parametric data are normally distributed (or nearly so) and *the magnitude of difference between the gradations of parametric data scales is consistent*. Whether the data are "interval scale" (data with no absolute zero, such as temperature in degrees C or F) or "ratio scale" (data with an absolute zero, such as temperature in degrees K, or age), this consistency of the data scale is always present. Parametric data have a dimension, a unit of measure (such as kilograms, meters, seconds, etc, … units that have a consistent level of magnitude everywhere on the data management scale) that can be subjected to dimensional analysis. To have dimension is a key way to distinguish parametric data from ordinal data, which are dimensionless.

Sullivan *et al.* reported their subjects' age in years, an example of ratio scale data (Table 27.2). There is a consistent meaning of an increment of *n* year(s) between any two possible uniformly-spaced ages. This consistency permits valid calculation of a mean and standard deviation, characterizations not valid for ordinal or nominal data.

Describing data [6]

Researchers can describe their data in terms of its "central tendency" and its "variability".

Central tendency and parametric data

Anyone who has ever computed an average has familiarity with "central tendency". For parametric data, three measures of central tendency exist. One is the mean, the arithmetic average of the data. Another is the median, the mid-most observation, which has half of the data points lying below it, and half lying above it. (Another way to describe median is to use the term "50th percentile") The final descriptor of central tendency is the mode, the most commonly observed data value. In the normal distribution, these three points are identical. However, in skewed distributions, where one

Table 27.2 Selected baseline characteristics of patients studied by Sullivan *et al.*

Characteristic	Prednisolone	No Prednisolone	Acyclovir	No Acyclovir Total	Total
Age (Years)	43.2 ± 16.2	44.9 ± 16.6	45.0 ± 16.6	43.0 ± 16.1	44.0 ± 16.4
House–Brackmann score	3.5 ± 1.2	3.8 ± 1.3	3.6 ± 1.3	3.7 ± 1.2	3.6 ± 1.3
Health Utilities Mark 3 score	0.80 ± 0.22	0.78 ± 0.21	0.79 ± 0.21	0.78 ± 0.22	0.79 ± 0.22
Derriford Appearance score 59	71 ± 37	75 ± 41	72 ± 39	74 ± 38	73 ± 39
Score on Brief Pain Inventory	10 ± 18	16 ± 21	12 ± 18	14 ± 21	13 ± 20

Source: Adapted from Sullivan *et al.* 2007 [2].

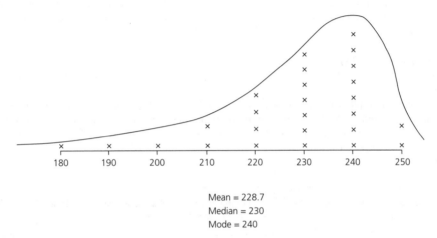

Mean = 228.7
Median = 230
Mode = 240

Figure 27.1 Systolic blood pressure in persons with renovascular hypertension. Mean, 228.7; median, 230; mode, 240. Source: Gaddis and Gaddis [6]; reproduced with permission from Elsevier.

"tail" of the distribution is longer than the other, the mean value lies toward the longer tail in a skewed distribution, compared to the median, while the mode lies at the "peak" of the skewed distribution (Figure 27.1).

Central tendency and ordinal data

For ordinal data, it is mathematically possible, yet methodologically incorrect, to use the individual data points to calculate an *apparent* mean value. It is inappropriate to calculate a "mean" of ordinal data, due to the lack of a consistent level of magnitude of difference between points on the data scale. Ordinal data is dimensionless. For example, Likert Scale data are not quantified in "Agreement Units", they are generally quantified as "Strongly Agree", "Agree", "Neutral", "Disagree" or "Strongly Disagree". There is no consistent order of magnitude of agreement or disagreement between the five points on the scale. This helps explain why such dimensionless data cannot have a mean. However, the median and the mode are appropriate descriptors of ordinal data.

Central tendency and nominal data

For nominal data, it is possible only to express the mode, the type of observation that was made most frequently in the study. With nominal data, there is no logical ranking of named data categories, so it is impossible to calculate a median.

Variability and parametric data

"*Standard deviation*" most thoroughly explains variability of parametric data. The standard deviation is the square root of a term called the "*variance*". The variance is the sum of squared deviations *from the sample mean*, divided by one less than the total number of observations:

$$\text{Variance} = \Sigma \left(x_i - \text{mean} \right)^2 / \left(n - 1 \right)$$

where n is the number of data points in the distribution and x_i is the value of each individual data point.

Deviations of each data point from the mean are squared in the variance calculation, so that a non-zero variability term is obtained. (If one calculated the difference between each data point and the mean in a normal distribution, the sum would be zero, because some data points fall above the mean, and the others fall below the mean.)

Another appropriate tool to express data variability is the *range*, a statement of the largest and smallest values observed.

Variability and ordinal data

Neither Standard Deviation nor variance can be computed for ordinal data because of the lack of a consistent size of difference of the units of the data scale, as previously described. Another way to express this is: Since ordinal data cannot correctly have a mean determined, ordinal data cannot have a variance or standard deviation correctly calculated, because the mean is used to calculate the variance. Variability of ordinal data is most commonly expressed by *"inter-quartile range"*, the range spanning the 25th to the 75th percentile values. Range can also be used to express variability of ordinal data.

Variability and nominal data

For nominal data, the only possible expression of data variability is to express the number of observations in each named category.

More detail regarding this topic is available elsewhere [6]. Sullivan *et al.* [2] expressed central tendency and variability for their data (Tables 27.1 and 27.2). They correctly used mean and standard deviation to describe subjects' ages, but incorrectly used mean and standard deviation to describe ordinal data that were studied as secondary outcomes. These ordinal scores included House–Brackman, Health Utilities Index Mark 3, Derriford Appearance Scale 59, and Brief Pain Inventory scores.

> By noting that mean and standard deviation were used inappropriately to describe the ordinal data in Table 27.2, you have just discovered a set of statistical errors in the esteemed *New England Journal of Medicine*!

Statistical inference, random sampling, bias and error [1]

A quirk but not a fatal flaw

Statistics permit researchers to infer a conclusion about an entire population based upon analysis of dependent variable data from samples of that population. Sullivan *et al.* inferred, from their patients with Bell's Palsy, that corticosteroids help increase the probability of full recovery from facial paralysis, but acyclovir does not [2].

This study was peculiar regarding how the authors assembled their study cohort. They went to the extraordinary step of establishing patient receiving centers at 17 hospitals, serving 88% of Scotland's population of 5.1 million persons, as their source for referrals. They nearly studied an entire population (Scots with Bell's Palsy), rather than a random sample. Usually, via random sampling, well-executed studies enroll a much smaller portion of the potentially eligible subjects.

If some factor unique among Scottish patients was to be likely to influence recovery from Bell's Palsy, the results that Sullivan's group obtained might not be applicable to other populations. However, many physicians would probably believe that Scotland supplied an appropriately representative population for study of treatment of Bell's Palsy, and the inferences from this study are broadly applicable.

The lack of random sampling and attempt to enroll nearly an entire population by Sullivan *et al.* thus constitutes a quirk, but not a fatal flaw that would suggest their conclusions were invalid. You will seldom read a manuscript for which the authors attempted to assemble an entire population or nearly an entire population. Random sampling is much more common, as it is less expensive and much easier from a practical perspective to study a random sample than to study an entire population.

Random sampling, a tool to decrease bias

Random sampling of a population is the tool that is usually employed to minimize bias in any study. *Bias* is any factor or attribute that can influence a study and make a particular conclusion more or less probable than would have been the case if that influence were not present. For example, if a researcher attempted to estimate the average height of

American males, and all study subjects were professional basketball players from the National Basketball Association, the non-random sample would be biased, because it should over-estimate the average height of American men.

All individuals in a population must have an equal chance of being a member of a study sample, if sampling bias is to be avoided. It is a matter of judgment to determine how much bias is introduced and how much influence on study conclusions exists when random sampling does not occur.

Numerous other aspects of a study's methodology can give rise to bias; space does not permit their enumeration here. (The reader is referred to other chapters in this book, especially Chapters 10 and 12.) As a result, all research studies risk stating erroneous conclusions [6]. The greater the degree of bias, the greater the probability of reaching erroneous conclusions.

Mechanics of statistical inference [7]

In any inferential study, two or more groups are compared for some trait during the testing of an hypothesis. An hypothesis that some type of difference between groups exists regarding this trait underlies most research. The hypothesis that a difference exists is known as H_1, *the alternative hypothesis*. H_1 does not specify the size of difference; it merely specifies that a difference is believed to exist. Because an infinite number of numeric sizes of difference are possible, H_1 contains an infinite number of hypotheses.

It is both impractical and mathematically impossible to attempt to test an infinite number of hypotheses. Researchers, therefore, must test the *"Null hypothesis" H_0*, the single hypothesis of zero difference between groups.

After collection of data and calculation of inferential statistics, the researcher can only reach one of two possible conclusions:

- One possible conclusion is that all groups studied appear to be statistically indistinguishable from each other (even though a numerical difference between groups is almost certain to be observed from the study data). This conclusion supports H_0. No *significant* difference appears to exist between the study groups. Statisticians would say that the null hypothesis is accepted as tenable.
- The only other possible conclusion is that the groups are inferred to appear to be different from each other, because a "significant" difference exists between the study groups. This difference is large enough that it is unlikely to have occurred due to chance. Statisticians would say in this case that the null hypothesis is rejected.

The statistical methods used to reach these inferential conclusions are rooted in probabilities. All inferential statistical methods yield a *"p-value"*, an expression of how probable the numerical difference(s) observed within the study were obtained due to chance alone. By convention, researchers deem any comparison between groups that appears to be less than 5% likely to have occurred due to chance alone as "statistically significant", and indicative of a probable difference between study groups. (This is the reason researchers often report, "Statistical significance was accepted if p<0.05.")

Type I and Type II errors

The fact that p <0.05 is deemed "statistically significant," leading the researcher to reject the null hypothesis, demonstrates a critical point. Statisticians and researchers inherently accept the fact that an erroneous conclusion, a conclusion that a difference appears to exist between groups when no true difference actually exists, can occur up to 5% of the time, which is to say, one time in 20. On the other hand, when the probability of difference by chance alone appears to be more than 5% or greater, statisticians say "the null hypothesis is accepted as tenable".

In summary, four possibilities exist with hypothesis testing:

- Biostatistics yield correct conclusions when the null hypothesis is supported as tenable, and the groups being compared do not differ from each other.
- Biostatistics yield correct conclusions when the null hypothesis is rejected, and the groups being compared truly differ from each other.
- Biostatistics sometimes suggest that a significant statistical difference exists between groups, when in fact the groups are not truly different. To reject the null hypothesis when the null hypothesis is true is to make a *"Type I" error*.
- Biostatistics sometimes suggest that no significant statistical difference exists between groups, when in fact the groups do differ from each other. To accept H_0 as tenable when it is false is to make a *"Type II" error*.

These possibilities are illustrated in Figure 27.2 (see Chapter 28, regarding statistical power, to learn more about how to decrease the probability of a Type II error).

		Truth/fact	
		Groups do not differ	Groups differ
Statistical inference	H_0 supported	Correct conclusion	Incorrect conclusion type II error
	H_0 rejected	Incorrect conclusion type I error	Correct conclusion

Figure 27.2 Correct conclusions, and Type I and Type II Error. Comparing possible findings of statistical inferential testing versus that which is actually true.

Matching the type of data to the appropriate inferential statistical test [8, 9]

When making comparisons between two or more groups, it is critical to use the proper inferential statistical test. It is a matter of using tools correctly! It is straightforward to list the appropriate statistical test to use, when certain data attributes are present [7, 8].

Inferential tests for nominal data

Most statistical testing of nominal data is performed using a *Chi-square test.* (The exception is that when a cell of a 2 × 2 contingency table has a frequency of four or less; then *Fisher's Exact Test* is used [7].) Chi-square testing compares observed versus expected outcome frequencies from each cell in a contingency table to derive a statistic with a numeric value. In this case, that statistic is called "Chi-square." Computer software can convert the value of the Chi-square statistic obtained directly from the data to the probability of obtaining that Chi-square value by chance, given the size of the contingency table developed by the experiment[7]. More about Chi-square testing is presented in Chapter 32.

Tests for ordinal data

For ordinal data, the appropriate test can be chosen after determining:

- Whether or not subjects participate in all treatment groups, as occurs in "cross-over" designs. Cross-over designs inherently decrease intersubject variability between groups. Thus, treatment effects can account for a relatively larger portion of the total variability between each individual subject's data.
- Whether or not "cumulative frequency grouping" occurs. Cumulative frequency grouping implies the use of a range of ordinal values within one outcome group. (For instance, grouping Glasgow Coma Scores of 3, 4, or 5 into one group is an example of cumulative frequency grouping.)
- Whether there are two, or more than two groups being compared. See Table 27.3 for a summary, which matches aspects of a study's design (whether or not a "cross-over" design is used) and the number of groups being studied to determine the proper inferential test for ordinal data.

Inferential tests for ordinal data require calculation of that test's statistic, such as the Mann–Whitney "U" for the Mann–Whitney test, or Friedman's "Q" for the Friedman test. From the numeric value of this statistic, calculated using the numbers that comprise the study data, the probability of obtaining the statistic result by chance can be determined. This process is highly analogous to how a Chi-square value for tests of ordinal data is used to determine the probability that the value of Chi-square could have occurred simply by chance. Statistical software performs these functions and provides the probability estimate ("p-value") that the researcher reports. For further detail regarding the underlying mathematical assumptions of these tests of ordinal data, or regarding the method of calculation of the test statistic for these tests and the translation of the value of the test statistic to a p-value, the reader is encouraged to consult a statistical text that addresses these matters.

Table 27.3 Picking the correct test for ordinal data.

Number of groups compared	Cross-over design?	Cumulative freq. distribution?	Correct test
2	No	No	Mann-Whitney "U (AKA Wilcoxon Rank Sum)
2	No	Yes	Kolmogorov-Smirnov
2	Yes	No	Wilcoxon Signed Ranks
3 or more	No	No	Kruskal-Wallis
3 or more	Yes	No	Friedman

For parametric data, the appropriate test to use depends upon the number of groups being compared. The *Student t-test* is used to compare two groups, and a form of *Analysis of Variance* (ANOVA) is used to compare three or more groups. Further, specific versions of the Student t-test can be used with cross-over experimental designs ("Paired t-test") and non-cross-over designs ("Non-paired t-test"). For more about ANOVA, see Chapter 32.

Multiple comparisons and Type I error rates

You may wonder why ANOVA, Friedman Tests, and Kruskal–Wallis tests are necessary and useful. These tests are specifically designed to determine, with a single test, whether or not a statistically significant difference exists among three or more treatment groups. The reason for their utility is clear to those who understand the impact of incorrectly making multiple inferential comparisons among three or more groups, using tests designed to compare two groups at a time.

The overall probability of committing a "Type I" statistical error, when making multiple comparisons between study groups, is $[1 - (1 - \alpha)^c]$, where "c" is the number of statistical comparisons made and α is the probability deemed to be "statistically significant" (Table 27.4).

For example, if a study has four treatment groups, six comparisons are possible…Group 1 vs 2, 1 vs 3, 1 vs 4, 2 vs 3, 2 vs 4, and 3 vs 4. Kruskal–Wallis and Friedman tests for ordinal data, and Analysis of Variance for parametric data, are designed to hold the experiment-wise Type I error rate constant at 5%, rather than being increased due to making the multiple possible intergroup comparisons. Contrast this 5% Type I error rate, when using inferential tests properly, to the probability of committing a Type I error that accrues from incorrectly making the six possible individual dual statistical comparisons. When setting p <0.05 to conclude a significant statistical difference for each individual test, the overall probability of making a Type I error rises to approximately 26.5%!

Sullivan *et al.* [2] reported a finding which clearly illustrates how a trial's Type I error rate increases with each additional statistical comparison that is made. They reported a statistically significant difference between groups for one of their secondary outcomes, which they discussed as a probable example of a Type I error.

Sullivan *et al.* reported 12 secondary outcome statistical comparisons for the three secondary variables they studied (Health Utilities Index Mark 3, Brief Pain Inventory, and Derriford Appearance Scale 59). Each of these was compared at three and at nine months after diagnosis of Bell's Palsy, for prednisolone versus no prednisolone and acyclovir versus no acyclovir groups.

The probability of making at least one Type I error when making 12 comparisons is approximately 46%. In Sullivan's study, 11 of the 12 secondary outcome comparisons were not statistically significant. However, one comparison yielded a statistically significant difference for quality of life (The Health Utilities Index Mark 3, when assessed nine months after onset of symptoms.) The data suggested that patients who did NOT receive prednisolone, and who were therefore less likely to have made a full recovery of facial nerve function, somehow had a higher quality of life at nine months after diagnosis than patients who received prednisolone. The data suggested an outcome that made no biologic sense.

The authors' discussion states the following, regarding this unexpected result: "Given that the secondary measures were obtained only in patients who had not recovered at three months, and *given the problem of multiple testing* (italics added), this result should be interpreted with caution" [2]. In other words, the authors dismissed a statistically significant difference between groups as unlikely to be correct, and they acknowledged that the greater the number of secondary outcomes compared in a study, the greater the probability of a Type I error.

This example also indirectly illustrates why most researchers and statisticians despise the practice of "data dredging," in which researchers will make numerous statistical comparisons, whether or not the comparisons make biologic sense, and whether or not the comparisons were planned before collecting data, in an effort to find something, anything, showing a statistically significant difference. "Data dredging" is a practice to be avoided, because it inherently requires multiple statistical comparisons to be made, while ignoring the fact that the probability of making a Type I error increases with multiple comparisons.

Table 27.4 Multiple comparisons impact the probability of a Type I error ($\alpha = 0.05$).

Number of comparisons	Type I error probability
1	0.0500
2	0.0975
3	0.1427
4	0.1855
5	0.2263
6	0.2649

The issue of multiple comparisons and the equation $[1 - (1 - \alpha)^c]$ also applies to evaluating the experiment-wise Type 1 error rate in studies that have primary and secondary outcomes. A study with one primary outcome and five secondary outcomes also makes six statistical comparisons. The probability of committing a Type I error when making six statistical comparisons is also approximately 26.5%! (Table 27.4)

Beware of studies with multiple secondary outcomes. They are reasonably likely to commit at least one Type I error. The fact that Type I errors are inherently more likely for secondary outcomes than for primary outcomes explains why secondary outcome findings that appear to be statistically significant should be restudied to determine whether a significant statistical association remains.

Summary

The prudent researcher and the prudent consumer of medical literature must be able to recognize the type of data being collected and analyzed in a study, in order to express study results correctly, in terms of characterizations of its central tendency and variability. Also, the type of data being analyzed must be known in order to pick the correct tool, the appropriate statistical test. Those who perform and read about research must also understand the concepts of Type I and Type II error, and the fact that experimental results are expressed as matters of probabilities, and not certainties.

KEY POINTS

- Three principal types of numeric data are reported in biomedical research.
- Appropriate methods are used to describe "central tendency" and "variability" of these types of data.
- Appropriate statistical tests are employed to make statistical inferences from these types of data.
- There is a relationship between the number of statistical comparisons reported in a manuscript and the probability that at least one instance of a "Type I" error will be committed, due to the number of tests done and not due to any error of application of statistical inferential techniques.

References

1 Gaddis, M.L. and Gaddis, G.M. (1990) Introduction to biostatistics: Part 1, basic concepts. *Ann Emerg Med*, **19**:86–89.
2 Sullivan, F.M., Swan, I.R.C., Donnan, P.T., *et al.* (2007) Early treatment with prednisolone or acyclovir in Bell's Palsy. *N Engl J Med*, **357**:1598–1607.
3 House, J.W. and Brackmann, D.E. (1985) Facial nerve grading system. *Otolaryngol Head Neck Surg*, **93**:146–147.
4 Gage, B.F, van Walraven, C, Pearce, L, *et al.* (2004) Selecting patients with atrial fibrillation for anticoagulation: stroke risk stratification in patients taking aspirin. *Circulation*, **110**:2287–2292.
5 Teasdale, G. and Jennett, B. (1974) Assessment of coma and impaired consciousness: A practical scale. *Lancet*, **2**:(7872):81–84.
6 Gaddis, G.M. and Gaddis, M.L. (1990) Introduction to biostatistics: Part 2, descriptive statistics. Ann Emerg Med, **19**:309–315.
7 Gaddis, G.M. and Gaddis, M.L. (1990) Introduction to biostatistics: Part 3, sensitivity, specificity, predictive value, and hypothesis testing. *Ann Emerg Med*, **19**:591–597.
8 Gaddis, G.M. and Gaddis, M.L. (1990) Introduction to biostatistics: Part 5, statistical inference techniques for hypothesis testing with nonparametric data. *Ann Emerg Med*, **19**:1054–1059.
9 Gaddis, G.M. and Gaddis, M.L. (1990) Introduction to biostatistics: Part 4, statistical inference techniques in hypothesis testing. *Ann Emerg Med*, **19**:820–825.

CHAPTER 28

Basic statistics: sample size and power: How are sample size and power calculated?

Manish Garg[1], Richard Harrigan[1], and Gary Gaddis[2]

[1] Temple University Hospital and School of Medicine, Philadelphia, PA, USA
[2] St. Luke's Hospital of Kansas City, MO, USA

> *"The day the power of love overrules the love of power, the world will know peace."*
>
> Mahatma Ghandi
>
> *"What about the love of sample size and power?"*
>
> Confused Researcher

Calculating an appropriate sample size to enable adequate statistical power is critical to planning any research study. A study that has an insufficient sample size and power will be unlikely to yield data that supports your hypothesis, even when that hypothesis is true. The consequence? Legions of readers will throw rotten tomatoes and lament "If only the study had been adequately powered to meet statistical significance!" Conversely, overly large sample sizes and power is not a good thing either. A study that is overly powered with astronomical sample sizes wastes resources because it could have been accomplished with fewer participants and less expense. Such studies are inherently able to deliver findings that may be statistically significant, but not clinically significant (e.g., think of cardiology registry studies where small changes in blood pressure show statistically but not clinically significant endpoints). So sample size and power is kind of like Goldilocks and the three bears – you want everything to be "just right."

In order to calculate the optimum sample size and power for your study, you need to understand the following research concepts:

- The purpose of sample size and power calculations.
- Important definitions relevant to sample size and power calculations.
- What is power?
- Factors that will influence sample size and power.
- When and how to calculate sample size and power.

The purpose of sample size and power calculations

Sample size and power calculations are estimates of how many participants are needed in a study [1]. Ideally, you would love to study a specific characteristic in the entire population, but this is rarely feasible. So instead, researchers measure the characteristic of interest in a select sample of the population and draw inferences about that population as a whole. Naturally, the greater the number of patients that are studied, the closer the measurements obtained in a study will approach the true value of those measurements in the entire population. We thus determine an estimation of sample size and power to figure out the minimum number of study participants needed to demonstrate a difference of a predetermined size or larger, without coming up short … and without expending the resources to study an excessive number of participants. (Remember Goldilocks; not too big, not too small, but just right.)

Doing Research in Emergency and Acute Care: Making Order Out of Chaos, First Edition. Edited by Michael P. Wilson, Kama Z. Guluma, and Stephen R. Hayden.
© 2016 John Wiley & Sons, Ltd. Published 2016 by John Wiley & Sons, Ltd.

Important definitions relevant to sample size and power calculations

You are an enthusiastic researcher who is attempting to answer a scientific question. You would like your study to be able to demonstrate a statistically-significant difference between groups, if indeed a difference is present. You wish to design a study that is unlikely to reach an erroneous conclusion. So let us first define the two types of hypotheses you must understand:

- The "**null hypothesis**" states that there is no difference between the two groups studied with respect to the variable(s) measured. The hypothesized size of difference between groups is exactly zero.
- The "**alternative hypothesis**" states that there is a non-zero difference between the two groups studied with respect to the variable(s) measured – and it is inferred that the observed difference is due to effect(s) of the treatment.

The alternative hypothesis is actually an *infinite number of hypotheses* from a mathematical standpoint because the size of difference is hypothesized to be a non-zero value. Since the null hypothesis is *a single hypothesis of zero difference*, it is the null hypothesis that is tested mathematically. Inferential statistical testing is used to estimate the likelihood that the size of difference observed between groups occurred due to chance. By convention, differences that are less than 5% likely to have occurred due to chance are deemed to be significantly different from a statistical and probabilistic perspective. This is why the expression "p<0.05" is used to denote a statistically significant difference between groups.

If the mathematics of hypothesis testing suggests that the numerical difference between the two groups you studied is not statistically significant (which is to say the numerical difference is 5% or more likely to have occurred by chance alone), you accept the null hypothesis. If the size of the numerical difference between the groups you studied is large enough that it is statistically significant (which is to say that the numerical difference is less than 5% likely to have occurred by chance alone), you accept the alternative hypothesis. Ideally, you would like to establish an alternative hypothesis that is clinically meaningful (clinically significant), that will make you the envy of the scientific community, and catapult you to unprecedented fame and glory.

Whoa tiger, settle down! You need to make sure you have planned your study so that you are unlikely to have committed one of these errors:

- A "**Type I error**" (a "false positive" represented by α) occurs when you *incorrectly reject* the null hypothesis (i.e., the null hypothesis is true, yet the inferential statistical tests applied to the study data led you to wrongly conclude that a statistically significant difference exists between study groups). By convention, researchers accept that most studies have a 5% chance of making this type of error. Type I errors can occur even though the researcher plans the study carefully and executes the study properly. One important means to decrease the probability of committing a Type I error is to minimize bias in a study's methodology. (Chapter 10 provides more information about bias.)
- A "**Type II error**" (a "false negative" represented by β) occurs when you *incorrectly accept* the null hypothesis (i.e., the alternative hypothesis is true, yet your inferential statistical test found no statistically different difference between study groups). By convention, via sample size planning, researchers accept a 10 or 20% probability of making these types of errors. So, Type II errors, like Type I errors, can occur even though the researcher plans the study carefully and executes the study properly. The most important means under a researcher's control to decrease the probability of making a Type II error is to study a sufficient number of participants.

What is power?

Now that you understand the hypotheses and types of error, let us introduce the concept of power. **Power** is the probability that the study will reject the null hypothesis when the alternative hypothesis is true (i.e., the probability of not committing a Type II error). As power increases, the chance of committing a Type II error decreases. Since the probability of committing a Type II error is the false negative rate β, **power is equal to $1 - β$** (which happens to be another formula for sensitivity; in other words, the sensitivity of the experiment to find a significant difference between study groups when the groups are in fact different).

Factors influencing sample size and power

So now that you have defined power, it is important to understand the following questions that will influence sample size and power in your study:

- What statistical test do you want to use?
- What is the measurement variance of the effect you are studying?

- What is the magnitude (effect size) of the measured difference delta (δ) for which you are looking? (And is it clinically or just statistically significant?)
- How important is the Type I or Type II error in determining your sample size?

Let us begin with the type of statistical test you want to use. It is important to note that the type of statistical test used affects how the sample size is calculated. Tests can be divided into parametric tests and non-parametric tests. **Parametric tests** deal with data that can be expected to be normally distributed and utilize the sample mean and the sample variance for their calculation. **Non-parametric tests** are used when the data are not normally distributed [like nominal (categorical) or ordinal (rank-ordered) data, *a* – see Chapter 27 for more information about this]. Parametric tests involve certain assumptions, such as that the data are normally distributed about the mean. If those assumptions are correct, parametric tests are more accurate and precise for determining differences between groups than non-parametric tests applied to the same data. (Parametric tests also have more power than non-parametric tests, but if the assumptions that underlie parametric tests are incorrect, those tests can deliver incorrect conclusions.) So, what does this mean for your study? Simple, you must determine if your data are likely to be normally distributed or not. If they are, you should choose a parametric test. If they are not, choose a non-parametric test, but realize that it will need more sample size than a parametric test to maintain power. The bottom line is that it is important to choose the right inferential test to analyze your data, and the characteristics of the inferential test will have an influence on the necessary sample size.

> An example of parametric data is the height of male Americans. The data are measured on a continuously distributed scale, where the size of a difference of one unit is always the same (e.g., an inch is always an inch; a centimeter is always a centimeter). The height of male Americans will be "normally distributed", which means that it will have a frequency distribution in the shape of a "bell curve."
>
> An example of ordinal data would be how those men respond to the statement, "I believe that the President is doing a good job." The men could be offered a survey and they could use Likert Scale data (Strongly Agree, Agree, Neutral, Disagree, Strongly Disagree) to rate the job performance of the President. These data are unlikely to be normally distributed and the size of difference between data points is not constant or discoverable.
>
> An example of categorical or nominal data would be the blood types of those men. How many are Type "A", Type "B" Type "AB", and Type "O"?

Another important factor influencing power and sample size is the **measurement variance**. Variance is mathematically related to the more commonly understood concept of standard deviation (which is the square root of variance). Variance measures how far a set of data points is spread out from the mean value. In your study, you are selecting a sample that will hopefully give you a probability distribution that accurately represents and includes the true value in the population. Now let's suppose you use a 95% confidence interval to describe the reliability of your sample while hoping the true mean value is not located far from your sample mean value.

> A 95% confidence interval defines the range of data values that are 95% likely to contain the true population mean, μ, as estimated from the sample mean $\bar{x}$.

Since the size of a confidence interval is inversely proportional to the number of participants studied, you want to maximize your sample size to reduce the negative effects of variance. What is the take-home message? A study with a small sample size will have large confidence intervals and will show statistical significance only if there is a large difference between groups; the same study with a larger sample size will have smaller confidence intervals and so will be able to demonstrate a statistically significant difference, when the groups being compared actually differ, even with a small difference between groups. Another way to say this is that larger sample sizes yield more narrow confidence intervals for expressing the range of values in which the true population value, as inferred from sample data, is likely to lie. Further, larger sample sizes will be able to discern relatively small sizes of difference between groups as significantly different.

The next question to ask yourself is: "Is the **magnitude** of the measured difference between groups both **statistically significant** and **clinically significant**? The magnitude of the difference is termed "delta" (δ). This magnitude is also referred to as the "effect size." Whereas you want a sample size that is sufficiently large to be powered to show a

Box 28.1 A tale of statistically versus clinically significant results.

An example of a statistical difference that many eventually came to believe did not provide a clinically useful effect is the example of administering corticosteroids to patients with acute spinal cord injuries. The National Acute Spinal Cord Injury Studies (NASCIS) II [2] and III [3] provided evidence that patients with complete or incomplete spinal cord injuries could achieve statistically significant gains in sensory and motor function if high-dose corticosteroids were administered promptly; these studies changed the way care was provided for these patients. Later, Nesathurai and Shanker [4] performed a critique of these studies, citing various methodological issues that cast doubt on the conclusions and, more importantly, highlighted that the clinical gains from high-dose corticosteroids were questionable. In addition, high-dose corticosteroids have widely recognized adverse effects, such as an increased probability of infections and avascular necrosis of bone. This has resulted in a change of recommendations from professional societies regarding high-dose steroids. The Congress of Neurological Surgeons has concluded that high dose corticosteroid therapy "…should be undertaken with the knowledge that the evidence suggesting harmful side effects is more consistent than any suggestion of clinical benefit" [5]. The Canadian Association of Emergency Physicians also no longer recommends this therapy as the standard of care in spinal cord injured patients. The 2013 guidelines issued by the Congress of Neurological Surgeons and the American Association of Neurological Surgeons recommend against the use of high-dose steroids early after an acute spinal cord injury, due to the lack of medical evidence for their efficacy and the probability of harmful adverse effects [6].

statistically significant difference, when a difference between groups is actually present, you also do not want to be overpowered, because you will waste time and resources. (You also potentially run the risk of finding a difference that is statistically but not clinically significant.) For example, registry studies (e.g., cardiology and trauma) at times involve thousands of patients that are typically retrospectively reviewed. Since the sample size and power in these studies are enormous, often very small findings (e.g., a few millimeters of mercury in a cardiology blood pressure registry study) can represent statistically significant differences between groups, which has minimal, if any, clinical significance. So if the mean blood pressure in a cardiology registry study is 150/80 in the treatment group, compared to a mean blood pressure of 154/84 in the placebo group, a numerical and statistical difference that is not clinically significant could result. Conversely, in an appropriately powered study with the right sample size, a blood pressure of 150/80 in the treatment group compared to a blood pressure of 165/100 in the placebo group that is (let us say) statistically significant would also represent a clinically significant distinction. What is the conclusion? An integral component of a sample size calculation is determining the size of difference between groups, δ, that you define as a clinically important difference. The sample size that is planned is the minimum sample size required, given the expected variances, to be 80 or 90% likely (depending on the power you choose) to find a difference between groups of size δ or larger (Box 28.1).

And what about the influence of Type I and Type II errors? This is very important. Remember, Type I error occurs when we incorrectly reject the null hypothesis (i.e., the false positive rate) and a Type II error occurs when we incorrectly accept the null hypothesis (i.e., the false negative rate). When determining an acceptable probability threshold for Type I error (denoted $p\alpha$), the industry standard is to choose a probability of <0.05. This means that, given a positive finding in a study, the chance of discovering this positive finding, or something greater, by chance, would occur on less than 5% of occasions. The $p\alpha$ of your study will be preset by you as you perform your sample size calculation (denoted, N). When determining an acceptable probability threshold for Type II error (denoted $p\beta$), the industry standard is to choose a probability of 0.8–0.9. This means that if there is a true difference in a study, we will find it 80–90% of the time. So how do you bring it all together? Statistical power is $(1 - p\beta)$ and represents the probability that the study will detect a true difference of size δ between two study entities, given a preset value of $p\alpha$ and a sample size, N.

When should you perform a sample size calculation?

The answer to the above question is (100%) before you start your study, and often during or after the study concludes. Ideally, you would love to have the foresight and vision to establish *a priori* your sample size and power calculations such that you could accurately estimate the needed sample size 100% of the time. However, the reality of any study is that before collecting data, the researcher must make certain assumptions about the desired effect size and variance, and your original study assumptions may not be totally accurate. For this reason you may wish to perform interim power calculations, using the size of the variance actually observed (rather than the estimated size used when planning the study) to see if you have the Goldilocks amount of sample size to find a difference of size δ. If your study finds a significant difference between groups, by definition your study was not underpowered. However, when the statistics support the null hypothesis, it is possible that the study was underpowered. The researcher should calculate power, given the number of participants studied, the size of difference δ between groups that is deemed to be clinically significant, and the variance observed from the data. Remember, you do not want to come up short with your numbers and you do not want too many data points (especially if time, resources, or potentially adverse outcomes are declaring themselves). It is important to mention that you should be able to calculate the sample size and power when you are evaluating someone else's work. That will let you know whether the large famous trial with "negative results" was likely to be due to the study being underpowered instead of a finding that should be trusted.

How do you perform a sample size and power calculation when testing for a possible difference between groups?

So let us put this all together with a concrete example and go through the mathematics. You probably will phone a statistician friend or order some specialized statistical software to perform your mathematical calculation for you (particularly if you are reporting categorical non-parametric data), but we can easily show an example of a comparative study that uses continuous normally distributed parametric data.

So, let us say you are trying to assist your emergency medicine colleagues from the scourge of rampant abscesses infesting the globe by studying a new antibiotic (RIFM) that is targeted against MRSA. From your previous pilot study and reviewing the literature, conventional antibiotics plus incision and drainage therapy takes, on average, four days to "heal" (which you will operationally define) with a standard deviation of three days. You believe RIFM (short for "**R**esistance **i**s **f**utile **M**RSA") plus incision and drainage therapy should demonstrate an improved healing time of two days which you believe is clinically important. What kind of sample size would you need for this study using conventional error and power set points? [1]

Organizing our thoughts onto paper:

What is the null hypothesis?	That RIFM will demonstrate no improvement in time-to-healing over conventional therapy
What is the alternative hypothesis?	That RIFM will demonstrate an improvement in time-to-healing over conventional therapy
What type of data, what statistical test?	Continuous normally distributed, t-test
pα level to avoid a Type I error?	0.05
pβ level to avoid a Type II error?	0.8
What is the clinically important difference δ?	2 day improvement in healing
What is the standard deviation?	From other studies, we ascertained 3 days

Now we need to calculate the effect size, also known as the "standardized difference." The equation for the standardized difference is:

$$\text{Standardized difference} = \frac{\text{Difference between the means}(\text{the clinically important difference})}{\text{Population standard deviation}}$$

So in our example the standardized difference = 2 days/3 days = 2/3 = 0.67. Next, to calculate our sample size we can either use a nomogram developed by Gore and Altman or a sample size formula. The Gore and Altman nomogram [7] is represented in Figure 28.1.

The Gore and Altman nomogram lists the standardized difference on the left vertical axis, the power on the right vertical axis, and the pα in the center (which will give you the sample size **N** which will need to be divided into two treatment groups). You make a line from the standardized difference to the power and "Eureka," you have your sample size. Let us plug in our numbers. Since the standardized difference is 0.67 and the power is 0.8, our line would intersect the sample size line at 70 participants – requiring 35 patients in the RIFM group and 35 patients in the conventional therapy group (plotted in Figure 28.2).

The other method of determining sample size is to use a sample size formula. The sample size formula [8] is:

$$N = \frac{2}{d^2} \times c_{p,power}$$

where "N" represents the number of participants required in each group, "d" represents the standardized difference, and $c_{p,power}$ represents a constant defined by the values chosen for the pα value and pβ (power). Commonly used values for $c_{p,power}$ are shown in Table 28.1.

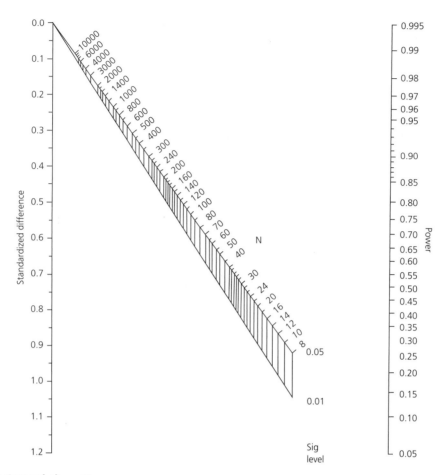

Figure 28.1 The Gore and Altman Nomogram.

Entering our values in the formula: $N = 2/(0.67)^2 \times 7.9$ (from pα of 0.05 and pβ of 0.80) = 35. Remember N = the number of participants required in each group, so you will need 35 patients in the RIFM group and 35 patients in the conventional therapy group. This is the same result as that obtained with the nomogram. You should practice adjusting the pα and pβ to understand the effect on your sample size.

How do you perform a sample size and power calculation when undertaking an equivalence or non-inferiority trial?

Our trial above, and really, the discussion for the entire chapter, has been about trying to prove that one drug is better than another. A non-inferiority trial is undertaken when a proposed new therapy represents less burden on the patient than the standard therapy. For example, consider a choice between two drugs to treat ventilator-acquired pneumonia. Clearly, if you wish to treat pneumonia, you want the drug that you pick to cure the patient, and you do not want the drug to cause adverse effects. Let us say that two drugs are options to use "Gentle-cillin," which recent data suggest seems effective, and "Gorilla-cillin," which has long been the current standard of care. If "Gorilla-cillin" has a high side effect profile, such as a high likelihood to cause *Clostridium difficile* colitis, and "Gentle-cillin" has less likelihood of causing this side effect, the question you should be asking is, "Is Gentle-cillin about as likely to cure the patient as Gorilla-cillin?" This is because you want to give the patient the best drug, the drug that is likely to enable a cure without causing adverse effects. The question of defining exactly what is meant by "about as likely to cure" involves subjective choices about what numerical difference of pneumonia cure rate is small enough to judge the differences between the two drugs

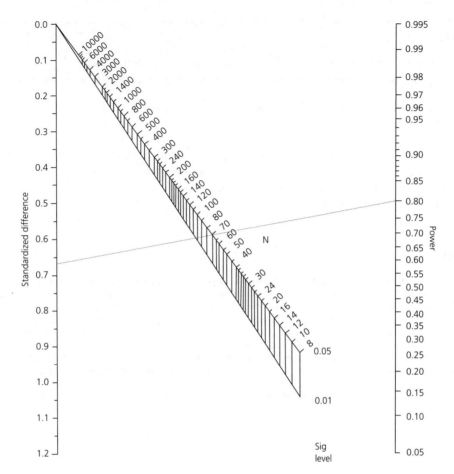

Figure 28.2 Sample size example.

Table 28.1 Common values for $c_{p.power}$.

pα	pβ			
	0.50	**0.80**	**0.90**	**0.95**
0.05	3.8	7.9	10.5	13.0
0.01	6.6	11.7	14.9	17.8

to be negligible. The assumptions that go into calculating the necessary sample size for such an equivalence or even non-inferiority trial (in which you are asking if one drug is "not worse" than another) are more complex than is the case for trials that look for a difference between treatments. If the reader wishes to learn more about sample size calculation for equivalence or non-inferiority trials, they are encouraged to consult a more comprehensive statistical text.

Summary

In summary, understanding and calculating sample size and power is critical to your study. You now have been given the power to determine one of the most important characteristics of your study – the sample size. What are you waiting for?

KEY POINTS

- Sample size and power calculations are estimates of how many participants are needed in a study.
- The "null hypothesis" states that there is no difference between the two groups studied with respect to the variable(s) measured.
- The "alternative hypothesis" states that there is a non-zero difference between the two groups studied with respect to the variable(s) measured.
- A "Type I Error" (a "false positive") occurs when you incorrectly reject the null hypothesis.
- A "Type II Error" (a "false negative") occurs when you incorrectly accept the null hypothesis.
- Power is the probability that the study will reject the null hypothesis when the alternative hypothesis is true.
- Variance measures how far a set of data points is spread out from the mean value.
- The best studies are both statistically and clinically significant.

References

1 Jones, S.R., Carley, S., and Harrison, M. (2003) An introduction to power and sample size estimation. *Emerg Med J*, **20**:453–458.
2 Bracken, M.B., Shepard, M.J., Hellenbrand, K.G., *et al.* (1985) Methylprednisolone and neurological function 1 year after spinal cord injury. Results of the National Acute Spinal Cord Injury Study. *J Neurosurg*, **63**(5):704–713.
3 Bracken, M.B., Shepard, M.J., Holford, T.R., *et al.* (1997) Administration of methylprednisolone for 24 or 48 hours or tirilazad mesylate for 48 hours in the treatment of acute spinal cord injury. Results of the Third National Acute Spinal Cord Injury Randomized Controlled Trial. National Acute Spinal Cord Injury Study. *JAMA*, **277**(20):1597–1604.
4 Nesathurai, S. (1998) Steroids and spinal cord injury: revisiting the NASCIS 2 and NASCIS 3 trials. *J Trauma*, **45**(6):1088–1093.
5 Hadley, M.N., Walters, B.C., Grabb, P.A., *et al.* (2002) Pharmacological therapy after acute spinal cord injury. *Neurosurgery*, **50**(Suppl):63–72.
6 Hadley, M.N. and Walters, B.C. (2013) Guidelines for the management of acute cervical spine and spinal cord injuries. *Neurosurgery*, **72**(Suppl 2):1–259.
7 Gore, S.M. and Altman, D.G. (2001) *How Large a Sample. Statistics in Practice.* BMJ Publishing, London, pp. 6–8.
8 Whitley, E. and Ball, J. (2002) Statistics review 4: Sample size calculations. *Crit Care*, **6**(4):335–341.

CHAPTER 29

Basic statistics: Means, P values, and confidence intervals

Daniel del Portal and Richard Harrigan

Temple University Hospital and School of Medicine, Philadelphia, PA, USA

Your friend, a non-physician, asks you if you have seen the latest episode of the popular television medical drama *Grey's Anatomy*. You laugh and tell him that you get enough medical drama at work. "Oh, come on, don't tell me doctors don't watch these shows," he says.

Confident that the physicians you know are too busy to indulge in trashy television, you bet him fifty dollars that doctors spend significantly less time watching medical dramas on television compared to, well … the rest of America. Citing the show's irresistible heartbreak and humor in every episode, your friend takes your bet.

You create a simple survey asking people to estimate the number of minutes they spent in the last month watching medical dramas on television. You distribute the survey to 30 of your physician colleagues at work, and you sample an equal number of people randomly in a public place. After you have collected all your data, you sit down to prove your friend wrong. It is only then that you realize you will need statistics.

Outlining your study

Firstly, you must define the characteristic on which you are comparing the two groups (physicians versus general public). In this case, that characteristic is the amount of time spent watching medical dramas on television.

Your friend is betting on the **null hypothesis**: he believes there is **no difference** between groups with regard to that characteristic. You have chosen an **alternative hypothesis** – the groups, in fact, do differ with regard to the characteristic – specifically that physicians spend less time than the general public watching medical dramas on television [1].

Describing your sample

How much television drama does each group watch? You sit down with your survey data and consider the various ways to describe the television watching habits of each group.

You need to decide which **measure of central tendency** to use to describe the distribution of values you have collected. The three most common measures of central tendency are the mean, median, and mode (see also Chapter 27).

- To calculate the **mean**, you sum all the reported values (minutes spent watching television) and divide them by the number of people in your sample.
- To calculate the **median**, you list each reported value in order from least to greatest and find the value right in the middle of your sorted list. This can be done easily by eliminating the first and last values on your sorted list. Do this again and again until only one value remains. This works well with samples that have an odd-numbered *n*. If your sample contains an even number of values, you will have to average the final remaining two values after eliminating from the top and bottom of the list. For example, in your sample of 30 people, the 15th and 16th values on your sorted list are averaged, and this is reported as your median (Figure 29.1).
- To determine the **mode**, you would list all the reported values and select the value most frequently reported. For example, if the most common answer were 30 minutes because that is the duration of the single medical drama that nearly everyone tunes in to, your mode would be 30 minutes (Figure 29.2).

Doing Research in Emergency and Acute Care: Making Order Out of Chaos, First Edition. Edited by Michael P. Wilson, Kama Z. Guluma, and Stephen R. Hayden.

Step 1: List all values in ascending order.

Step 2: Cross off the lowest and highest values one by one.

Step 3: Repeat until you are left with one number. That is the median. If there are two numbers remaining (as in this example), they are averaged.

$$\frac{29+30}{2} = 29.5 \text{ (median)}$$

The list of values: 3, 7, 8, 10, 10, 11, 15, 15, 20, 22, 23, 25, 25, 28, 29, 30, 30, 30, 30, 35, 36, 38, 42, 45, 45, 55, 60, 60, 72, 99.

Figure 29.1 Calculating the median.

Some people watch a lot of television and some watch very little. Most people cluster somewhere in the middle. This is your classic **normal distribution.** In a normal distribution, the mean, median and mode are all very close to one another (Figure 29.3) [2].

The more outliers you get (people who watch either a lot more or a lot less television than the rest of the sample), the more your distribution may be **skewed** in one direction or another. This might happen, for example, if you had sampled your retired aunt and a few of her friends in the nursing home who religiously tune in to every medical drama while your aunt proudly boasts that her nephew is a doctor. The high number of television minutes they report pulls the mean higher, but it may not substantially affect the median or mode, which could more accurately reflect watching habits for the entire sample and would, thus, be better measures of central tendency (Figure 29.3). This is important, because many statistical tests can only be used if your data is not particularly skewed [2]. If it is, you will need the help of a good statistician!

The mode is the value in your data set that occurs most *frequently*.

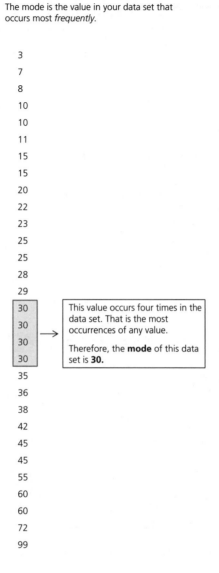

3

7

8

10

10

11

15

15

20

22

23

25

25

28

29

30
30
30
30

This value occurs four times in the data set. That is the most occurrences of any value.

Therefore, the **mode** of this data set is **30.**

35

36

38

42

45

45

55

60

60

72

99

Figure 29.2 Calculating the mode.

Comparing groups

You now have data for two groups, physicians and the general public, and you want to compare them to see if they are **significantly different** in terms of time spent watching television drama. When comparing two groups for differences, you must decide on whether you are running a **one-tailed comparison** or a **two-tailed comparison**.

A two-tailed comparison is used when you want to prove that two groups are different with respect to the characteristic you are studying. In our example, you would use a two-tailed comparison if you do not care which group watches more television. You just want *to show that the two groups are not the same* in the amount of television they watch [2].

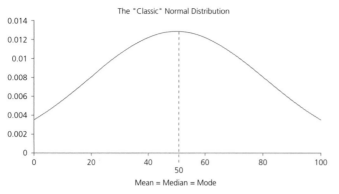

The "Classic" Normal Distribution

In the "classic" normal distribution, the *mean*, *median*, and *mode* are equal.

The y-axis represents the frequency in your data set (or in the population) of the corresponding value on the x-axis.

Mean = Median = Mode

Rarely will your own data perfectly fit a normal distribution. Let us look at the data you collected regarding minutes of TV watched by the general public.

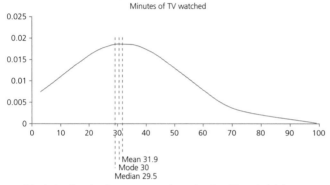

Minutes of TV watched

Your data set roughly follows a normal distribution. Although there are some outliers, the *mean*, *median* and *mode* are very close to one another.

Mean 31.9
Mode 30
Median 29.5

What is the effect of outliers on measures of central tendency? Let us include in our data set one person who watches 300 minutes of television…

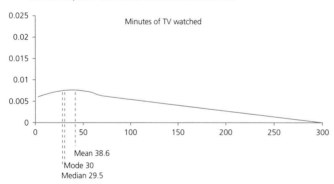

Minutes of TV watched

Outliers can *skew* the distribution. In this case, the inclusion of a single outlier who watches 5 hours of television daily has *skewed* the distribution. This pulls the *mean* higher but does not affect the *median* or the *mode*, which are therefore better measures of *central tendency*.

(Note the scale of the x-axis has been modified to include the outlier.)

Mean 38.6
Mode 30
Median 29.5

Figure 29.3 The normal distribution and measures of central tendency.

However, the way you phrased your bet, you win *only* if you show that physicians spend *less* time watching television than the general population. If it turns out physicians watch *more* television than everyone else, you still lose the bet. Therefore, you are only interested in whether there is a difference in one direction. In the language of statistics, you are performing a one-tailed, or *directional*, comparison. It is harder to meet statistical significance using a one-tailed comparison, a fact that you will remember next time you make a bet like this!

Accounting for chance

> *"Even a broken clock is right twice a day."*
>
> Stephen Hunt

Let us say that after reviewing the data you collected, you find that physicians do, in fact, watch fewer minutes of medical drama on television when compared to the general public. You want to *reject the null hypothesis* (that the two groups do not differ in amount of television watched). But what if your findings were just a result of chance and not really reflective of a true difference between groups?

The statistical concept that comes into play is that of the **p value**. This is the probability that the difference you observed between groups was due to chance alone. The more extreme the true difference between groups is, the lower the p value will be. In medical research, a common threshold for **statistical significance** is a p value less than 0.05. This means the difference you observed between groups would happen by chance less than 5% of the time, or 1 out of 20 times. Another threshold for significance may be chosen when the context supports it.

Most often, the p value is calculated using statistical software. When practical, increasing the sample size can increase **power** (Chapter 28) and decrease your p value when a true difference does exist.

The problem with P values

Your friend, it turns out, is married to a statistician and, after obtaining a brief consultation, he throws you a curve – he objects to your reporting statistical significance merely with p values! He suggests you employ **confidence intervals**, saying that this is a much better way to report significance and will add value to your conclusions.

Although for years p values were the principal and final common pathway on the road to reporting statistical significance, statisticians raised questions about their ability to do the job. Several criticisms have been offered. p values only reveal whether there is a statistically significant difference with regard to the characteristic of interest. However, p values:

- Do *not* reflect the **magnitude** or **precision** of the difference.
- Do *not* help you to decide if you can **generalize** the results beyond the sample you have studied.
- Do *not* address how the results might vary if the study were performed repeatedly.

Thus, confidence intervals have been used increasingly over time in the scientific literature in an attempt to address these pitfalls [3]. Confidence intervals help to quantify and give information about the certainty of your conclusions.

Confidence intervals: Another statistical weapon

There is a "more for your money" benefit when using **confidence intervals**. They will reveal if there is a statistically significant difference *and* they will give you information about that difference – the size, the precision, and the practical significance of the results. Moreover, even if there is no statistically significant difference between groups with regard to the characteristic of interest, confidence intervals allow a glimpse of the possibility that there may be a clinically important difference – one you might have detected had your sample size been larger (Chapter 28). Sounds like your friend's wife might be right!

Simply stated, confidence intervals are two numbers, reflecting *upper and lower limit* values, between which the "true" value for the population can likely be found; these limits include the result from your study sample. Similar to p values, they are expressed as probabilities; 95% confidence intervals have a 5% chance that the confidence interval does not contain the "true" value for the population; 99% confidence intervals have a 1% chance that the confidence interval does not contain the "true" value; and so on. Stated another way, if the "true value" lies outside your 95% confidence interval, *your data* would be expected to produce *this result* less than 5% of the time [4].

Returning to our example, let us say the non-physicians watched a mean of 480 minutes of medical dramas per month while the physicians tuned in for a mean of 320 minutes per month. That seems like a big difference … and let us suppose that analyzing your data showed that difference between means – 160 minutes – to be statistically significant for a sample size *n* at *p* < 0.05. But there is another way to look at this data: you can use a statistical package to calculate confidence intervals. For the sake of simplicity's, say that *your mean difference of 160 minutes* has a *95% confidence interval of 140–180 minutes* (or 160 minutes, +/– a confidence interval of 20 minutes). That means that if you repeated this study 100 times, the mean difference would fall in the range 140–180 minutes in 95 out of those 100 iterations of the study.

Interpreting confidence intervals

Several points can be gleaned from confidence intervals [5, 6]; these include not only statistical significance, but also clinical significance.

- If the confidence intervals **do not span zero** (with continuous data) then the difference is **statistically significant**.
- If they **do cross zero** (e.g., mean difference 160 minutes, confidence intervals –10 minutes to 330 minutes) then the difference between groups is **not statistically significant** – that difference could include 0, which means no difference between groups (you accept the null hypothesis), and it could run all the way to –10, which means the doctors watched *more* minutes of medical drama than their non-medical counterparts.
- If **95% confidence intervals include zero** within their range, this means the difference between groups is **not significant at a p value of 0.05**.
- The **width of the confidence interval** tells you something about the strength of your study's result. Narrow confidence intervals imply that your result is within a tight range of where the "true" result lies; this allows you to feel more confident that your result is close to the "real" result. But is it meaningful?
- **Narrow confidence intervals may show statistical significance, but may not be clinically important**. Back to our example – if you had an extremely large sample size and your study showed the mean difference between groups to be eight minutes, with a confidence interval of 6–10 minutes, then it *is* statistically significant, but … is eight minutes (or really, some value between 6 and 10 minutes) *really a meaningful difference* of time spent watching medical dramas?
- Conversely, wide confidence intervals may still be of use – for example, whereas the low end may be at or below zero, the high end of the range is equally likely to be where the "true" result lies. **Wide confidence intervals may encourage you to simply gather more subjects if you judge this possible effect to be potentially important – if not statistically significant at this time**. Restated, confidence intervals allow you to look at a "negative study" (confidence interval includes zero, not statistically significant) and decide if there might still be a *clinically* important difference (look at the upper end of the interval and decide if that difference would be clinically important).
  So, you agree to use confidence intervals, perhaps in addition to p values, when you report your data.

Application to clinical research

Suppose instead of comparing something as mundane as television watching time, you wanted to study something clinical, such as whether adding phenobarbital to a lorazepam-based sedation protocol affects the need for ICU admission in emergency department patients with acute alcohol withdrawal. This is precisely what Rosenson *et al.* did in a study published in *The Journal of Emergency Medicine* in 2012 [7].

In this study, Rosenson *et al.* compared two groups – alcohol withdrawal patients treated with phenobarbital versus those treated with placebo, with regards to a *characteristic of interest*, rate of ICU admission. Each group received either phenobarbital or placebo in addition to the standard lorazepam given by protocol. The *null hypothesis* in this case would be that both groups have similar rates of ICU admissions. The researchers, however, hypothesized that patients treated with phenobarbital would have lower ICU admission rates than patients who received placebo (the *alternative hypothesis*). They analyzed the results for 102 participants, 51 in the treatment group and 51 in the placebo group.

Rosenson *et al.* found that patients that received phenobarbital had fewer ICU admissions (8%) than patients who received placebo (25%), with p <0.05. They reported a 95% *confidence interval* of 4–32. This indicates a 5% chance that the difference in ICU admissions was either less than 4% or greater than 32%. Thus, with 95% confidence, the study demonstrated *at least* a 4% decrease in ICU admissions for the phenobarbital group. It also suggests that the reported decrease in ICU admissions (25% – 8% = 17% difference) may not fully demonstrate the true difference between groups, which could be as much as 32% fewer ICU admissions, again with 95% certainty.

An understanding of means, p values, and confidence intervals is fundamental to basic research statistics. Whether making a casual bet with friends or setting out to demonstrate the efficacy of a drug, you need to know how to describe your results in the most basic terms. Now you do.

Onward to the next topic…

KEY POINTS

- The *null hypothesis* states there is no difference between groups.
- *Mean, median and mode* are three measures of *central tendency* used to describe a sample or population.
- A *one-tailed comparison* looks for differences only in a specific direction when comparing groups with respect to a characteristic. A *two-tailed comparison* looks for whether two groups differ, but does not specify in which direction.
- The *p value* expresses the likelihood that a difference between groups is the result of chance.
- *Confidence intervals* not only show the presence or absence of a statistically significant difference due to the treatment(s) in question, but also give information on the magnitude and precision of that effect.

References

1 Jones, J. (2000) Research fundamentals: statistical considerations in research design: a simple person's approach. *Acad Emerg Med,* **7**:194–199.
2 Dawson, B. and Trapp, R.G. (2004) *Basic and Clinical Biostatistics,* 4th edn. McGraw-Hill.
3 Gardner, M.J. and Altman, D.G. (1986) Confidence intervals rather than P values: estimation rather than hypothesis testing. *BMJ,* **292**:746–750.
4 Wang, E.W., Ghogomu, N., Voelker, C.C.J., *et al.* (2009) A practical guide for understanding confidence intervals and *P* values. *Otolaryngol Head Neck Surg,* **140**:794–799.
5 Young, K.D. and Lewis, R.J. (1997) What is confidence? Part 1: The use and interpretation of confidence intervals. *Ann Emerg Med,* **30**:307–310.
6 Young, K.D. and Lewis, R.J. (1997) What is confidence? Part 2: Detailed definition and determination of confidence intervals. *Ann Emerg Med,* **30**:311–318.
7 Rosenson, J., Clements, C., Simon, B., *et al.* (2013) Phenobarbital for acute alcohol withdrawal: a prospective randomized double-blind placebo-controlled study. *J Emerg Med,* **44**:592–598.

CHAPTER 30

Basic statistics: Assessing the impact of therapeutic interventions with odds-ratios, relative risk, and hazard ratios

Jesse J. Brennan and Edward M. Castillo

Department Emergency Medicine, University of California San Diego, San Diego, CA, USA

> *"The best thing about being a statistician is that you get to play in everyone's backyard."*
>
> John Tukey

So you just had a brilliant idea for an intervention trial and you are feeling quite happy with yourself (as you should), but how will you determine if the intervention had any impact on the main outcome? Here we describe some simple but informative approaches to assess the impact of your intervention. By the end of this chapter, you will be able to answer the following questions:

- What is relative risk?
- What is an odds ratio?
- Which one should I use?
- Time as a factor: What is a hazard ratio?
- How do you interpret statistical significance?

Before we dive in, let us first address your most pressing question: *"Why in the non-statistical world must I be subjected to math"?* Given the availability of popular statistical software programs with point and click options, as well as free on-line statistical calculators, that is a fair question. The answer is not so you will literally be able to do it by hand (or by calculator), because quite frankly you will likely never need to. However, we highlight the different methods by which each is calculated so that you might better understand the subtle differences between relative risks and odds ratios. To this end, we must both "do the math".

Hypothetical study example

To illustrate how a relative risk and odds ratio is calculated, we will be referring to a hypothetical example of a randomized clinical trial targeting patients at risk for returning to the emergency department (ED) for repeated care (Table 30.1). Patients in the intervention group are treated with what we hope is the proverbial magic pill (or in this case a heavy dose of case management) while patients in the control group receive the standard of care. The outcome of interest is whether the patient returns to the ED for repeated care within 30 days of the initial visit (*Yes* or *No*).

Doing Research in Emergency and Acute Care: Making Order Out of Chaos, First Edition. Edited by Michael P. Wilson, Kama Z. Guluma, and Stephen R. Hayden.

What is relative risk?

Simply put, relative risk is a ratio of two event probabilities. In the context of an intervention trial, we might say that it is the risk of an event (or outcome) occurring in the intervention group compared to the risk of that event occurring in the control group. However, determining the risk (or probability) of the event occurring in each group is not as complicated as you might imagine. For this purpose, probability is equivalent to a proportion. Thus, calculating the relative risk is "relatively" simple. We simply divide the proportion of patients in which the event occurred in the intervention group by the proportion of patients in which the event occurred in the control group. The resulting relative risk value can then be used to interpret both the directionality and magnitude of the relationship; that is, whether the risk of the event occurring in the intervention group is more or less likely to occur than in the control group, and to what extent. A value of one implies identical risk for both groups; whereas, a value smaller than one indicates less risk of an event occurring in the intervention group compared to the control, and a value larger than one indicates more risk. For example, a value of 0.5 would indicate half the risk; while a value of 2.0 would indicate twice the risk.

Referring to the example in Table 30.1, the relative risk can be calculated as the proportion of patients in the intervention group with a 30-day visit ($15 \div 100 = 0.15$) divided by the proportion of patients in the control group with a 30-day ED visit ($20 \div 100 = 0.20$) (Box 30.1). So we find that the risk of coming back to the ED within 30 days for patients receiving case management is lower than the risk (or 0.75 times the risk) for patients receiving the standard of care ($0.15 \div 0.20 = 0.75$) (Box 30.1). Simple as π.

What is an odds ratio?

In its simplest form, an odds ratio is a ratio of the odds of an event occurring in two different groups. In the context of an intervention trial, we might say that it is the odds of an event (or outcome) occurring in the intervention group compared to the odds of that event occurring in the control group. This may sound similar to the definition of relative risk, but in this context the odds of an event occurring and the probability of an event occurring are not derived in the same manner.

To calculate the odds ratio, we first determine the odds of a 30-day visit separately for each group. For example, referring to the example in Table 30.1, the odds of a 30-day ED visit in the intervention group is equivalent to the

Table 30.1 Number of patients with a 30-day ED visit by study group.

Study Group	Outcome (30-day ED Visit)		
	Yes (not desired)	No (desired)	Total Patients
Intervention (enhanced case management)	15 (a)	85 (c)	100 (a + c)
Control (standard of care)	20 (b)	80 (d)	100 (b + d)

Box 30.1 Calculating a relative risk using the hypothetical study example in Table 30.1.

1 Proportion of patients in the intervention group with a 30-day visit:
$$a \div (a+c) = 15 \div (15+85) = 15 \div 100 = 0.15$$
2 Proportion of patients in the control group with a 30-day visit:
$$b \div (b+d) = 20 \div (20+80) = 20 \div 100 = 0.20$$
3 Proportion of patients in the intervention group with a 30-day visit divided by the proportion of patients in the control group with a 30-day visit:
$$\text{Relative Risk} = \left[a \div (a+c)\right] \div \left[b \div (b+d)\right] = 0.15 \div 0.20 = 0.75$$

Box 30.2 Calculating an odds ratio using the hypothetical study example in Table 30.1.

1 Odds of a patient in the intervention group returning to the ED within 30 days:

$$\left[a \div (a+c)\right] \div \left[c \div (a+c)\right] = a \div c = 15 \div 85 = 0.18$$

Note that "(a + c)" in the numerator and denominator cancel each other out, leaving us with a simple formula of "a ÷ c".

2 Odds of a patient in the control group returning to the ED within 30 days:

$$\left[b \div (b+d)\right] \div \left[d \div (b+d)\right] = b \div d = 20 \div 80 = 0.25$$

Note that "(b + d)" in the numerator and denominator cancel each other out, leaving us with a simple formula of "b ÷ d".

3 Odds of a patient in the intervention group returning to the ED within 30 days divided by the odds of a patient in the control group returning within 30 days:

$$Odds\,Ratio = (a \div c) \div (b \div d) = 0.18 \div 0.25 = 0.71$$

probability of the event occurring ($15 \div 100 = 0.15$) divided by the probability of the event not occurring ($85 \div 100 = 0.85$), or 0.18. Similarly, the odds of a 30-day ED visit in the control group is equivalent to the probability of the event occurring ($20 \div 100 = 0.20$) divided by the probability of the event not occurring ($80 \div 100 = 0.80$), or 0.25 (Box 30.2). Again, it is important to note here that the probability of the event occurring or not occurring is simply the proportion of patients in which the event does or does not occur. After we have determined the odds separately for each group, we can calculate the odds ratio by simply dividing the odds of a 30-day visit in the intervention group (0.18) by the odds of a 30-day visit in the control group (0.25). So we find that the odds of a patient returning to the ED within 30 days after receiving case management is less than (or 0.71 times) the odds of a patient returning to the ED within 30 days without case management (Box 30.2).

Similar to relative risk, interpretation of directionality and magnitude of the relationship also centers on the value of one. A value of one implies that the odds of an event occurring are identical for both groups; whereas, a value smaller than one indicates lower odds of an event occurring in the intervention group compared to the control, and a value larger than one indicates higher odds.

Which one should I use?

Generally, an odds ratio can be used in any type of study design whereas relative risk is reserved for either retrospective or prospective cohort studies. For instance, it is often preferable to use relative risk in a cohort study in which we might compare similar groups of patients who have either been exposed or not exposed (to treatment) in relation to the occurrence of an event or outcome. For example, if the goal is to simply describe which group is more or less likely to have a 30-day ED visit in relation to patient exposure to the intervention, the relative risk is straight forward and often easier to interpret than the odds ratio. Intuitively, it is just easier to speak to the *likelihood* of a 30-day visit than it is to the *odds*.

However, there is a specific type of study design, commonly referred to as retrospective case–control design, in which the use of relative risk is generally ill-advised. Imagine, for example, we wish to study potential risk factors for obesity in adulthood, such as being overweight as a child. Using a case–control design to address this question, we might first select an adult group of clinically obese patients and an adult group of non-obese patients, then assess the number of patients in each group who were overweight as early as five years of age. In such a design, in which group membership has been assigned based on the outcome rather than exposure, the probability of obesity (or non-obesity) in adulthood is more of a reflection of the number of patients assigned to each group than anything else, which simply makes the relative risk uninformative.

Finally, regardless of which type of study design is used, it is preferable (easier) to use an odds ratio if there is a need to account for (control for) additional factors (confounders) that might be related to the outcome. In such a case, more complex statistical analyses are employed, such as multiple logistic regression analyses. The resulting odds ratios are referred to as *adjusted* odds ratios, as they describe the independent association with the outcome with consideration to other covariates in the model.

So at this point you might be thinking: "The relative risk and odds ratio in this example are almost identical. Does it *really* matter which one I use?" Keep in mind that an odds ratio is often used to estimate true risk when true risk cannot be directly estimated; it is an approximation of relative risk. It just so happens that in most cases involving trials in a clinical setting, the outcomes under study are relatively infrequent (death, adverse event, etc.), in which case there is little difference, either literally or theoretically, between an odds ratio and a relative risk. However, the larger the initial probability of the outcome (i.e., the larger the proportion of patients with 30-day ED visits), the more dissimilar the odds ratio will be to the relative risk. For example, using the example in Table 30.1, consider that the proportion of patients with a 30-day ED visit was 0.60 in the intervention group and 0.80 in the control group (instead of 0.15 and 0.20, respectively). The relative risk would still be equal to 0.75 (0.60 divided by 0.80); however, the corresponding odds ratio would be approximately 0.38 (the odds of 30-day visit in intervention [0.60 divided by 0.40 = 1.50] divided by the odds of 30-day visit in control group [0.80 divided by 0.20 = 4.00]). In such a case, the odds ratio becomes over-inflated in relation to the relative risk.

Regardless of which statistic you decide to use, this last point is critical to understanding how assuming that the relative risk and odds ratio are equivalent to one another can lead to confusion and misinterpretation. From a clinical perspective, it would be appropriate to interpret the relative risk estimate of 0.75 to mean that the intervention reduced the risk of a 30-day visit by 25% (1 − relative risk). However, based on the corresponding odds ratio of 0.38, it is not appropriate to say that the intervention reduced the risk of a 30-day visit by 62% (we just determined that it is 25%). The confusion arises in the literature, for example, when an odds ratio is described as an outcome being *twice as likely* to occur in group A as group B, rather than *twice the odds*. Based on this language, we are likely to infer that researchers are actually describing relative risk, which we know is not the same. Although, even in such a case, if the relative risk and odds ratio were similar, are we really at terrible risk of reaching a different conclusion in our study (i.e., the intervention did or did not have an impact)? No, not really. We are likely to reach the same conclusion even if they are not similar. However, the more dissimilar these estimates are the more caution we need to take in interpreting an odds ratio in relation to effect size; that is to say, the impact of the intervention.

Time as a factor: What is a hazard ratio?

Now that we have described the difference between the relative risk and odds ratio, it is worth mentioning an additional approach that can be used when studying the timing of the event in addition to whether the event simply occurred or did not occur. For example, say we are not only interested in the risk of repeat ED visits within 30 days, but we are also interested in this risk over time; such as time to a repeat ED visit as measured by 3, 7, 14, 21, and 30 days from the initial visit. In this instance, we can examine a cumulative risk associated with each time point as well as relative risk for the entire study period taking time to outcome into consideration. This is what is referred to as the hazard ratio. While calculation of the hazard ratio is beyond the scope of this chapter, it can be generated using Cox proportional hazard regression analyses provided by most statistical software programs. In addition, you can visually inspect the relative proportion of patients who do and do not have a repeat ED visit over time (survival if you will) using a Kaplan-Meier plot. If, for example, the time to a 30-day ED visit for patients who received case management was longer than patients who received standard of care, it will be apparent on the plot and the hazards ratio will likely reflect a value greater in magnitude than our original relative risk obtained at 30-days, taking time to 30-day visit into consideration (Figure 30.1).

How do you interpret statistical significance?

The final piece to this puzzle is to determine whether the relative risk (or odds ratio) we find can be considered meaningful in the context of our intervention. To interpret statistical significance, we rely on the 95% confidence interval (CI). Essentially, if the 95% CI includes the value of one, then the estimate is not statistically significant, meaning that the probability of finding a relative risk (or odds ratio) of this magnitude by chance alone is greater than 5% (see also Chapter 29). For instance, in our study example shown in Table 30.1, the 95% CI for a relative risk of 0.75 includes the value of 1.0 (0.41–1.38). In this case, we would conclude that our intervention did not significantly impact 30-day ED visits, or that the risk of a 30-day ED visit for patients receiving case management was equivalent to patients who received standard of care. However, holding constant all other factors that contribute to a methodologically sound study, keep in mind that statistical significance is related to the power of a study to find a treatment effect if it truly exists. For example, if sample size is very large, a relative risk (or odds ratio) close to 1.0 may be considered statistically significant, but it does not necessarily mean it is clinically relevant. Similarly, if sample size is very small a relative risk

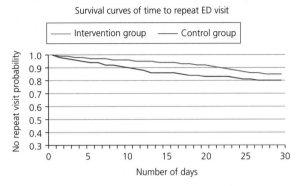

Figure 30.1 Hypothetical survival curves of time to repeat ED visit.

much higher (or lower) than 1.0 may not be considered statistically significant, but it does not necessarily mean that the treatment had no effect (see also Chapter 28).

Unless you are a contestant on a television game show, "p value <0.05" does not have to be your final answer. The p value simply informs us of the likelihood that the difference (or effect size) we are seeing between two groups may or may not be due to chance alone. However, if you have planned ahead of time you should already know whether your sample size is sufficient to detect a meaningful difference, and how large of an effect size you would need to reach statistical significance. If you do not have a lot of experience with statistics, do not be shy about consulting with someone who does before you begin collecting data. It will not matter how much data you collect or how well you collect it if in the end you cannot properly evaluate your study.

> *"To call in the statistician after the experiment is done may be no more than asking him (her) to perform a postmortem examination: he (she) may be able to say what the experiment died of."*
>
> Ronald Fisher

Final thoughts

Hopefully you will leave this chapter with a better understanding as to why the odds ratio and relative risk are not interchangeable and should not be interpreted as such, as well as how and when to use these tools to describe the results of your study. If not, you can always ask a statistician to do it!

KEY POINTS

- Relative risk is a ratio of the probability of an event occurring in two different groups (ratio of proportions).
- Odds ratio is a ratio of the odds of an event occurring in two different groups (ratio of odds).
- Odds ratio and relative risk are calculated differently and are not interchangeable.
- Odds ratio and relative risk values reflect both directionality and magnitude of the relationship being examined.
- The 95% confidence interval is used to interpret statistical significance.

Further reading

1 Chernick, M.R. (2011) *The Essentials of Biostatistics for Physicians, Nurses and Clinicians.* John Wiley & Sons Ltd.
2 Lachin, J.M. (2010) *Biostatistical Methods: The Assessment of Relative Risks,* 2nd edn. Wiley Series in Probability and Statistics, John Wiley & Sons Ltd.
3 Rudas, T. (1998) *Odds Ratios in the Analysis of Contingency Tables.* Sage University Paper Series on Quantitative Applications in the Social Sciences, 07-199, Sage Publications Ltd.

CHAPTER 31

Basic statistics: Assessing the impact of a diagnostic test; choosing a gold standard, sensitivity, specificity, PPV, NPV, and likelihood ratios

Stephen R. Hayden

Department of Emergency Medicine, UC San Diego Health Systems, CA, USA

> *Novice Medical Student:* "I am seeing a 23-year-old woman with shortness of breath and non-productive cough. She denies fever, smokes a pack a day, and takes birth control pills. I want to order a CBC, BMP, CXR, and D-dimer..."
> *Wise Attending Physician:* "Tell me how the results of the CBC, BMP and D-dimer will affect your clinical decision making in this patient?"

Diagnostic tests rarely establish the presence of a medical condition with certainty; instead, a physician uses test results to help strengthen their estimate that a disorder is either likely or less likely in an individual patient [1]. If a test is not going to inform decision making in this manner, clinicians should question why it is necessary to obtain it in the first place.

Our estimate of disease probability before knowing the result of a diagnostic test is called the pretest or prior probability and the estimate after knowing the test result is termed the post-test or posterior probability of disease. The degree to which pretest probability is modified to obtain an estimate of post-test probability is determined by the characteristics of the test. These characteristics are classically measured and reported in a number of ways and provide an idea of the *impact* the results of a diagnostic test will have on your clinical decision making. In this chapter the following characteristics of diagnostic tests are discussed as they commonly apply to acute care research:

- Sensitivity
- Specificity
- Accuracy
- Positive and negative predictive value
- Likelihood ratio.

Before considering these elements, however, it is worth mentioning what we mean by a "gold" standard. When designing or appraising a study on how good a particular diagnostic test is at distinguishing between patients that have the disease of interest and those that do not, the test needs to be compared to a standard or criterion that reasonable clinicians would agree makes the definitive diagnosis or defines the target disorder [2]. In other words, the accuracy of a diagnostic test is best determined by comparing it to the "truth" or as close to it as we can come. It is likewise important that ALL subjects that have the test of interest performed also have the gold (or "criterion") standard test completed [2]. This may not always be as straightforward as it seems. For example, in the early studies of the utility of computed tomography (CT) scanning for appendicitis, findings on CT were compared to presence of inflammation on the pathological specimen removed at operation. However, it is not only impractical but also unethical to design a study that unnecessarily subjects some patients to surgery they may not need. These early studies included only those patients already selected for surgery and so represented a skewed patient population (selection bias). The true practical

Doing Research in Emergency and Acute Care: Making Order Out of Chaos, First Edition. Edited by Michael P. Wilson, Kama Z. Guluma, and Stephen R. Hayden.

value of a test is established only in a study that closely resembles clinical practice and not just patients with severe disease. It is important to include an appropriate number of patients and spectrum of disease to assess the test in real life circumstances. Later studies looking at CT in appendicitis used a combined outcome of surgical pathology results or clinical follow up at 30–90 days as a criterion standard against which to compare CT results.

There are two other important aspects to consider when designing a study to evaluate a diagnostic test. Firstly, the interpretation of both the criterion standard as well as the new test should be *independent* and *blinded* to important clinical information or outcome [2]. This is especially important for tests that require integration or analysis such as radiological imaging. Secondly, the results of the test being evaluated cannot influence the decision to perform the criterion standard for comparison [2], otherwise the properties of the test will be artificially inflated; this is called verification bias. An example of this would be a study on patients with suspected acute coronary syndrome and exercise stress testing where patients with positive stress testing are more likely to undergo angiography (criterion standard) than those with negative stress testing.

> *"There is nothing like blinding a radiologist to ensure that an emergency physician will get an accurate result from a study evaluating the efficacy of a CT scan."*
>
> Stephen R. Hayden, MD

Test results when two outcomes are possible

In the acute care setting, diagnostic tests are often reported as "positive" or "negative" (binary outcomes), even if the actual data represent a number on a continuous scale. In the latter case a cutoff point is chosen above which the result is considered positive, below which it is negative; this is called dichotomization of continuous data. An example is quantitative D-dimer testing for pulmonary embolism in which a cutoff point of 500 µg/L is used for a commonly performed assay in patients under age 50 years. When results are reported this way, test characteristics can be described using *sensitivity, specificity, positive predictive value (PPV), and negative predictive value (NPV)*. These values are simple to calculate and understand using a classic 2 × 2 table (Figure 31.1).

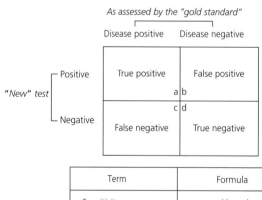

Term	Formula
Sensitivity	a / (a + c)
Specificity	d / (b + d)
Positive predictive value	a / (a + b)
Negative predictive value	d / (c + d)
Accuracy = Proportion of correct diagnosess divided by total #	(a + d) / (a + b + c + d)

Figure 31.1 A 2 × 2 Table for a diagnostic test.

Sensitivity and specificity

Sensitivity is the ability of a diagnostic test to reliably predict the presence of disease. It answers the question, "Of all people who have disease, what proportion is test positive?" Mathematically, it is calculated as the true positives divided by the sum of the true positives plus false negatives, or from the 2 × 2 table: a / (a + c). It is sometimes referred to as a "vertical" property of a 2 × 2 table, meaning that the values do not vary significantly with changes in the prevalence of disease in the population, whereas the positive and negative predictive values do. *Specificity* refers to the ability of a test to reliably predict the absence of disease. It answers the question, "Of all people who do not have disease, what proportion is test negative?" It is calculated as the true negatives divided by the sum of the true negatives plus false positives, or from the 2 × 2 table: d / (b + d). Like sensitivity, specificity is also referred to as a vertical property and does not vary much with prevalence of disease.

Two rules of thumb that are useful to remember in applying sensitivity and specificity are SPin and SNout. SPin refers to the situation in which a test with a very high specificity can help the clinician "rule in" disease if the result is positive, while SNout refers to the circumstance where a test with a very high sensitivity can help "rule out" disease if the test result is negative.

SPin: A test with a very high *Specificity* will "rule in" disease if positive.

SNout: A test with a very high *Sensitivity* will "rule out" disease if negative.

Take the example of a 23-year-old woman who presents with shortness of breath and non-productive cough for one day. She is otherwise healthy, denies chest pain except when she coughs, and takes no medications other than birth control pills. She has no recent immobilization or surgery, no history of deep vein thrombosis (DVT) or pulmonary embolus (PE), no history of cancer, and her examination is normal including normal oxygen saturation and no signs of a DVT. You feel she has a low probability of PE but cannot completely exclude it as a possibility. Consequently, you wonder if a D-dimer would help inform your clinical decision making. In this situation, you want to modify your estimate of pretest probability from low to extremely low; so low, in fact, that no further work-up is necessary and you can exclude PE in favor of an alternate diagnosis. This would require that D-dimer have a very high sensitivity (SNout). You are able to locate a very recent systematic review in the *British Medical Journal* from 2013 in which the pooled sensitivity from over 5500 patients in the age group less than 50 years is 97.6 (95% CI: 95.0–98.9) and feel confident that a negative D-dimer in your patient would exclude a PE [3].

Positive and negative predictive value

The positive predictive value (PPV) of a test relates to how likely a test will be positive when disease is truly present. PPV helps answer the question, "Of all the people who are test positive, what proportion will actually have the disease?" and is calculated as the true positives divided by the sum of the true positives plus the false positives, a / (a + b). Likewise, the negative predictive value (NPV) of a test reflects how likely a test will be negative when disease is truly absent. NPV helps answer the question, "Of all the people who are test negative, what proportion will not have the disease?" and is calculated as the true negatives divided by the sum of the true negatives plus the false negatives, d / (c + d). PPV and NPV are sometimes termed horizontal properties of the 2 × 2 table and ultimately vary with prevalence of disease in a population of patients.

Accuracy of a diagnostic test

The accuracy of a diagnostic test refers to its overall ability to predict both the presence and absence of disease. It is calculated as the sum of the true positives plus the true negatives divided by the total. Interestingly, this measure of a test is often not reported in many research studies; most probably because it loosely combines sensitivity and specificity, which often have an inverse relationship. In other words, in studies where continuous data are being dichotomized and a cutoff point is being determined, one must sacrifice sensitivity in order to maximize specificity and vice versa.

Likelihood ratio

Is your head swimming yet? If so, you are not alone. These concepts are not intuitive for clinicians in the acute care setting. While we are familiar with the terms sensitivity, specificity, NPV, and PPV, discussions about true positives, false negatives, and how NPV varies with disease prevalence are not practical at the bedside. Another disadvantage to these measures is that they can only be used in situations where test results are binary. For tests in which more than two results are possible, sensitivity, specificity, PPV, and NPV are no longer applicable. A classic example of this is the ventilation perfusion lung scan (or VQ scan) for pulmonary embolism. Results from this test are often reported as normal, low probability, intermediate, or high probability, and so do not fit neatly in a 2 × 2 table as in Figure 30.1. A *Likelihood Ratio (LR)*, however, does not suffer from this limitation and can be calculated and applied to any test result, whether binary, multiple, interval, or continuous data.

A LR also allows a clinician to more directly estimate post-test probability from pretest probability of disease. For many clinicians it is a more intuitive measure of the impact of a diagnostic test and helps answer the important question, "What are you going to do with the result of that test?"

Likelihood ratio for dichotomous test results

In the situation where two test results are possible, usually reported as positive or negative, the LR is referred to as either the LR positive or LR negative. The LR(+) is the probability of a *positive test result* in patients *with disease* divided by the probability of a *positive test result* in patients *without disease* [1]. It is the probability of the test result, NOT the probability of disease! Similarly, the LR(−) is the probability of a *negative test result* in patients *with disease* divided by the probability of a *negative test result* in patients *without disease*.

Mathematically, LRs can be calculated from a 2 × 2 table just like other measures of diagnostic tests and should be reported in studies evaluating a new diagnostic test or strategy (Figure 31.2).

A likelihood ratio is the probability of the test result; not the probability of disease.

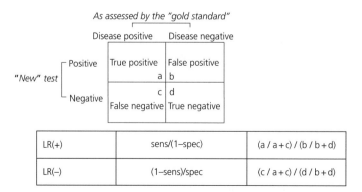

Figure 31.2 2 × 2 Table; likelihood ratios.

Rules of thumb [1]

- LR of 1 means test result does not change probability of disease = no impact.
- LR of 2–5 or 0.5–0.2 = modest impact on clinical decision making.
- LR of 5–10 or 0.2–0.1 = moderate impact.
- LR of >10 or <0.1 = major impact.

Consider the example of 27-year-old-man presenting to the ED with lower abdominal pain for one day. Initially his pain was poorly localized but now it seems it is worse in his periumbilical region. He denies fever, has mild nausea but no vomiting, and is able to tolerate oral foods but his appetite is diminished. He has a history of kidney stones but states this is different. His vital signs are normal and his examination is normal except for mild tenderness to palpation in the midline, lower abdominal area without overt rebound tenderness or guarding. You order a urinalysis and laboratory tests and suggest that an abdominal CT be obtained. The patient expresses concern that he has already had two CT scans in the past two years for recurrent kidney stones and asks if an ultrasound (US) might be an alternative?

In order to answer this question, you need to know the test characteristics of US for the diagnosis of suspected appendicitis in the acute care setting and what impact it would have on your estimate of this patient's pretest probability of appendicitis. This is easily answered by knowing the LR(+) and LR(−) of US for appendicitis in patients presenting to the ED with abdominal pain. In a multicenter study published in *Radiology* in 2013 by Leeuwenburgh *et al.*, the reported sensitivity and specificity of graded compression US was 77% and 94% respectively, the LR(+) was 12 and the LR(−) was 0.25 [4]. Knowing the sensitivity and specificity in this case does not help you as much in your clinical

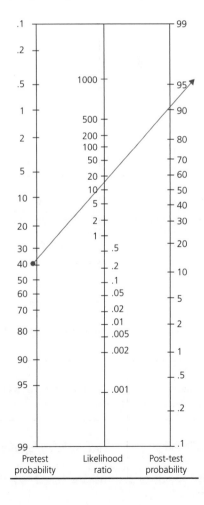

Figure 31.3 Fagan Nomogram[5].

decision making. You estimate your patient's pretest probability of appendicitis is in the low to moderate range, therefore the sensitivity is not high enough to rule out disease without further information or testing, and the specificity of 94% does not necessarily "rule in" disease with enough precision. However, starting from a low to moderate pretest probability of approximately 40%, if the US is positive for appendicitis, knowing the LR(+) is 12 allows a direct estimate of post-test probability of 90% using a simple nomogram [5], (Figure 31.3). Given the clinical scenario, and a probability of appendicitis of 90% or more, most surgeons would take this patient to the operating room. Conversely, if the US is negative, a LR(–) of 0.25 means his post-test probability of appendicitis is still 10–12% and further testing is necessary. Interestingly, in the same study by Leeuwenburgh *et al.*, immediate MRI was compared to the criterion standard if US was negative and the LR(+) for MRI was 15, and LR(–) was 0.04 [4].

Likelihood ratios for interval or continuous data

By nature, most laboratory information is quantitative. Interpretation, therefore, often depends on the *degree* of positivity or negativity of a result, not just qualitatively whether the result is positive or negative alone. Grouping together quantitative data into two arbitrary groups based on a cutoff point loses both information and the ability to more precisely discriminate between groups. Intuitively, though, clinicians would agree that there is a difference in likelihood that a PE is present in a patient with a D-dimer of 501 and a D-dimer of 5000, when 500 is used as the level to define positivity.

	Disease +	Disease –	Total
Test interval 1	a	b	a+b
Test interval 2	c	d	c+d
Test interval 3	e	f	e+f
Total	a+c+e	b+d+f	a→f

LR interval 1	(a / a+c+e) / (b / b+d+f)
LR interval 2	(c / a+c+e) / (d / b+d+f)
LR interval 3	(e / a+c+e) / (f / b+d+f)

Figure 31.4 Calculating interval likelihood ratios.

Likelihood ratios can be calculated for test results that are reported in any number of intervals, but it is most useful to define the intervals in such a way to stratify patients into groups where decisions make clinical sense. A classic example might be a test that reports results in terms of low probability/risk, moderate risk, or high risk such as a VQ scan. Intervals can be defined and a contingency table can be set up as in (Figure 31.4).

KEY POINTS

- Clinicians use test results to help strengthen their estimate of disease probability in individual patients.
- Sensitivity is the ability of a diagnostic test to predict the presence of disease.
- Specificity refers to the ability of a test to predict the absence of disease.
- A test with a very high Specificity will "rule in" disease if positive.
- A test with a very high Sensitivity will "rule out" disease if negative.
- Likelihood ratio allows a clinician to more directly estimate post-test probability from pretest probability.
- LR is the probability of a *given test result* in patients *with disease* compared to the probability of the same *test result* in patients *without disease*.

References

1 Hayden, S.R. and Brown, M.D. (1999) Likelihood ratio: A powerful tool for incorporating the results of a diagnostic test into clinical decision making. *Ann Emerg Med*, **33**:575–580.
2 Jaeschke, R., Guyatt, G.H., Sackett, D.L., *et al.* (1994) User's guides to the medical literature, III: How to use an article about a diagnostic test. *JAMA*, **271**:703–707.
3 Schouten, H.J., Geersing, G.J., Koek, H.L., *et al.* (2013) Diagnostic accuracy of conventional or age adjusted D-dimer cut-off values in older patients with suspected venous thromboembolism: systematic review and meta-analysis. *BMJ*, **346**:f2492.
4 Leeuwenburgh, M.M., Wiarda, B.M., Wiezer, M.J., *et al.* (2013) Comparison of imaging strategies with conditional contrast enhanced CT and unenhanced MR imaging in patients suspected of having appendicitis: A multicenter diagnostic performance study. *Radiology*, **268**(1):135–143.
5 Fagan, T.J. (1975) Nomogram for Baye's theorem (C). *N Engl J Med*, **293**:257.

CHAPTER 32

Advanced biostatistics: Chi-square, ANOVA, regression, and multiple regression

Gary Gaddis

St. Luke's Hospital of Kansas City, MO, USA

Introduction

When my wife and I were in graduate school, learning to become medical scientists, we were subjected to weekly statistical critiques of recent biomedical literature by the late Dr Hal Morris, a Professor in the Department of Health, Physical Education, and Recreation at Indiana University. Dr Morris taught several very good biostatistics classes. As the only two future medical scientists in these classes, we would cringe as he reveled in sharing recently published medical manuscripts from leading medical journals that nonetheless contained biostatistical errors. However, he unwittingly jump-started our interest in biostatistics. The lessons in this chapter can help you to avoid being singled-out for making biostatistical errors in a similar fashion by one of Dr Morris' current kindred spirits.

Chi-square testing [1]

Background

Chi-square tests are used with nominal data to make statistical inferences. Nominal data are rates, proportions, or frequencies of named events that are observed for individuals in different treatment groups (see Chapter 27 to learn more about nominal data). Two types of Chi-square testing exist:

- The Chi-square test of independence.
- The Chi-square goodness of fit test.

Both tests statistically compare rates or proportions. The more commonly utilized "test of independence" compares data from two or more groups studied simultaneously, to determine whether they appear to differ statistically from each other. The "goodness of fit" test compares a new sample's data against proportions observed from a previously studied comparison group. The test determines if the new sample differs statistically from the comparison group.

For any Chi-square test, a column of the data matrix is reserved for each named outcome and a row of the matrix is reserved for each group of subjects. The junction of a row and a column is called a "cell". The data matrix of all of the cells is called a "contingency table". The simplest contingency tables have two rows and two columns, to portray two possible outcomes in two treatment groups. However, Chi-square tests can be carried out for data from experiments with three or more groups and/or three or more named classifications of outcomes.

Example

As an example, Aguilar *et al.* [2] studied several clinical outcomes during the introduction of prehospital Continuous Positive Airway Pressure (CPAP) into an urban emergency medical service (EMS) system. One outcome was whether continuation of CPAP in the emergency department (ED), after it was started by prehospital EMS, impacted the probability of need for ICU admission. 18 of 65 subjects whose CPAP was discontinued in the ED and 40 of 109 whose CPAP was continued in the ED required ICU admission.

Doing Research in Emergency and Acute Care: Making Order Out of Chaos, First Edition. Edited by Michael P. Wilson, Kama Z. Guluma, and Stephen R. Hayden.
© 2016 John Wiley & Sons, Ltd. Published 2016 by John Wiley & Sons, Ltd.

Table 32.1 ICU admissions. Observed numbers (percentages) as obtained by Aguilar *et al.* [Expected values for each cell are in brackets] and [expected values if ICU admission was equally likely in both groups, that is, were a randomly occurring event].

	ICU Admission	No ICU Admission	Row Total
CPAP Discontinued	18	47	65
[Expected value]	[21.67]	[43.33]	
CPAP Continued	40	69	109
[Expected value]	[36.33]	[72.67]	
Column Total	58	116	174

Box 32.1 Calculation of Chi-square.

- Place the data into a contingency table; rows for Groups and columns for Outcomes.
- Determine the row and column totals.
- The expected frequency for each cell in the contingency table is the associated row total times the column total, divided by the total number of subjects. *In the matrix above, these expected frequencies are noted in brackets.*
- For each cell, the difference between observed and expected frequencies is squared and then divided by the expected frequency for that cell. For the data in Table 30.1, these values are:
  ○ 13.47/21.67; 13.47/43.33; 13.47/36.33; and 13.47/72.67.
  ○ These values are then summed to calculate Chi-square.
- Thus, Chi-square equals the sum, from each cell of the matrix, of the squared deviations between observed and expected values, divided by the expected value for that cell.
- Most statistical software permits the user to construct the Chi-square matrix and input cell frequencies. The software computes Chi-square and determines the probability of that value of Chi-square occurring by chance alone. This is the p value that statistical software will report.

Source: Aguilar *et al.* 2013 [2]. Reproduced with permission of Elsevier.

With this data, let us determine whether discontinuation of CPAP in the ED was associated with a greater likelihood of ICU admission? The ICU admission frequencies can be used to construct Table 32.1, which shows the resulting Chi-square contingency table.

For this contingency table, $X^2 = 1.485$, and p = 0.223. The ICU admission rate did not differ significantly between historical controls and the current sample[1]. There is a 22.3% chance of obtaining the numbers in this contingency table by chance alone.

How to calculate Chi-square

No matter the size of the contingency, Chi-square tests compare the observed frequencies in the contingency table against the expected frequencies that would be observed by chance. Box 32.1 shows how this is accomplished.

Yates' correction for continuity

With 2 × 2 tables, Chi-square testing is slightly biased toward leading the researcher to make a Type I error. The reason lies in the math underlying Chi-square testing (Chi-square testing yields discrete values, but the Chi-square statistic is continuously distributed). The Yates' correction was developed to decrease the probability of making a Type I error from data in a 2 × 2 contingency table.

Yates' correction is to subtract 0.5 from the absolute value of [observed value – expected value] differences for each cell, then square these corrected values, to obtain the numerator for calculation of the Yates'-corrected Chi-square. The denominator remains the same expected cell frequency as calculated without the correction. As with an uncorrected Chi-square test, these values are then summed to calculate a corrected Chi-square value. The Chi-square statistic that results after applying Yates' correction will always be smaller than the uncorrected value and the resulting p value will be always be larger. This is how Yates' Correction decreases the probability of a Type I error.

[1] Aguilar *et al.* [2] erroneously stated the p value for this comparison was 0.012. The correct p value of this matrix is 0.223 for this contingency table. The researchers erroneously concluded that discontinuation of CPAP in the ED increased the probability of a need for ICU admission.

Fisher's exact test

For some 2 × 2 contingency tables, there may be a cell size of four or less in the table. When this occurs with just one cell, Fisher's exact test is used. Fischer's exact test directly calculates a statistical probability for the contingency table. When a cell size of four or less occurs for two or more cells, the researcher must collect more data until statistical inference can be made. Most basic biostatistics texts cover Fisher's exact test.

Summary

When comparing rates or proportions of named outcomes between two or more groups, Chi-square testing is generally indicated. Yates' correction should be applied when $p < 0.05$ in a 2 × 2 table. Fisher's exact test is reserved for direct calculation of p for 2 × 2 contingency tables with one cell frequency of four or less.

Analysis of variance (ANOVA) [3]

When to use ANOVA

Analysis of variance (ANOVA) is the right test to pick when the researcher makes inferences from parametric data obtained from three or more study groups.

When not to use ANOVA

The Student t-test is utilized when there are only two study groups and the data is parametric[2]. If the study data are ordinal, consult Chapter 27, which summarizes how to select the correct test to draw statistical inferences from ordinal data.

Why not to use the Student t-test to compare multiple groups?

Novice researchers quickly learn that when an ANOVA F-ratio reveals a statistically significant difference, it does not yet reveal which of the three or more groups being compared differ significantly from each other. They therefore wonder why they should not perform multiple Student t-tests to make direct statistical inferences with these data. The answer lies in the consequence of making the multiple comparisons between groups that repeated t-tests require. The more study groups there are, the greater the number of intergroup comparisons that must be made to make all possible comparisons. The performing of multiple intergroup comparisons causes a greater probability of a Type I error. The link between multiple comparisons and Type I error is discussed at the end of Chapter 27.

How to calculate an ANOVA F-ratio

ANOVA is calculated using means (measures of central tendency) and variances (measures of variability). ANOVA partitions variances that result from the two sources of variability in a study's dependent variable.

Consider a study with results from three groups of five individuals. Numerically identical results for all five subjects *within* any study group would be highly improbable, because of interindividual biologic variability and because of possible imprecision or inaccuracy of the measurements. For ANOVA, this interindividual variability is the source of "within groups" variance. This is used toward determining the denominator of an F-ratio calculation.

Variability of data values between groups is partitioned into "between groups" and "within groups" variances. Variability due to a treatment's effects causes "between groups" variability. Intersubject variability is also still present, due to "within groups" variability as described above. Thus, "between groups" variability and "within groups" variability both contribute to the numerator term in an ANOVA F-ratio.

Moving from an "F-ratio" to an estimate of probability

Following application of ANOVA, the resulting "F-ratio", or "F" calculated from ANOVA, can be expressed as a point on a continuously distributed F-ratio curve. This curve has a specific shape and equation, dependent on the number of degrees of freedom of the numerator and the denominator used to calculate "F" (see the following example). The process of translating an "F-ratio" to a statistical probability by use of the F-distribution is conceptually similar to how a Z score can be translated to a probability value by using the properties of the normal distribution. When "between-groups"

---

[2] It would be unconventional, but not incorrect, to calculate an F ratio for a two group comparison. The Student t-test delivers the same p value as an ANOVA would deliver, with less calculation steps.

variance is markedly larger than "within-groups" variance, F becomes larger. The larger the value of "F", the less likely different values in the treatment groups occurred by chance alone.

Example

Most readers will probably find it easier to work through a step-by-step example than to understand a conceptual written description of how to calculate "F". Using the data set shown in Table 32.2, the following simple example is provided to facilitate the reader's understanding of the mechanics of calculation of an F-ratio. Note that few real data sets will have such an extremely high F-ratio and such an extremely low probability of occurring by chance alone. Also note that few data sets will have so few subjects in each group, in order to assure sufficient statistical power (Chapter 28).

For this data set:

1 Calculate the grand mean of all data points, and the mean for each group:
(a) Grand mean = 28; Mean (Litter 1) = 38; Mean (Litter 2) = 28; Mean (Litter 3) = 18.
2 Calculate the sum of squared deviations from Grand Mean for all 15 puppies:
(a) In this example, sum of squared deviations from Grand Mean of 28 for all 15 points in the Table = 1000.
(i) $36-28=8; 8^2=64$. $39-28=11; 11^2=121$; etc.
(ii) The sum for all 15 points = 1000.
(iii) This value will be used toward calculation of the numerator of the F-ratio.
3 Calculate the sums of the squared deviations within each group (cell value – group mean) [2]:
(a) Squared deviations for the five dogs within Litter 1 = 6.
(i) $36-38=-2; -2^2=4$. $39-38=1; 1^2=1.4+1+0+1+0=6$.
(b) Squared deviations for the five dogs within Litter 2 = 10.
(c) Squared deviations for the five dogs within Litter 3 = 4.
4 Calculate sum of squared deviations from Step 3 for the individual litters:
(a) 6 + 10 + 4 = 20.
(b) This term will be used toward calculation of the denominator of the F-ratio.
5 Determine the appropriate number of degrees of freedom (df):
(a) Between groups df = 2 (number of groups – 1).
(b) Within groups df = 12 (total number of data points – number of groups).
6 Determine the numerator and denominator of "F" using variance and degrees of freedom:
(a) Numerator = 1000 / 2 = 500.
(b) Denominator = 20 / 12 = 1.667.
7 Calculate "F":
(a) F = 500 / 1.667 = 300.
8 Finally, the statistical software will translate this "F" into a probability value, appropriate for the number of groups and number of subjects in the study:
(a) $p=5.68\times10^{-11}$.
9 Conclusion: This distribution is highly unlikely to have occurred due to chance alone. There is a difference of body mass between the three litters of pups.

Steps after a significant "F-ratio" is observed

Once a "significant" F-ratio has been obtained, the question arises of where, within the data, the difference exists. Using the example of masses of the three breeds of dogs in Table 32.2, is Breed 1 different from Breed 2, Breed 3, or both? Is Breed 2 different from Breed 3?

Table 32.2 Data set for the calculation of an "F-ratio". (Weight of dogs (kg) at age 6 months. Each litter is from a different mother.)

	Litter 1	Litter 2	Litter 3
Dog 1	36	29	17
Dog 2	39	26	19
Dog 3	38	28	18
Dog 4	39	30	17
Dog 5	38	27	19

- These questions are resolved by "*post hoc*" tests.
- At least seven different *post hoc* tests exist.
- The choice of "*post hoc*" tests to use after a significant "F-ratio" has been obtained is beyond the scope of this chapter, but *the specific test to be used to analyze the data should be chosen a priori, when the study is being designed*, not once the data has been analyzed. Most basic biostatistics books cover this topic.

Other Important points regarding ANOVA

- *Multiple nominal independent variables and Factorial Design ANOVA:* The example illustrated in Table 32.2 had one independent variable (dog breed) and one parametric dependent variable (dog mass). Sometimes, research designs may include more than one independent variable. If the researcher studied the three dog breeds in the example, but also examined males versus females, there would be two independent variables, and neither is numeric. In such a situation, breed and gender are both called "factors". A study design with two genders and three breeds would be called a "2 × 3 Factorial" design. Specific ANOVA calculations exist for factorial design ANOVA.
- *Crossover designs and repeated measures ANOVA:* The researcher can decrease the degree of variability between subjects in all three treatment groups if each subject "acts as their own control" and undergoes all three treatments in random order. This is termed a repeated measures design, or a "crossover" design. The resulting within-groups variability is less than would occur without a crossover design. Treatment effects contribute proportionately more to inter-subject data variability than any "within-groups" effects with repeated measures designs. This permits studies to require fewer subjects to achieve adequate sample size and statistical power.
- *Covariates of the independent variable and ANCOVA:* Several numeric covariates of an independent variable, such as body mass index, or age, may influence a dependent variable such as blood pressure. Analysis of Covariance (ANCOVA) can be used when there is at least one numeric covariate and one dependent variable, to evaluate for the influence of covariates upon the dependent variable. ANCOVA simulates the outcome on the dependent variable "Y" if the amount of covariate "X" were held constant between subjects[5]. (However, researchers could also choose to use multivariate regression to attempt to predict the "Y" that would result due to the combined influence of the independent variable, along with the influence of covariates. An overview of multivariable regression is given at the end of this chapter.)
- *Multiple numeric dependent variables and MANOVA:* If researchers did not use a "crossover" design, and did randomize subjects to receive one of three blood pressure medications for five years, they may wish to evaluate not only diastolic blood pressures but also left ventricular wall thickness. Multivariate Analysis of Variance (MANOVA) techniques exist to permit the researcher to accommodate such a study design with one independent variable and two or more numeric dependent variables.
- *Multiple numeric dependent variables, multiple covariates of the independent variable, and MANCOVA:* In a prospective randomized non-crossover study of three blood pressure medications administered for five years, the independent variable would be the type of medication received. However, age and body mass index are numeric covariates that could impact the value of the dependent variable of blood pressure. If a researcher studied the numeric dependent variables of blood pressure response *and* left ventricular wall thickness with such a design, they would use Multivariate Analysis of Covariance (MANCOVA) for statistical inference.

Summary

Unlike the case for incorrect use of multiple Student t-tests, ANOVA techniques permit comparison of parametric data from three or more different groups while keeping the experiment-wise Type I error rate at the desired level. The ANOVA F-ratio is a ratio that considers the effects of "between groups" variance plus "within groups" variance toward calculation of its numerator, and "within groups" variances toward calculation of its denominator. Various special ANOVA tests exist for multiple factor and for crossover study designs. Variations of ANOVA also exist to permit statistical comparisons when evaluating multiple independent variables, multiple dependent variables, or both.

Regression [4–6]

Background

Medical researchers and clinicians often want to create a model to describe systems and to be able to predict the value of a dependent variable once the value of an independent variable is known. Regression analysis enables this to be done.

Single variable regression techniques permit determination of the "line of best fit" between an independent variable and a dependent variable, when variation of the value of the independent variable seems likely to cause variation of the value of the dependent variable. The general equation of a straight line is Y = a + bX, where "a" is the Y-intercept and "b" is the line's slope.

This section presents a brief overview of how single variable linear regression analysis permits determination of "a" and "b". Regression reveals the equation for that straight line that most precisely describes the relationship between a single independent variable and a single dependent variable. Linear regression is the simplest form of regression analysis.

Two caveats must be noted:

- Sometimes more than one independent variable influences the value of a dependent variable. Regressions can be performed to account for multiple independent variables. The topic of multiple regression is considered at the end of this chapter.
- A visual inspection of the plot of all data points should be done before performing a regression analysis. Sometimes, non-linear relationships can become evident simply by inspection and techniques other than linear regression should be applied. For example, an object dropped from a height will continuously accelerate, so the line of best fit for velocity (dependent variable) versus time (independent variable) is not a straight line, it is a parabola. A curvilinear relationship exists, and curvilinear regression should be used to determine the equation of the parabola that describes the relationship between velocity and time.

Linear regression example

Consider the relationship between change of body mass (dependent variable) versus caloric intake (independent variable) in a population of young adolescents (Table 32.3).

The principal determinant of mass change over time is the average caloric intake per day. (Other factors can also influence this relationship; they are noted in the section on Multiple Regression).

Calculation of the regression line

The general equation of a line is Y = a + bX, where "a" is the Y-intercept and "b" is the slope. The slope of a line "b" is a form of covariance, in that any change in "X" is expected to cause a change in "Y".

- The equation to solve for "b" is determined using every individual "i" value of "X" and "Y":
  - $b = \Sigma (X_i - \text{mean of all X values})(Y_i - \text{mean of all Y values}) / \Sigma (X_i - \text{mean of all X values})^2$
  - Because Y = a + bX, and therefore a = Y – bX, the equation for "a" is simply:
  - a = (mean of all Y values) – b * (mean of all X values)

Strength of association

A regression line does not completely explain the variability of values of the dependent variable "Y", as the value of independent variable "X" changes, unless all values of "Y" fall on the regression line. Such an event is nearly impossible. The strength of association between "X" and "Y" is determined by the size of the Pearson correlation coefficient "r". Most standard statistical texts cover the calculation of "r". The value of "r" can range from –1 to 1. From "r", the Coefficient of Determination, r^2, is easily determined. The value of r^2 conveys how much of the variation of "Y" is explained by the variation of "X".

Patient	Mean caloric consumption per day	Mass change per month (lb)
1	1200	0.0
2	1500	0.5
3	1800	0.5
4	2000	1.5
5	2500	4.0
6	1800	1.0
7	2500	3.0
8	2000	2.0

Table 32.3 Caloric intake and change of body mass.

Notable characteristics of the regression

The line of best fit that results from linear regression analysis is the line that has the minimum possible value for the sum of the squared deviations along the y-axis for every data point. In other words, for any value of "X", the regression line predicts:

- A value for "Y-bar" for all individual X_i values between the minimum (X_{min}) and maximum (X_{max}) value of X used to calculate the regression line, or
- A value for $\hat{Y}$ (Y-predicted) by the line of best fit when extrapolating beyond X_{min} or X_{max} values used to derive the regression line.

For each individual "i" data point, at any "X_i", there is a point "(X_i, Y_i)" that is unlikely to lie exactly at X_i, Y_i-bar (for X between X_{min} and X_{max}) or $X_i, \hat{Y}_i$ (for X not between X_{min} and X_{max}). The mathematics that underlies regression analysis permits determination of the equation of the line for which the sum of all individual "i" values of $(Y\text{-bar} - Y_i)^2$ to be the minimum possible value.

Note that some data points will lie above the regression line and others will lie below the line (Figure 32.1 [4, Figure 4]). If numerous individual data points were obtained for different subjects at any value of "X_i", the frequencies of observing different values of "Y_i" would be normally distributed (Figure 32.2 [4, Figure 3]). For Figure 32.2, the normal distributions of values of "Y" are oriented in the "z" axis perpendicular to the "x" and "y" axis. Figure 32.2 graphically conveys the fact that with regression, there is always an error term, and the points used to construct the regression do not fall exactly on the regression line. However, these points are likely to fall near the regression line.

Testing a regression for statistical significance

Given that a sum of squared deviations is used to determine the regression line, and that squared deviations are also used to calculate the F-ratio in ANOVA, it should not be surprising that significance testing for a regression is performed in a fashion highly analogous to ANOVA. The objective of statistical testing of a regression analysis is to determine whether or not the slope of the regression line differs significantly from zero. Also, more than one regression lines can be compared to determine whether their slopes differ significantly from each other. Further explanation is available [5, 6].

Summary

Linear regression is a modeling tool. Individual data points can be used to determine a simple linear regression line to model any process where variation of a single independent variable results in linear variation of the value of a dependent variable. The slope of the regression line is an expression of covariance; an expression of how much the value of "Y" can be expected to vary, for a given size of variation of the value of "X". The value of the coefficient of determination r^2, which is the square of the correlation coefficient, conveys the strength of association between "X" and "Y". Testing for statistical significance with regression analysis evaluates whether or not the calculated slope "b" differs from zero.

Multiple regression [5, 6]

Background

Most dependent variables are influenced by more than one independent variable. For example, the change of body mass for any person over time could be expected to depend not only upon their average daily caloric intake, but also upon their lean body mass (which impacts basal metabolic rate), their gender, and their daily activity level and caloric expenditure. Therefore, a tool to permit an expression of how multiple independent variables influence a dependent variable is highly useful to medical scientists.

Multiple regression techniques permit the use of more than one independent variable to predict the value of a dependent variable. These techniques have come into widespread use along with the revolution in microcomputers that can handle the complex and time consuming calculations involved in multiple regression statistical techniques. These techniques are being utilized more often because their ability to use more than one independent variable to predict a dependent variable models biological systems better than regression equations for only one independent variable.

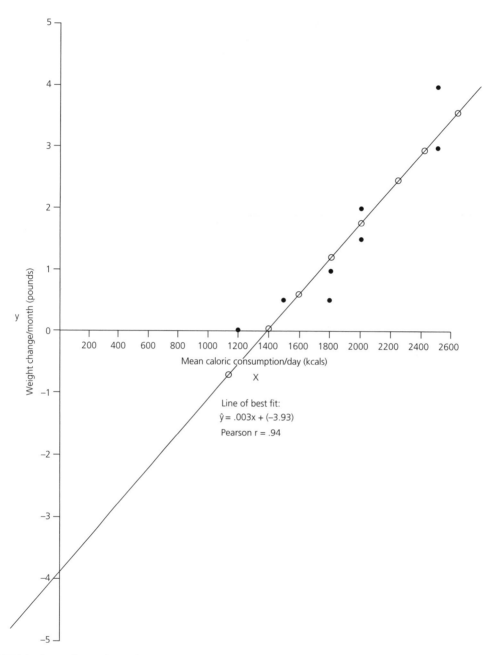

Figure 32.1 Weight change (lb/month) as a function of mean caloric consumption (Kcal/day). This graph displays the individual data points from Table 32.3 and shows the resulting regression line. (Source: Gaddis and Gaddis 1990 [4]. Reproduced with permission of Elsevier.)

General format of multiple regression equations

The general format of a multiple regression equation for "n" independent variables is:

$$Y = a + m_1X_1 + m_2X_2 + m_3X_3 + \ldots m_nX_n$$

This equation does not yield the equation for a line, but it does permit prediction of the value of a dependent variable once the relative weights of "m_i" and the values of all "X_i" that significantly influence "Y" have been determined.

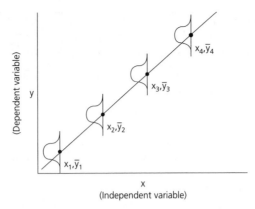

Figure 32.2 For a given value of the independent variable (X), there will be a subpopulation of dependent variables (Y) that displays a normal distribution. The mean value of each subpopulation will form a point on the regression line. (Source: Gaddis and Gaddis 1990 [4]. Reproduced with permission of Elsevier.)

Conceptual overview

There is insufficient space in this text to discuss the many issues and nuances of multiple regression techniques. If you wish to become more informed regarding multiple regression, you will need to consult well-written statistical texts [6]. The following concepts are most crucial to understand:

- The independent variables with multiple regression can be numeric or nominal, while the dependent variable is numeric. A technique called "dummy coding" permits nominal variables to be included in a numeric multiple regression equation. (A biologic example includes use of plasma creatinine levels, gender, and mass to estimate glomerular filtration rate.)
- The multiple "R" serves the same function in multiple regression as the Pearson "r" in simple linear regression. The value of R^2 tells how much of the variation of the dependent variable is accounted for by the multiple regression equation.
- Multiple regression can be performed in one of several stepwise fashions, each of which are done rapidly by microcomputing software, but each of which would require lengthy calculations if done by hand. In general:
  - With *"forward selection"*, independent "X" variables are added to a regression one at a time. The first independent variable utilized in the equation is the one with the highest correlation with "Y". The next "X" variable added is the one that increases R^2 by the greatest amount. Additional independent "X" variables are added, until adding an additional variable does not cause a statistically significant increase of R^2.
  - With *"backward elimination"*, all "X" independent variables studied are initially included in the regression, and then the "X" variables which reduce R^2 by the smallest amount are sequentially removed, one at a time, until the removal of an "X" variable causes a significant reduction of R^2. The "X" variable that significantly reduces R^2, and the other "X" variables which remain, are included in the multiple regression equation.
  - *Stepwise regression* uses both forward selection and backward elimination. New "X" variables are added to the regression equation as is done with forward selection, but after forward selection, all previously added "X" independent variables are checked to determine whether they would significantly reduce R^2. Those that would significantly reduce R^2 if removed from the model are retained, and those that would not significantly reduce R^2 if removed from the model are eliminated.
  - A discussion of the advantages and disadvantages of each option is beyond the scope of this chapter but is available in advanced biostatistics texts.

Summary

Multiple regression techniques are highly useful mathematical modeling tools, which require complex calculations best accommodated by microcomputers and statistical software. A large number of multiple regression techniques exist. All multiple regressions permit evaluation of the influences of numeric or nominal independent variables, or

---

KEY POINTS

This chapter has provided an overview of selected important traits of and the correct application of the following statistical inferential tests:

- Chi square
- Analysis of variance
- Linear regression
- Multiple regression.

---

both, upon numeric or nominal dependent variables. It is not possible to concisely summarize in this chapter this broad topic in a manner that approaches the more concise summaries of Chi-square, ANOVA, and simple regression.

References

1 Gaddis, G.M. and Gaddis, M.L. (1990) Introduction to Biostatistics: Part 5, statistical inference techniques for hypothesis testing with nonparametric data. *Ann Emerg Med*, **19**:1054–1059.
2 Aguilar, S.A., Lee, J., Castillo, E., *et al.* (2013) Assessment of the addition of prehospital continuous positive airway pressure (CPAP) to an urban emergency medical services (EMS) system in persons with severe respiratory distress. *J Emerg Med*, **45**:210–218.
3 Gaddis, M.L. and Gaddis, G.M. (1990) Introduction to Biostatistics: Part 4, statistical inference techniques in hypothesis testing. *Ann Emerg Med*, **19**:820–825.
4 Gaddis, M.L. and Gaddis, G.M. (1990) Introduction to biostatistics: Part 6, correlation and regression. *Ann Emerg Med*, **19**:1462–1468.
5 Dawson-Sanders, B. and Trapp, R.G.(1994) *Basic and Clinical Biostatistics*, 2nd edn. Appleton and Lange, Norwalk, CT; Chapter 12, Statistical methods for multiple variables.
6 Vach, V. (2013) *Regression Models as a Tool in Biomedical Research*. CRC Press, Boca Raton, FL.

CHAPTER 33

Can I combine the results of this study with others? An introduction to systematic reviews

Brian H. Rowe

Department of Emergency Medicine and School of Public Health, University of Alberta, Edmonton, AB, Canada

Patient scenario

A 22-year-old female undergraduate student presented to the emergency department (ED) with gradual onset of headache, nausea, vomiting, and photophobia. She is an otherwise healthy woman with a history of similar migraines. She does not smoke, drinks alcohol occasionally, and is studying for her nursing final examinations. She takes no medications and denies fever, rash, or a headache different from her past presentations. At triage, she was speaking in short sentences, her eyes were covered by dark sunglasses, and she occasionally retched into a basin. She was alert although anxious, and had the following vital signs: pulse = 104 beats per minute; respiratory rate: 20 breaths per minute; temperature = 36.8°C; SaO_2 = 95%. Her neurological examination was entirely normal.

In the ED, she was triaged as urgent and received intravenous (IV) normal saline (1 liter), IV metoclopramide (Maxeran/Reglan) 10 mg, and IV ketorolac (Toradol) 30 mg. She was placed in a quiet area of the ED and reassessed in an hour, at which time her headache was rated as 1/10 and her nausea had abated. Given pending examinations, she requested treatment to reduce the risk of her headache recurring and your resident suggested dexamethasone. The resident cites an article that demonstrates an impressive reduction of headache relapse after discharge [1], although at journal club another article was reviewed that suggested no effect [2].

Introduction

The above scenario is common in emergency medicine and acute care practice for a variety of reasons. Firstly, in many acute care disciplines such as emergency medicine, funding is difficult to obtain and researchers are often forced to conduct small site-specific research studies. Large cardiology-like mega-trials are generally uncommon in this field. Secondly, small samples often fail to have the power to detect important differences between or among treatments, so vote-counting of published results is often misleading (e.g., 3 studies show no effect and 2 studies show a positive effect – what to do?). Thirdly, a publication bias exists in the health field, so positive results are published more frequently than negative ones and some are ***never*** published [3]. This results in an over-estimation of many treatment effects. Finally, acute care clinicians are involved in managing many common diseases, so pooled analyses of small studies often provides important information that would not be possible for the common practitioner to garner through medical speed-reading.

This chapter focuses on summarizing the evidence in acute care when there are multiple studies on the same topic. Using the approach outlined herein will enable clinicians and scientists to assess the evidence to avoid missing important treatment benefits and potentially harmful effects. Moreover, it will provide you with a feeling of superiority over your peers and consultant teachers.

Doing Research in Emergency and Acute Care: Making Order Out of Chaos, First Edition. Edited by Michael P. Wilson, Kama Z. Guluma, and Stephen R. Hayden.

© 2016 John Wiley & Sons, Ltd. Published 2016 by John Wiley & Sons, Ltd.

Terminology

Overall, many terms have been used to describe the process of systematic reviews (SRs). In the past, BOGSAT (i.e., **B**unch of **O**ld **G**uys **S**itting **A**round a **T**able) was a common way to develop consensus on a management issue. This failed for a variety of reasons, mostly because the "old guys" (i) were not up to date, (ii) failed to conduct a systematic search for the evidence and had a biased selection process, (iii) often did not grade the evidence, and (iv) failed to use any statistical tests to determine an effect estimate and the precision of that estimate. Clearly, there are potential ways bias can be introduced into the SR process and clinicians need the evidence to be of the highest quality.

Nowadays, the approach to combining the results from similar studies to determine an overall or average effect is to conduct a SR. Not all SRs are created equally and one of the criteria of a good SR is the rigor of the methods applied to determine the results. Systematic reviews can be quantitative or qualitative and the decision to pool data in a review is a critical one; both have value and quantitative/pooled results do not necessarily produce a better review.

How do you start?

The most important starting point for a systematic review is the design of an appropriate clinical question. If you are looking for light reading around a topic to understand it better, grab a text book (but good luck staying awake)! Alternatively, if you have a focused question, a SR may be the best way to obtain an answer. A high quality question compartmentalizes the topic area and describes the design of studies to be included. All questions should include focused details on the **P**opulation, **I**ntervention (and comparison treatment), and **O**utcomes associated with the question. Many people add a descriptor of the **D**esign to the question, and so this approach is often abbreviated as PICO-D. However, these are only some of the components necessary for developing the question. Examples of each component used to construct focused questions are illustrated in Table 33.1.

Methods: What are the keys to a "good" systematic review?

There are now widely accepted methods for completing high quality systematic reviews. These are summarized briefly in Table 33.2 and explained here.

Who is driving the bus and what are the directions? (Developing a protocol)

Nobody would ever consider starting a randomized controlled trial without a protocol, would they (once again, I am talking to myself)? Similarly, a systematic review should not "emerge" after you have sifted through a few articles! You need a protocol. If possible, it should be registered (http://www.crd.york.ac.uk/prospero) [4].

Table 33.1 Example of PICO-D methodology for developing clinically appropriate questions (based on Patient Scenario presented in the text).

Population	Intervention/ Control	Outcome	Design	Topic
Patients with acute headache in the ED	Clinical decision rule	SAH	Prospective cohort	Diagnosis
Patients with acute migraine headache in the ED	IV fluid bolus vs restricted fluids	Pain relief VAS of pain	RCT	Therapy
Patients with acute migraine headache in the ED	IV metoclopramide vs standard care	Pain relief VAS of pain	RCT	Therapy
Patients with acute migraine headache in the ED	IV ketorolac vs standard care	Pain relief VAS of pain	RCT	Therapy
Patients with acute migraine headache in the ED	IV narcotics vs standard care	Pain relief VAS of pain Sedation Addiction	RCT	Therapy / Safety
Patients with acute migraine headache discharged from the ED	Dexamethasone vs placebo	Prevention of relapse of migraine headache	RCT	Prevention
Adult patients	Migraine headaches	Increased incidence of stroke	Prospective cohort	Prognosis

ED = Emergency Department; IV = intravenous; RCT = randomized controlled trial; SAH = subarachnoid hemorrhage; VAS = visual analog scale.

Table 33.2 Criteria to consider when reviewing or conducting a systematic review.

Item	Low quality	High quality
Protocol	Not registered or unavailable	Registered or available
Question	Unfocused or general question	Focused PICO-D question
Search	Limited electronic database search and/or poorly described	Search of multiple electronic databases and well described; methods filters used
	Excludes unpublished and foreign language manuscripts	Includes unpublished and foreign language manuscripts
	No search of the gray literature	Comprehensive search of the gray literature
Selection	Single reviewer without any assistance	Multiple independent reviewers
		Multiple-step process
		Process for adjudication of disagreements
Quality assessment	Poorly developed or invalid tool used	Validated tool used
	Poorly described or reported	Well described and reported
Data extraction	Minimal data extraction and poorly described	Exhaustive data extraction and well described results
		Independent extractors
		Process for adjudication of disagreements
Study characteristics	Minimally reported and/or poorly described studies	Comprehensive and well described studies
Pooling of evidence	Unjustified	Justified
	Poorly described techniques and cannot be reproduced	Well described techniques and reproducible
	Precision variably or un-reported	Precision reported
Heterogeneity	Not examined or reported	Comprehensive reporting and discussion of heterogeneity
	Heterogeneity not explored.	Comprehensive and well described *a priori* subgroups and sensitivity analyses
Conclusions	Exceed the findings of the review.	Correspond to the evidence contained within the review.

A needle in a haystack (Locating the evidence)

Searching for evidence is a complex and time-consuming task. The reasons for these difficulties are multifactorial and may be as trivial as the manner in which the manuscript was coded in the National Library of Medicine (NLM) or as serious as *publication bias.* Publication bias arises when a project with positive results is published (at all, sooner, in a higher impact journal, etc.) compared to a similar project with negative results. This is an important bias to avoid, as its existence can most often over-estimate the efficacy or effectiveness of a treatment.

The solution to the problem is an exhausting search using multiple approaches. For example, to ensure that one has identified all relevant possible citations pertaining to a clinical problem, simple searching is often ineffective. Searching MEDLINE, the bibliographic database of the NLM, for randomized controlled trials using a non-comprehensive search strategy will miss nearly half of the relevant publications. In addition, by not adding other electronic databases (e.g., EMBASE) in the searching, clinicians may be missing an additional 40% of the available evidence [5].

Gray ("hard to find") literature searching is another option for reviewers. For example, hand searching has been shown to increase the yield of randomized controlled trial searches. Unpublished and foreign language literature may contain important information relevant to your PICO-D question and should not be excluded. Given the volume of literature, the search strategies required, and the need to be multi-lingual detective work, it is hardly surprising that clinicians find it difficult to obtain all of the relevant articles in a particular topic area. Several strategies can be used to address this issue. One strategy is to target searches, using designated filters (Table 33.2). Another, and the choice of this author, is to search for high quality systematic reviews and primary research using the Cochrane Library to answer the PICO-D question [6]. Finally, the inclusion of a specialized health librarian on the team as a critically important strategy.

Is that a red apple, green apple, or an orange? (Selecting the evidence)

Once the searches are completed, high quality systematic reviews will document their efforts to avoid *selection bias.* For example, if the professor is the only one selecting articles or if he/she is looking over your shoulder all the time, it is likely that potentially relevant articles will be missed and irrelevant ones may be included. Some of my Canadian colleagues who help on reviews will do their screening while relaxing during commercials and watching their favorite ice hockey team on television – obviously, we need to ensure their work is checked!

Overall, the best approach is to have a multiple-step process, designed to avoid missing anything that is potentially relevant. Most importantly, the selection should be independent and conservative and a process for resolving disagreements should be developed. High quality SRs clearly describe these processes and SRs produced by a single reviewer should be interpreted with caution. Finally, SRs completed by those employed by or influenced by drug companies should be interpreted with **extreme** caution.

Garbage in–garbage out (Grading the evidence)

No matter how strong the methods are in a SR, they cannot salvage poor quality research. Readers need to know whether included articles are "good" (e.g., are they all high quality studies with limited risk of bias) or are they "rubbish" (e.g., are they all low quality studies with high risk of bias). After reviewers have identified relevant studies for inclusion, critical appraisal of these studies must be performed. Ultimately, the evidence is only as good as the individual included trials and strong reviews use a validated tool, report the results, and attempt to explore any heterogeneity, if present.

Many methods have been employed, ranging from user-specific forms, the Jadad score [7], the Newcastle–Ottawa tool [8], and recently, the Cochrane Risk of Bias (RofB) tool [9]. While the risk of bias tool is gaining widespread acceptance, it appears to be most important to select the appropriate tool and apply it in practice, and report the results to the audience.

Making sense of it all (Describing the evidence)

High quality systematic reviews make explicit decisions about what data to extract from the study, the extraction tools to use, and, specifically, the primary and secondary outcomes to report. These decisions are made *a priori* to avoid "fishing expeditions" (e.g., *post hoc* analytic changes) and should reflect clinically important measures of effect (e.g., pain scores and relapse in migraine headaches) rather than numerical values loosely linked to important outcomes (e.g., pulse rate). Once again, high quality reviews report these features and display the main findings of the extraction in a summary table so readers can review the important features of the included studies.

To pool or not to pool, that is the question (Meta-analysis)

One of the most important decisions a reviewer must make and defend is the decision to statistically pool results among studies. High quality reviews painstakingly evaluate similarities among studies with respect to population/setting, intervention/exposure, control, outcomes, and study design *prior* to pooling. Despite these robust efforts, included studies still may not be sufficiently similar to justify pooling. Such situations demand researchers avoid the temptation to pool and mandate a qualitative approach to synthesis. In situations where studies are sufficiently similar, reviewers should employ and report explicit and appropriate methods for data synthesis wherever possible. For example, in reviews published in leading emergency medicine journals, only 48% of reviewers reported the methods used to combine the findings of the relevant studies [10].

Not many of us are statisticians, and my bank manager claims
I am not very good with numbers

The good news in systematic reviews is that you do not need to be a statistician to produce or understand pooled analyses. For dichotomous outcomes (e.g., admissions, relapse), most reviewers report relative risks (RRs), odds ratios (ORs), or risk differences (RDs) with associated 95% confidence intervals (CI) for both the individual trials and their overall pooled estimate. Increasingly, therapy SRs use RR as a method of reporting results, since it is most appropriate for the RCT designs employed. In practical terms, the "weight" of each trial's contribution to the overall pooled result for dichotomous outcomes is largely a function of sample size (and to a certain extent the event rate). For example, the larger the trial, the greater influence it has on the pooled estimate. In such settings, the convention is that the effects favoring the treatment in question (e.g., less relapses of migraine in the treatment group) are located to the left of the line of unity (1.0 Studies 4 and 6 in Figure 33.1) while those favoring the control or comparison arm (more relapses of migraine in the treatment group) are located to the right of the line of unity (Studies 4 and 6 in Figure 33.2). When the 95% CI crosses the line of unity, the result is considered non-significant (Studies 1, 2, 3, and 5 in Figure 33.1).

For continuous variables with similar units (e.g., weight, airflow measurements, pulse), individual study and pooled mean differences (MD) are generally calculated. In practical terms, the "weight" of each trial's contribution to the overall pooled MD for continuous outcomes is based on the standard deviation (SD) and sample size. For example, the smaller the SD and the larger the sample size, the greater the study's influence on the pooled estimate. For continuous measures with variable units (e.g., quality of life measures by two different instruments), standardized mean difference (SMD) can be calculated. For both the SMD and a MD, effects favoring the treatment in question are located to the

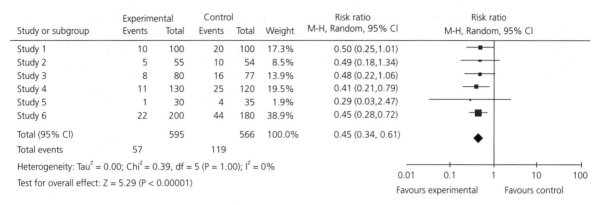

Figure 33.1 Homogeneity of study results from a fictitious meta-analysis.
Note: Results demonstrate visual homogeneity (all point estimates to the left of the neutral line {RR = 1.0}, overlapping 95% CIs, same direction of effect) which statistical tests confirm (p = 1.00; I2 = 0%).

right of the line of unity (0) while those favoring the control or comparison arm are plotted to the left. Once again, when the 95% CI crosses the line of unity, the result is considered non-significant.

Heterogeneity is your friend (we do not get out much)

It is important to recognize that despite efforts to pool similar studies (using PICO-D), there are always slight differences among studies in one or all of the main domains associated with PICO-D. If all of the studies were performed in *exactly* the same manner, by chance there could still be some variability in results. Rather than have a full-blown anxiety attack, many believe heterogeneity is good and should be explored, again as part of the SR protocol.

Statistical tests can determine if the degree of variability among studies is greater than that expected by chance. This type of variability is called statistical heterogeneity. If statistical heterogeneity exists, the pooled result should be viewed with caution and reasons for the identified variability should be explored. The apparent reasons for statistical heterogeneity are explored using the PICO-D approach (e.g., look for differences in patient populations, severity of disease, interventions, etc.).

For the researcher, there are a variety of issues to consider when examining heterogeneity. Firstly, after all of this work finding, selecting, grading and extracting the data, do the studies still represent the same PICO-D? If so, then it is safe to assume there is theoretical clinical homogeneity and a clear rationale to combine the data. Secondly, visual inspection of scatter plots will reveal homogeneity versus heterogeneity (Figure 33.2). Finally, statistical tests, such as the I-squared (I^2) statistic, have been used to detect statistical heterogeneity [11].

One way to explore heterogeneity is through subgroup (patient characteristics such as age, sex, etc.) and sensitivity (non-patient characteristics such as study quality, dose and delivery of medication, comparison treatments, etc.) analyses. Because fishing expeditions (e.g., looking for a positive p value) are common here as well, explicit criteria have been developed for valid subgroups (and as a corollary to sensitivity analyses). For example, subgroups are considered more valid if they are developed *a priori*, produce a statistically and clinically important effect size, are one of a few subgroups, if indirect evidence exists, if both within versus between study differences exist, and if subgroup consistency can be demonstrated within the field [12].

Interpreting the evidence for clinical practice

Once completed, the SR results need to be translated into terms understandable to the common end-user (e.g., patients, clinicians, decision and policy makers, etc.). This can be challenging, since grading the evidence has changed frequently over the past two decades. Currently, the Grades of Recommendation, Assessment, Development and Evaluation (GRADE) is the most widely accepted approach applied for this area of reviews [13].

In the clinical scenario in question, there is a systematic review that addresses the issue and partially resolves the question [14]. Using a comprehensive search strategy to avoid publication bias and techniques to avoid selection bias, multiple reviewers combine results from seven trials to demonstrate that dexamethasone reduces relapse after discharge (OR = 0.74; 95% CI: 0.60, 0.90).

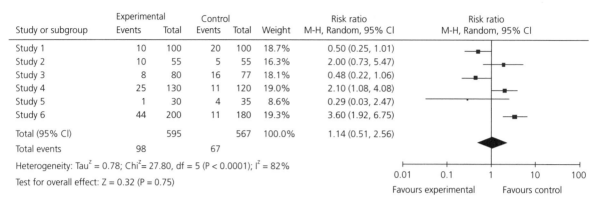

Figure 33.2 Heterogeneity of study results from a factitious meta-analysis.
Note: Results demonstrate visual heterogeneity (point estimates to the left and right of the neutral line {RR = 1.0}, non-overlapping 95% CIs, variability in the direction of effect) which statistical tests confirm (p < 0.0001; I2 = 82%).

Where can you find good SR evidence?

When I first started practicing medicine, there were not personal computers, the "cell phone" was visualized as a shoe phone on the Get Smart TV series, systematic reviews were rare, and Bachman-Turner Overdrive (BTO) was still a viable band (do not get me wrong, their music still resonates, if you catch my drift). Anyway, the "good old days" were not so good for clinicians or patients, let me tell you. Since that time, systematic reviews have now populated the medical field (and some might say polluted it)! There are often more systematic reviews on a topic than there are primary studies in the review. Fortunately, several highly respected resources to help clinicians are now available and described here. (Note: this is a selective list.)

Cochrane Library (International)
The Cochrane Library is comprised of several databases, three of which require some description here. The Cochrane Central Register of Controlled Trials (CENTRAL) is an extensive bibliographic database of controlled trials that has been identified through structured searches of electronic databases and searching by hand by Collaborative Review Groups (CRGs). Currently, it contains thousands of references (CL, Version 2, 2015) and can function as a primary literature searching approach with therapeutic topics. The Database of Abstracts of Reviews of Effects (DARE) consists of critically appraised structured abstracts of non-Cochrane published reviews that meet standards set by the Centre for Reviews and Dissemination at the University of York, UK. The last and perhaps most important resource is the Cochrane Database of Systematic Reviews (CDSR), a compilation of regularly updated systematic reviews with meta-analytic summary statistics. Contents of the CDSR are contributed by CRGs, representing various medical topic areas (e.g., Airways, Stroke, Heart, Epilepsy, etc.). Reviews are produced using *a priori* criteria, adhere to rigorous methodological standards (Table 33.2), and undergo peer review prior to publication. Regular "updates" are required to capture new evidence and address criticisms and/or identified errors.

AHRQ (USA)
The Evidence-based Practice Centers (EPCs) funded by the Agency for Healthcare Quality and Research (AHRQ) are experienced research groups who employ methodologically rigorous standards to predict both scoping and large reviews. These reports are cited in the electronic databases and available on-line (http://www.ahrq.gov).

NICE (UK)
The National Institute of Health and Care Excellence (NICE) produces rigorous systematic reviews and health technology assessments. These reports are cited in the electronic databases and available on-line (www.nice.org.uk).

Conclusions

Overall, acute care practitioners, especially emergency clinicians, have come to rely on systematic reviews to inform their diagnosis, treatment, and prevention of disease. Systematic reviews are an important source of high-level health evidence and many are directly relevant (e.g., In a 22-year-old athlete, should we perform a radiograph to rule-out a significant ankle fracture in the ED?) or indirectly relevant (e.g., Does an ankle support prevent future ankle sprains after the ED in the same athlete?) to the practice of emergency medicine [15]. Not all systematic reviews are created equally and whether producing or consuming (as a learner) a systematic review, there are well-accepted steps in the process of development outlined in this article that form the foundation for a high quality evidence synthesis product. Good luck!

KEY POINTS

If performing a systematic review:
- Find some friends and a librarian – you need help and they will keep you honest.
- Develop a focused, clinically relevant research question using the PICO-D format.
- Develop an *a priori* protocol (and register it).
- Develop comprehensive electronic and gray literature searches by consulting an experienced medical librarian.
- Use a multiple step, independent process for study selection and describe how differences will be resolved.
- Grade the quality of the evidence using the appropriate tool.
- Describe the rationale and techniques for pooling of studies.
- Report point estimate and precision of the primary and secondary outcomes.
- Report and explore heterogeneity using subgroups and sensitivity analyses.
- Conclusions should be congruent with results.

If evaluating and using a systematic review:
- Evaluate the PICO-D question (Is it relevant to my practice? Is it important?)
- Search for evidence of an *a priori* protocol (preferably registered).
- Evaluate the search strategy for *publication bias*.
- Evaluate the selection strategy for *selection bias*.
- Evaluate the validity of data extraction and quality assessment.
- Was the pooling of studies described and appropriate?
- Was the precision of the estimates of outcomes reported?
- Where heterogeneity exists, were subgroup and sensitivity analyses performed?
- Are the outcomes congruent with the text?

Acknowledgements

The author would like to thank Ms Jessalyn Frost (Department of Emergency Medicine) for her assistance with the production of this chapter. Dr Rowe is supported as a Tier I Canada Research Chair in Evidence-based Emergency Medicine through the Canadian Institutes of Health Research (CIHR) from the Government of Canada (Ottawa, ON). Dr Rowe Co-Directs the University of Alberta's Evidence-based Practice Centre (EPC), funded by the Agency for Healthcare Quality and Research (AHRQ), in Bethesda, MD, USA. He has participated in ED-based research in the past two years funded by industry partners; however, he is not a paid employee or consultant to any company.

References

1 Innes, G.D., Macphail, I., Dillon, E.C., *et al.* (1999) Dexamethasone prevents relapse after emergency department treatment of acute migraine: a randomized clinical trial. *Can J Emerg Med,* **1**(1):26–33.

2 Rowe, B.H., Colman, I., Edmonds, M.L., *et al.* (2008) Randomized controlled trial of intravenous dexamethasone to prevent relapse in acute migraine headache. *Headache,* **48**:333–340.

3 Ospina, M.B., Kelly, K., Klassen, T.P., and Rowe, B.H. (2006) Publication bias of randomized controlled trials in emergency medicine. *Acad Emerg Med,* **13**(1):102–108.

4 Straus, S. and Moher, D. (2010) Registering systematic reviews. *Can Med Assoc J,* **182**(1):13–14.

5 Lefebvre, C., Manheimer, E., and Glanville,J. (2011) Chapter 6: Searching for studies. In: J.P.T. Higgins and S. Green (eds) *Cochrane Handbook for Systematic Reviews of Interventions Version 5.1.0* (updated March 2011). The Cochrane Collaboration, www.cochrane-handbook.org (last accessed 15 May 2015).

6 Rowe, B.H. and Alderson, P. (1999) The Cochrane Library: A resource for clinical problem solving in emergency medicine. *Ann Emerg Med,* **34**:86–90.

7 Jadad, A.R., Moore, R.A., Carroll, D., *et al.* (1996) Assessing the quality of reports of randomized clinical trials: is blinding necessary? *Control Clin Trials,* **17**(1):1–12.

8 Wells, G.A., Shea, B., O'Connell, D., *et al.* (2014) The Newcastle–Ottawa Scale (NOS) for assessing the quality of nonrandomised studies in meta-analyses. http://www.ohri.ca/programs/clinical_epidemiology/oxford.asp (last accessed 15 May 2015).

9 Higgins, J.P. and Altman, D.G. Chapter (2011) Chapter 8: Assessing risk of bias in included studies. In: J.P.T. Higgins and S. Green (eds) *Cochrane Handbook for Systematic Reviews of Interventions Version 5.1.0* (updated March 2011). The Cochrane Collaboration, www.cochrane-handbook.org (last accessed 15 May 2015).

10 Kelly, K.D., Travers, A., Dorgan, M., *et al.* (2001) Evaluating the quality of systematic reviews in the emergency medicine literature. *Ann Emerg Med,* **38**:518–526.

11 Higgins, J.P. and Thompson, S.G. (2002) Quantifying heterogeneity in a meta-analysis. *Stat Med,* **21**(11):1539–1558.

12 Oxman, A.D. and Guyatt, G.H. (1992) A consumer's guide to subgroup analyses. *Ann Intern Med.,* **116**(1):78–84.

13 Guyatt, G.H., Oxman, A.D., Vist, G.E., *et al.* (2008) GRADE: an emerging consensus on rating quality of evidence and strength of recommendations. *BMJ,* **336**(7650):924–926.

14 Colman, I., Friedman, B., Brown, M., *et al.* (2008) Dexamethasone to prevent migraine relapse after discharge from the emergency department: A systematic review. *BMJ,* **336**(7657):1359–1361.

15 Emond, S.D., Wyer, P.C., Brown, M.D., *et al.* (2002) How relevant are the systematic reviews in The Cochrane Library to emergency medical practice? *Ann Emerg Med,* **39**:153–158.

CHAPTER 34

How to write a scientific paper for publication

Stephen R. Hayden

Department of Emergency Medicine, UC San Diego Health Systems, CA, USA

> *"Vigorous writing is concise. A sentence should contain no unnecessary words, a paragraph no unnecessary sentences, for the same reason that a drawing should have no unnecessary lines and a machine no unnecessary parts. This requires not that the writer make all his sentences short, or that he avoid all detail and treat his subjects only in outline, but that every word tell"*
>
> Strunk and White, *The Elements of Style* [1]

Introduction

Scientific writing in order to get a paper accepted to a major journal differs from other forms of writing, such as essays, textbook chapters, or even creative writing. While the latter often involves description of sentiments, situations and fiction, the former requires delivery of facts without editorial comment or extraneous detail. The purpose of this chapter is to provide some suggestions for inexperienced scientific writers, from the point of view of a journal editor or reviewer. This chapter should hopefully increase the chances your manuscript will get reviewed and minimize the chances that harsh criticism will suppress your intellectual curiosity to pursue future clinical research.

How do you choose a journal to submit to?

This is an often overlooked initial aspect of the scientific writing process. However, it may have nearly as much impact on the ultimate success of submission as the quality of the research itself! As a first time, or inexperienced author, you must be realistic because your projects are rarely accepted to top tier journals. It is just too hard right out of the gate to engage in the kind of research that will qualify for top tier journals. The key is to find the best fit for your project and not simply be seduced by the most prestigious journal. Go to the journal web site and identify the target audience; see if it matches the intended audience for your work. This is also a place where the advice of an experienced research mentor can be invaluable.

Journals that are indexed in PubMed can be found at http://www.ncbi.nlm.nih.gov/sites/entrez. Many journals do not require the author to pay for publication. There are other "open access" journals, however, where the author pays for publication to ensure the widest audience (not just subscribers). Publication costs in these journals may be as much as $1600–1800 per article, although many are far cheaper. Some open access journals may only exist in an on-line version.

The reason it is so important to choose the journal first is to follow their instructions to authors very carefully in order to format your manuscript correctly. The importance of this cannot be overemphasized. Most journals have an administrative screening process. If your manuscript does not follow the specific journal's format faithfully, it may be returned or even rejected summarily. For example, if you are submitting to an emergency medicine journal, use the terms emergency physician (EP), emergency department (ED), or emergency medicine (EM). Do not use emergency room physician, emergency room, ER physician, EM physician, or even ED physician. The first time you use common terms like ED, spell them out and abbreviate them in parentheses. Thereafter, to save space, use the abbreviation. Tables, figures, and abstracts are exceptions to this requirement, as tables and figures are often removed from the

Doing Research in Emergency and Acute Care: Making Order Out of Chaos, First Edition. Edited by Michael P. Wilson, Kama Z. Guluma, and Stephen R. Hayden.

manuscript and placed in a separate file. If so, the figures and legends will still need to be clear. Abstracts as well are often read in isolation, as readers will generally perform on-line literature searches to retrieve abstracts independent of the full text electronic version of the article. Consequently, an abstract must also stand alone with all abbreviations defined first (abbreviations must then be defined again in the text of the manuscript of course).

Rules of the road from an editor's perspective

The overriding principle of scientific writing is to be concise! A manuscript should be readable right from the start. The landmark paper, "Molecular Structure of Nucleic Acids" by Watson and Crick [2] was a page and a half! Clearly, a paper need not be loquacious to be important.

The following is an example from an actual submission to the *Journal of Emergency Medicine:* "In emergent department, emergent physicians should to be knowledge about the mechanism of injury. Vital sign, complete neurological examination, ophthalmologic and radiological examination should first to survey in emergent department. To prevention of secondary brain injury, hypotention and hypoxia should be avoided." Authors should have a native English speaker proofread their manuscript prior to submission, as a submission with mistakes like this will not be passed on for review, no matter what the quality of the content is.

In another example, "In addition, emergency physicians must be familiar with the current post-PCI anticoagulation recommendations in order to detect and intervene when such patients, either because of non-compliance or error, are under treated, as early cessation of this vital therapy is the greatest predictor of subsequent deadly thrombotic events." If a reviewer or editor has to read a sentence more than once in order to understand it … it is too confusing.

Avoid the "physician guilt trip"

Many authors will conclude a case report submission with the following language or something similar; "Even though this may be the first reported case of X condition in the medical literature physicians MUST know about this (even though authors likely did not know about it until they decided to write it up) or patients will suffer some terrible outcome." This places an impossible burden of knowledge on practicing physicians and should be avoided. Instead, it is much more practical and honest to say, "We present this case to increase awareness among physicians of the clinical presentation of X…"

Scientific writing should be understandable to non-scientists. Avoid medical jargon such as the recently popular term "high index of suspicion" when the intended meaning is really high level of suspicion. Similarly, avoid using medical terminology when a simpler lay term is precise enough. For example, it may be preferable to use "venous thromboembolism" rather than blood clot, as the latter has many meanings, but "pulmonary" has little advantage over "lung." A few characters may make a difference to an editor or publisher concerned with page and word limits for a given journal issue. The aim should be to convey a concept in the fewest words possible.

Use a clear writing style

Outline your paper before you begin to write it. The included template (Appendix 34.1) incorporates the main elements for a good research paper. Consider varying your sentence length to enhance readability. If a process is detailed and requires a long explanation with parenthetical phrases and multiple qualifiers, follow it with a short sentence. Your reader will be grateful. Avoid run-on sentences. Instead, simply divide the sentence into two. Paragraphs should have a minimum of three sentences and rarely more than five or six. These include a topic sentence, paragraph body, and a concluding sentence. If there are only two sentences, incorporate these into the previous or following paragraph.

When you have completed your first draft, have another person outside of your specialty or not involved in medicine at all read the manuscript before submitting it. If they are able to understand it, then most readers of medical journals will also be able to understand it. As my colleague Mark Langdorf (editor of the *Western Journal of Emergency Medicine*) once said, "The goal is to not write in a language called 'medicine,' but rather in plain English."

Section-by-section considerations

The title

Titles should be headlines and should answer the question posed by the research. It should describe the design when applicable: that is, prospective, randomized trial, cohort study, retrospective, case series, report, survey, and so on. There should be a balance between brevity and accuracy. The title should contain no abbreviations and it should grab the reader's attention to entice them to read the article in greater detail. For example, "Intramuscular Ziprasidone 20 mg is effective in reducing acute agitation associated with psychosis: A double-blind, randomized trial."

Structured abstract

A structured abstract is important because many users of the medical literature will perform an electronic search and scan the abstracts retrieved. The key information must be easy and efficient to acquire and a structured abstract facilitates this. The abstract needs to include the major findings of the study. Typical sections in a structured abstract for an interventional study include:

- Background or introduction: two sentences at maximum.
- Objective or aim: one sentence.
- Methods: 2–3 sentences.
- Results: major results only; begin with the most important finding and then 1–2 secondary outcomes at most.
- Conclusion: one sentence.

Readers may read and rely upon the abstract or sometimes only the "conclusion" sentence by itself. Therefore, the abstract section must stand alone with the reporting of both positive and negative results. Be aware that some journals limit the total word count of the abstract. Many authors write the abstract long before the manuscript is complete; if this is your habit, make sure you go back and check that the information contained in the abstract section still matches that contained in the body of the paper once it is complete.

Some journals require a structured abstract for all manuscripts, including papers of other than interventional design. In this case the following generic structure may be used:

- Background or introduction: two sentences at maximum.
- Discussion: 4–5 sentences with subheadings as appropriate.
- Conclusion: one sentence.
  A special situation may arise if a structured abstract is required for a paper involving a case report:
- Background: defines entity or frames issue; why is this case important?
- Case Report/Summary: describe in 2–3 sentences the essence of the case.
- Conclusion: "What can a practicing physician learn by reporting this case?"
  - (remember to avoid the "physician guilt trip")

The above are generic suggestions. Most importantly, remember to follow the "Instructions to authors" for the specific journal you intend to submit your paper to.

Introductory section

The introductory section for most research papers is typically four paragraphs in length. The first paragraph should describe the historical background and significance of the topic to the medical literature or practicing clinician. The second paragraph should include a brief review of prior pertinent literature. It should not be an exhaustive literature review. Only cite references in the introduction that properly frame the research question, as other citations belong in the discussion section. The third paragraph should identify gaps in current knowledge and state the rationale for the current study. The final paragraph details how the current study attempted to fill in these knowledge gaps. The last sentence of the final paragraph of the introduction should clearly state the overall objective of your study. This is where readers expect to find the phrase, "we hypothesized," or "our objective was…" or "we sought to…" or similar words.

The methods section

The methods section should follow a coherent structure that parallels the design of the study. Make very transparent for the reader what was done and why. Take the general approach that your methods should be described in sufficient detail and clarity as to permit replication. Describe setting and participants and be specific about inclusion and exclusion criteria. How were subjects identified and allocated? This is important information; it enables readers of your paper to know how well the population being studied matches the patients in their clinical practice and, therefore, how well the results will apply to their practice setting. Identify the study design (randomized controlled trial, cohort, observation, retrospective chart review) and be specific. Clearly state the interventions you made, whether blinding occurred (patients, providers, assessors of outcome, investigators, etc.). Clearly label your primary and secondary outcome measures, as sample size or power calculations are based on the primary outcome measure. Identify how you gathered, recorded, analyzed data, and the safeguards that you put in place to protect integrity and security. State what statistical tests and programs you used and any assumptions you made. Provide an assertion whether Institutional Review Board approval or exemption was obtained. Having a biostatistician or senior researcher review this portion of the manuscript can be extremely helpful in avoiding mistakes that may lead to delays in review or even rejections. If the study is a retrospective chart review, the methods section should comply with the elements promoted by Gilbert and Lowenstein [3] or Worster and Bledsoe [4] (see also Chapter 14).

The results section

In most interventional research papers that include human subjects, by convention Table 1 reports patient demographics and important characteristics. More recently, journals are discouraging reporting p values when comparing groups of patients for the simple reason that multiple comparisons could falsely elevate the chance of finding a significant difference by chance alone (Chapter 27). Report demographics honestly and let the readers decide if an age difference between groups for a given outcome is significant or not. Furthermore, when reporting patient demographics and the numbers of patients included in your study, it is very important to include not only the number actually included, but also the number of patients that were eligible for inclusion during the study period as well as all patients that were included but lost to follow up. This may be best represented by a flow diagram.

In the remainder of the results section present the primary outcome measure first, followed by secondary outcomes devoting a minimum of a paragraph to each. If there are more than four or five related results, it is better to report these in a graph or table. Results from tables should not be repeated in text but instead include a general synopsis of the tabular results. Results should generally be stated in absolute, not relative, terms. For example, "The absolute risk reduction was 4% (8% to 4%)" rather than, "The relative risk reduction was 50%." This is a more honest way to report results and avoids artificially inflating the benefit of an intervention. When comparing groups, include 95% confidence intervals around measures such a p values, and cite the number-needed-to-treat (NNT) and to harm (NNH). This provides the reader with information to assess the practical importance of the results of your study. If your research involves the utility of a diagnostic test, then report the likelihood ratio associated with it in addition to the typical sensitivity, specificity, and positive/negative predictive values. Readers may then more directly modify an estimate of disease probability using the Fagan nomogram [5].

Be wary of the difference between statistical significance and clinical significance. For example, in an emergency department triage study it was found that time to disposition decision decreased by six minutes from 260 to 254 minutes (95% CI −12 to 0, p < 0.025). This result was statistically significant and the authors went on to conclude that their triage intervention should be adopted by other emergency departments. However, most clinicians (and patients) would not see a six minute difference in the course of a 4–5 hour visit to be clinically important. As an author, do not overstate your conclusions.

When it comes to pictures or figures, while it may seem obvious to you, do not assume all readers will be able to identify key findings so annotate them with arrows for the sake of greater clarity.

The discussion section

The discussion should emphasize the key findings first, following the order of interventions in the methods and results sections. Present the primary outcome followed by a discussion of the secondary outcomes. This section is the place to offer your opinion regarding the importance of your study and how it could change practice or inform clinical decision making. As previously pointed out, however, be humble and do not overstate the impact of your results. This section should be limited to 5–6 items, each with 1–2 paragraphs. Previous literature is commonly cited in the discussion section and the current study should be placed into this context and identify how it addresses the knowledge gap. Do not offer opinions or address issues that were not studied, rather keep the discussion focused on the specific objectives and research question.

By convention the limitations section includes the last few paragraphs of the discussion section. This section is vitally important and can increase the likelihood a paper will be successfully reviewed and ultimately accepted for publication. It is much better for you to be intellectually honest about the shortcomings of the paper; the more limitations you point out the fewer you leave for reviewers to discover. If reviewers and editors feel you have been honest and thorough in identifying limitations and dealing with them the best you could, they will be more forgiving and likely to recommend acceptance for what can be learned from the paper. The limitations section should generally be 1–2 paragraphs and acknowledge major flaws, such as small sample size, subjects lost to follow up, retrospective design, bias, lack of blinding, limited applicability, and so on.

The conclusions section

Performing the perfect study is virtually impossible; therefore, avoid the temptation to overstate your conclusions. Use modifiers such as "it appears" or "from these data" to tone down statements and make them specific to the populations and settings studied. For example, "In adults..." or "In emergency department patients with chest pain it appears that..." Calling for further investigation is nearly always warranted. Remember that retrospective studies cannot show causation, only demonstrate associations, and so use this word in summary statements when indicated. When writing a case report the conclusion should highlight what physicians should learn by reading it. Avoid statements such as, "The physician must know about this condition..." and instead use phrases like, "We present this case to increase awareness among physicians of the presentation of..."

The references

The most important issue to remember for references is to follow the instructions for authors for the journal you are submitting to. Moreover, do not forget to do a final literature search before submission, as new references may have recently been published that you will want to include.

Conclusion

Scientific writing is both rewarding and challenging. By following these rules of the road you will enhance your chances of getting your paper reviewed and ultimately accepted to the journal of your choice.

KEY POINTS

- Follow instructions to authors carefully; this cannot be overemphasized.
- Articles must be concise and readable.
- There is elegance in brevity;
  - Every word should *tell*!
- Ask for help; collaborate and network; find a good research mentor.
- Have fun and don't let abstracts or work go without being written up!

References

1 Strunk, W. (1999) *The Elements of Style*. W.P. Humphrey, Ithaca, NY (1918) / Bartleby.com (1999).
2 Watson, J.D. and Crick, F.H.C. (1953) A structure for deoxyribose nucleic acid. *Nature*, 171:737–738.
3 Gilbert, E., Lowenstein, S., Koziol-McLain, J., *et al.* (1996) Chart reviews in emergency medicine research: Where are the methods? *Ann Emerg Med*, **27**:305–308.
4 Worster, A., Bledsoe, R.D., Cleve, P., *et al.* (2005) Reassessing the methods of medical record review studies in emergency medicine research. *Ann Emerg Med.*, **45**:448–451.
5 Fagan, T.J. (1995) Letter: Nomogram for Bayes theorem. *N Engl J Med*, **293**(5):257.

Appendix 34.1

Manuscript Publication Template
(From the UC San Diego Emergency Medicine Residency)

TITLE SECTION
- Descriptive title
- Authors
- List of author selected key-words
- Source of financial support for study (if applicable)
- Acknowledgments
- Address for reprints

ABSTRACT SECTION (use structured format)
- Purpose of study or study objective
- Methods including
  - Study design
  - Setting
  - Participants – identify study/control groups if applicable
  - Interventions
  - Measurements – clearly specify primary outcome measure
  - Statistical tests applied
- Results
- Conclusions

INTRODUCTION SECTION
- Historical background
- Significance of study
- Review of prior pertinent literature
- Identify gaps in knowledge and state rationale for current study
- Clearly state in final paragraph study hypothesis or objective

METHODS SECTION
- Note human subjects/IRB approval, consent procedures
- State study design – method of randomization, blinding if appropriate
- Setting
- Participants – specify in detail inclusion and exclusion criteria
- Interventions – describe in sufficient detail to permit replication
- Measurements – identify clearly primary and secondary outcome measures
- Consider use of a flowchart to describe patient flow
- Data collection and analysis – specify statistical tests, sample size calculation

RESULTS SECTION
- Note number of total eligible patients during study period
- State number of patients excluded and why
- Number of patients enrolled by group
- Indicate completeness of follow up by group. What happened to every patient? Use flow chart.
- Include basic patient demographics and comparison of groups in "Table 1"
- Report results for primary outcome measure followed by secondary outcomes
- Include a power analysis for sample size.

DISCUSSION SECTION
- Discuss how current findings relate to prior studies
- Cite relevant prior literature
- Note specifically how current findings are new or different from prior reports
- Discuss implications of current findings
- Discuss limitations of current study
- Note future questions or areas needing further research

CONCLUSIONS
- State important conclusions – must be supported by specific data
- Do not overstate conclusions
- Limits on applicability (ability to generalize) conclusions

REFERENCE SECTION
- List in order they appear in text – use required journal format

APPENDIX SECTION
- Description of special procedures too detailed for body of paper
- List of definitions, codes, diagnostic criteria, etc.
- Sample data forms, questionnaires, etc.

CHAPTER 35

How do I make reviewers happy? The review process: What do reviewers look for in a manuscript? What is the review process?

David J. Karras and Jacob W. Ufberg

Department of Emergency Medicine, Temple University School of Medicine, Philadelphia, PA, USA

Introduction

Congratulations on the birth of your new manuscript! After an exciting conception, meticulous planning, arduous execution, painstaking analysis, agonizing writing, and endless revisions, you are finally ready to submit your study manuscript for publication. Just like every proud parent, you are firmly convinced that your manuscript is spectacularly beautiful and will be regarded as a masterpiece by any journal editor or reviewer lucky enough to behold it.

Now it is time for a reality check. You have spent so much time fussing over every detail of your study, that it is likely that you are blind to its flaws. And there will be flaws, ranging from small details to potentially fatal issues. Editors and reviewers may not understand your study premise, may disagree with your methodology and statistical techniques, or may object to your conclusions outright. Sometimes reviewers just do not think your study is interesting enough for publication. Reviewers' comments inevitably seem cruel, simply because they point out study limitations that you did not anticipate and they do not appreciate your hard work.

Your task at this stage is to objectively reassess your manuscript from a reviewer's viewpoint. You need to "sell" your manuscript by persuading readers that the topic is relevant to the specialty, that you have chosen an appropriate method and that your conclusions are sound. Just as importantly, you need to avoid "overselling" your manuscript by trumping up its importance. This chapter will help with your reality check, review the most common problems cited by editors and reviewers, and help you bullet-proof your paper for critical review.

Part 1: What to expect when submitting: A step-by-step guide to the review process

Most peer-reviewed print journals follow a similar process for assessing whether a manuscript is suitable for publication. While the following is a general guide, it is critical to review the "Information for Authors" page or web site where each journal spells out its unique process and requirements. This point is so important it bears repeating: Follow the instructions to authors carefully! Most journals have a screening process and nothing will delay your article being sent out for review more surely than not following the journal's directions. Many journals have a step-by-step checklist that must be followed to the letter before they will even look at your manuscript.

Technical review

The journal's non-editorial staff initially reviews manuscripts to assure that the submission meets the journal's specific requirements. The staff may return manuscripts that are improperly submitted. While fixing the formatting and resubmitting your manuscript will not put you at a disadvantage for acceptance, it obviously lengthens the review process unnecessarily. Be sure to read and follow every instruction for submitting the manuscript. You can call or e-mail the

---

journal's staff with specific questions, but do not expect them to make exceptions or to tell you anything other than what's explicitly stated in the "Information for Authors".

Editor assignment
After the manuscript is successfully submitted, an editor is assigned. At smaller publications, the editor-in-chief might take responsibility for all submitted manuscripts. At larger journals the task is divided among several editors, who may be referred to as deputy, associate, or decision editors. These editors may be assigned to manuscripts that meet their own area of interest or expertise, or may simply take manuscripts in rotation.

Initial review
The editor will usually perform an initial review of the manuscript to determine whether further peer review is warranted. Editors may reject manuscripts out-of-hand if the subject matter is beyond the journal's domain or unlikely to interest the readers, if the methodology is clearly flawed, or if the writing is so bad that it is impossible to understand. While this sounds autocratic, a fast rejection is often preferable to a long wait for a review of a manuscript that is clearly not suitable for publication in a given journal.

Peer review
Most manuscripts are sent to reviewers for comment. Reviewers may be assigned randomly or matched to the manuscript's subject matter according their own interests and area of expertise. Some journals ask authors to suggest reviewers; this option appears to be getting less common as journals try to increase the objectivity of the reviews they collect. Editors may also assign statistical reviewers to comment specifically on the methodology, statistical analyses, and results.

Reviewers are expected to read the entire manuscript in exquisite detail. They note whether the authors have clearly defined their goals, explained their methods, thoroughly reported their findings, and justified their conclusions. Reviews may comment on the grammar and readability, but only when they interfere with comprehension. Some journals provide scoring rubrics and pose detailed questions to the reviewers, while others simply ask reviewers to provide overall impressions and suggestions. Reviewers are usually asked to recommend whether the manuscript should be accepted, revised, or rejected. They may also be asked to provide separate, confidential comments for the editor that will not be shared with the authors.

The blinded review process
Many journals request that authors submit a blinded copy of the manuscript. While the editor will know the authors' identity for purposes of communication, the reviewers are blinded to this information. Other journals forego this step, citing evidence that blinding does not impact reviewer objectivity.

Authors are often concerned that reviewers may reject their manuscript due to personal or professional bias. They fear that reviewers may have a strong interest in the topic and object to others publishing in their field or contradicting their results. Authors may also be concerned that a reviewer will recognize them and be biased personally against them. In our experience, editors and reviewers usually do an admirable job of performing objective reviews, and often take pains to minimize potential biases. Reviewers with conflicts of interest may disqualify themselves from performing a review, but usually they provide a critique and identify their potential biases. These individuals are often truly experts in their field and generally provide excellent comments and balanced analyses. In the end, the editor will consider all reviewers' comments, and manuscripts are rarely rejected based on negative comments from a single reviewer.

Consensus review
The editor is responsible for providing a global assessment of the manuscript's suitability for publication, based on the reviewers' comments and his or her own impressions. The editor may compile a consensus review, summarizing the most salient comments and suggestions, resolving conflicting criticism, and making specific recommendations for improvement. Alternatively, the editor may simply forward each reviewer's comments to the author. While the latter approach may appear more objective, it often presents the author with widely divergent and contradictory opinions and suggestions.

Decision options
The editor may accept the manuscript without revision. This is rare at selective peer-reviewed publications – less than 10% of submissions receive this decision – as even the best manuscripts have some issues that need to be resolved before publication. Some journals provide editors with an option to conditionally accept a manuscript, requiring only minor revisions. More often, the editor will inform the author that the manuscript will be reconsidered after the reviewers'

concerns have been addressed in a formal revision. This is known as "revise and reconsider". Finally, the editor may decide that the reviewer's comments warrant rejecting the manuscript without providing an opportunity for revision.

Revisions and final decisions

The "revise and reconsider" option may be difficult for authors. The editor may simply have minor concerns about the study that can be easily addressed. Sometimes, however, the editor has serious concerns regarding the study's methodology, execution, data interpretation, or presentation. The conclusions or even the entire focus of the manuscript may need to be modified, requiring major revisions. Occasionally the reviewers may state that study is fatally flawed, but the editor decided to grant the author an opportunity to justify the methodology or analysis.

When major revisions are requested, the authors need to decide whether to comply with the suggestions, explain why the suggested revisions are unnecessary, or concede that the manuscript cannot be revised. There is no guarantee that the manuscript will be accepted if the revisions are made. The editor may send the manuscript to the same reviewers for reconsideration, or may render a final decision independently.

Turn-around times

The time frame for receiving the editor's decision varies widely by journal and circumstances. Out-of-hand rejections may take only a few days. It generally takes a month for a study to be sent for full review. If a "revise and reconsider" decision is rendered, the authors will be given a specific deadline to submit their revisions, usually a few weeks to a month from the time the decision is rendered. If the revision is not received by the deadline, the editor will assume that the authors do not want their manuscript reconsidered and will close the file.

Part 2: Bullet-proofing your manuscript

Some studies are so important and methodologically sound that editors and reviewers can barely contain their excitement to accept the manuscript. Conversely, some studies are seriously flawed and no amount of revision can render them suitable for publication, at least in the authors' preferred journal. The majority of studies fall in between these extremes: they have merit, but they also have limitations that impact their validity. Authors of these middle-ground manuscripts need to take an honest look at the study's potential problems, anticipate the reviewers' concerns, and openly address the limitations. Bullet-proofing the manuscript can be the essential difference between a quick rejection and ultimate publication.

Follow "Instructions for Authors" to the letter

This is self-evident. Editors are busy and will not look favorably on manuscripts that do not adhere to the journal guidelines for content and format. Editors may overlook these issues for exceptionally strong manuscripts, but they are more inclined to reject a marginal manuscript if the authors appear to have trouble following instructions.

Unsympathetic feedback

Getting honest feedback from a reliable disinterested party is an important proactive step. Your independent reviewer should be knowledgeable about the field, but not necessarily expert in the specific topic. Ideally, he or she will have experience as a reviewer for a medical journal and knows how to pick apart a manuscript. If possible, choose someone who is your senior and will not be worried about offending you. Be sure to specify that you want critical comments; there is little value to a polite cursory review.

Style points

It is not just what you say, it is how you say it. Editors and reviewers are supposed to be blind to grammar and spelling, but it is human nature to look negatively at poorly written manuscripts. Editors and reviewers are already working hard to gauge the scientific merit of your study; making them struggle to understand your grammar will not garner a sympathetic audience. If a reviewer or editor has to read a sentence or paragraph twice to understand it then it is not clear and concise enough; this will impact negatively on the review. Be concise. All journals have page limits and editors want to pack as many articles in an issue as they can. In the same way that a diagram should have no unnecessary lines, a sentence should have no unnecessary words and a paragraph should have no unnecessary sentences. Ask a second disinterested party to review your manuscript for style and grammar; this reader does not need to be a medical professional.

Make it interesting to the non-expert

You're an expert in your subject matter, but the editors, reviewers, and readers are probably not. One of the editor's most important decisions is determining whether your topic is interesting to the majority of the journal's readers, not just those immersed in a narrow field. Beyond picking an appropriate journal, making your manuscript interesting is largely a function of writing style. Your introduction should persuade the "casual" journal reader that your topic is relevant. Do not assume that the reader already knows the study background, clinical relevance, and prior investigations. Many manuscripts are ultimately accepted not because the study itself is profound, but because the authors have written an interesting and engaging discussion that addresses a question that is relevant to the journal's readers.

Know your limitations

Every study has some flaws, either because of design oversights or due to the inevitable compromises that were necessary along the way. Do not try to convince yourself – and the reviewers – that the limitations are not important. The reviewers will identify every potential weakness in your study and will include it in their criticism. Rather than having to justify your study's limitations in revisions, proactively address *every* potential objection to your methodology and conclusions in the "Limitations" or "Discussion" section, as appropriate to the journal. Think of it as a game: the goal is to identify more potential limitations than the reviewers can. Be intellectually honest, but you do not need to apologize. It is fine to state that execution did not go exactly as planned or that another methodology might have been appropriate. Your goal is to show reviewers that you understand your study's deficiencies and stand by your conclusions. Editors will quickly reject a manuscript that ignores, refuses to acknowledge, or minimizes important limitations. A study that is honest about its limitations, does not overstate its conclusions, and paints an accurate portrait of the its value is more likely to be accepted in the end.

Choose an appropriate journal and audience

Choose a journal based not its impact factor or perceived prestige, but based on the best match between your topic and the journal's target audience. Look carefully at the types of articles a journal publishes, see where articles similar to yours appear, and read the journal's mission statement, aims, and scope. Some outstanding manuscripts are rejected by selective journals because the topic is too esoteric for their readers. Conversely, marginal manuscripts may be accepted by journals that are eager to publish studies addressing particular topics. A "Call for Manuscripts" is an outstanding opportunity to publish a manuscript that might be marginal in other circumstances – it tells you that a journal is actively looking to promote the visibility of a particular topic, and may lower the bar for accepting manuscripts in this field.

Data dredging

Editors and reviewers hate fishing expeditions: manuscripts with vague or non-existent objectives, voluminous data collection, multiple statistical analyses that do not address a specific hypothesis, and conclusions that have nothing to do with the study goals. Failure to define a specific study objective is a common reason for rejection. Secondary objectives are fine, but the entire manuscript needs to be framed by a *principle* hypothesis or goal. A common error is to frame an observational study as a hypothesis-testing trial, including statistical analyses of results that were only noticed after *post hoc* inspection and analysis of the data. Such analyses are invalid and reviewers pick up on this issue quickly. An observational study can report such findings only with the caveat that the results may have value if validated by further study.

Abstract problems

Write the abstract last. The abstract should contain only information already discussed in the body of the manuscript. A common error is to submit abstracts that present data or conclusions that do not appear anywhere else. While this is probably an oversight, it does not reflect well on the author. Make sure the numbers in the abstract are the same numbers presented in the body of the manuscript. Also, remember that many journals require a structured abstract and this may be the only thing that thing an end user may see when performing an electronic search. Your abstract should be clear enough and well crafted to present the key interventions and results, and should stand alone in an electronic format.

Only one chance to make a first impression

Just as you were taught in high school, your introduction needs to set the stage and grab the readers' attention. Reviewers are likely to lose interest if the introduction is poorly written or does not make the study seem relevant to the specialty. A great introduction states what is known about a subject, explains why further investigation is necessary, and concisely tells the reader what the authors have set out to do – all in a few paragraphs. By convention, you should clearly state the study objective in the last sentence of the final paragraph in the introduction section.

Results: Just stick to the facts

The "Results" section is not the place to opine on the implications of your research or defend your study methodology. This should be factual analysis of your data, framed entirely by the study objectives and based only on the statistical methodology you have already specified. Secondary results should not be overemphasized. Avoid introducing results that were never part of the study question. "Interesting findings" from unplanned analyses may just be statistical artifacts; *post hoc* analyses should be clearly stated as such, if mentioned at all. Overstating the importance of secondary or unplanned analyses is a common and serious flaw.

A picture is worth a thousand digits

Editors and reviewers like pretty pictures. Replace tables with graphs whenever possible, and avoid putting long iterations of statistical results in the body of the manuscript. Use graphs appropriately. Bar graphs and line graphs portray different kinds of data. Three-dimensional graphs must be reserved for data that has three dimensions. Do not use figures to distort your data; reviewers will spot these manipulations.

Discussion: fair and balanced

The discussion should revisit the introduction: you have already set the stage, now explain how your study adds to our body of knowledge. A nice way to organize the discussion section is to present your interpretation of the main outcome measure or key results first, then secondary outcomes in the same sequence you presented them in the results section. The key to an effective discussion is being even-handed in reviewing the relevant literature and assessing the implications of your research. Outline avenues for future investigation; if you are really organized, you have already started your follow-up study.

Conclusions

Reread your study goals and hypothesis before writing your conclusion. The conclusions should specifically and exclusively address the study objectives. It is permissible to qualify your conclusions in light of the study's limitations; this makes you appear forthcoming and rarely diminishes prospects for publication. Never try to cast the result of *post hoc* analyses as a principal conclusion. Additionally, do not overstate your conclusions. You may think your work is worth a Nobel Prize and will change practice tomorrow. In reality, only about 2% of studies published in peer-reviewed journals influence clinical practice. Be honest about what the reader can take away from your research.

References

You probably cannot cite every study relevant to your manuscript. References should cite a representative sample of important work in your field. In a further effort to be even-handed, whenever possible cite studies that reach different conclusions from yours. Obviously, all publications explicitly mentioned in the text must be referenced. Be sure to check the instructions for authors and use standard reference formatting. Improperly formatted endnotes make reviewers question the author's credibility.

Part 3: Responding to the decision

The job of the reviewer is to detect imperfections in your study design, your statistical methods and analysis, and the inferences you have made based on your result. Many will even comment on your syntax, grammar, and writing style. Expect suggestions, criticisms, requests for clarification, and even requests for additional analyses of your data. You need to develop a thick skin before going any further down this road.

What was the decision?

As mentioned above, the decision types may differ slightly between journals, but generally fall into four rough categories – Accept, Revise and Accept, Revise and Reconsider, or Reject. If your decision is "Accept" or "Revise and Accept", the journal has decided to publish your manuscript as-is or with very minor alterations. A "Reject" decision is the end of the line for that particular journal. Remember, a rejection may not be a condemnation of your research;

it is often it is a matter of finding an appropriate venue for your manuscript. A rejection can be a blessing in disguise; reviewers often provide thorough analysis of your manuscript and useful commentary that guides your revisions for resubmission elsewhere.

"Revise and Reconsider": Reading between the lines

A "Revise and Reconsider" decision is the toughest outcome to handle, as you are usually asked make significant changes to your manuscript without the guarantee of publication. Read the editor's letter and reviewers' comments carefully; these are your guides to deducing what is expected for further consideration. Go through the comments on a point-by-point basis. You may find that you can easily address the concerns and queries without compromising the spirit of your manuscript and your conclusions. At times it may be difficult or impossible to revise your manuscript to meet the suggestions. Reviewers may ask for additional data that you did not collect or suggest additional statistical analyses. Occasionally reviewers suggest a totally different study design or make similarly unhelpful comments.

Know when to hold, know when to fold

You are now faced with a key decision: whether to comply with revision requests, to respectfully disagree with the suggestions, or to walk away from the journal. The revision process is a major and often painful undertaking. Consensus decision letters should provide a clear understanding of the journals' major concerns with the manuscript. You will need to make every requested revision or provide a detailed explanation of your justification for not doing so. When a consensus review asks for revisions you are unable or unwilling to make, it is probably time to choose another journal.

The issue is trickier in journals that do not provide consensus letters. The "raw" reviewer comments have not been consolidated by the editor and often conflict with one another. The editor may not expect you to make every change suggested by each reviewer, but you will still need to respectfully respond to each comment. If a single reviewer makes demands that seem unreasonable, you may still have a fighting chance for successful resubmission to journal.

What if you think the reviewer is just wrong?

Reviews often contain suggestion with which you strongly disagree. While it may not be necessary to modify your manuscript to satisfy each reviewer comment, you will need to provide sound justification for declining to make suggested revisions. The editor may not agree with your assessment and may insist that you adhere to the reviewers' suggestions. This may be a deal-breaker if you are unwilling or unable to make the revision.

On occasion, editors will ask you to make changes to your manuscript that, in your opinion, significantly change the spirit of the manuscript and the conclusions that you are trying to convey. These require a value judgment: do you want to see the manuscript published by this journal the way they want it written, or would you rather see the manuscript published to your satisfaction in another journal? This decision requires soul-searching and discussion between all contributing authors.

Corresponding with the editor

It is not usually necessary to correspond with the editor as you complete your revisions. On occasion, however, you may not understand what is being asked of you or the reviewers may have provided conflicting suggestions. The decision letter (usually an e-mail) will provide the editor's name and contact information. Most editors are happy to correspond by e-mail to clarify the expectations for revision. Editors may be far more sympathetic in personal correspondence than in formal communication and can work with you to resolve the reviewers' concerns in a mutually satisfactory way. You can pose direct questions to the editor about whether declining to make a specific revision would be a deal-breaker. This can save an enormous amount of time in the end and permit you to move on and submit your manuscript elsewhere. If you would prefer a telephone discussion, it is best to e-mail the editor and set up a time for discussion.

Submitting revisions

The decision letter will contain detailed instructions for submitting a revised manuscript. You may be required to submit a manuscript with changes highlighted, or to use an automated tracking function to identify your revisions. Again, it is imperative that you follow these instructions to the letter.

Most journals require that you provide a detailed cover letter outlining your responses to the queries and suggestions provided in the initial review. You will need to supply a point-by-point response to each reviewer or consensus comment, query, and suggestion. If you have made a requested revision, it is sufficient to state, "changed as suggested." If you choose not to make a suggested revision, or if you disagree with a suggestion, you will need to justify your decision.

At times this requires an in-depth discussion of your statistical methods or the rationale for your methodology. Be clear and succinct.

It is just business

It is easy for authors to become personally offended by reviewer's comments and suggestions. After all, some stranger has insulted your precious offspring. It is critical to address the editor and the reviewers' comments with utmost professional respect. Even if you feel belittled by a comment, attacking the reviewer will damage your chances for acceptance on further review. Remember that the editor has endorsed the suggestions, at least passively, by passing on the reviewers' comments. The editor and the reviewers are working on the same team; you do not want to become their adversary. Instead of simply refusing to make a modification, offer to clarify your manuscript to addresses their concern. Thank the reviewers for their suggestion, even if you disagree with it. In short, your spirit and tone should be that of a partner in a mutual effort to improve your manuscript for publication.

Summary

Understanding important rules and customs of manuscript preparation and submission can greatly enhance the chances of seeing your study published in your journal of choice. Necessary steps include knowledge of the editorial process and timeline, ensuring that your manuscript is concise, accurate, and well written, meeting the target journal's requirements, and understanding potential editorial decisions and how best to respond to them.

KEY POINTS

- Choose your journal carefully based upon the best match between your topic and the journal's target audience.
- Read the journal's instructions for authors and follow them to the letter.
- Write the manuscript as clearly and concisely as possible.
- Write a manuscript that is interesting to the non-expert.
- Acknowledge your study's limitations – every study has them.
- Get honest feedback from at least one reliable, disinterested party prior to submission.
- Understand the editorial process and timeline to avoid anger, disappointment, or impatience.
- Respond to any requests from the editors quickly, professionally, and accurately.

Further reading

1 DeBehnke, D.J., Kline, J.A., and Shih, R.D. (2001) Research fundamentals: Choosing an appropriate journal, manuscript preparation, and interaction with editors. *Acad Emerg Med*, **8**:844–850.
2 Ezeala, C., Nweke, I., and Ezeala, M. (2013) Common errors in manuscripts submitted to medical science journals. *Ann Med Health Sci Res*, **3**:376–379.
3 Kibbe, M.R., Sarr, M.G., Livingston, E.H., *et al*. (2014) The art and science of publishing: reflections from editors of surgery journals. *J Surg Res*, **186**(1):7–15.
4 Lewis, L.M., Lewis, R.J., Younger, J.G., and Callaham, M. (1998) Research fundamentals: I. Getting from hypothesis to manuscript: an overview of the skills required for success in research. *Acad Emerg Med*, **5**:924–929.
5 Schriger, D.L. and Cooper, R.J. (2001) Achieving graphical excellence: suggestions and methods for creating high-quality visual displays of experimental data. *Ann Emerg Med*, **37**:75–87.
6 Singer, A.J. and Hollander, J.E. (2009) How to write a manuscript. *J Emerg Med*, **36**:89–93.

CHAPTER 36

How do I write a grant?

Zachary D.W. Dezman and Jon Mark Hirshon

Department of Emergency Medicine, University of Maryland School of Medicine, Baltimore, MD, USA

Dr Stevenson is an aspiring young researcher who is writing a grant to support his research into the impact of anticoagulants on trauma patients. However, he has little knowledge or experience about developing and organizing a successful proposal. After much work, he submits a National Institute of Health (NIH) K23 grant (a grant that supports research that has direct patient contact), which goes unscored because it should have been submitted as a NIH K08 (a grant without direct patient contact). He resubmits a revised version as a NIH K08 and is successful! In the process he learns – understand the details of the RFA (request for applications) when submitting a proposal.

Introduction

Writing a successful grant combines art, skill, science, self-confidence and a touch of salesmanship. This chapter provides a brief introduction to grant writing in order to impart some key ideas and concepts. Creating a fundable proposal is a complex task requiring many steps and multiple components. A key early step of successful grant writing is finding an experienced mentor, both to help guide you through the funding process and to show the funding agency that you have knowledgeable expert support. There are many other components that go into successful grant writing: showing you have the appropriate collaborators (research is a team activity); institutional resources and environment (equipment, statistical support, appropriate space, etc.); appropriate financial structure and support; and appropriate ethical considerations (either human subjects or animals). Any application will contain instructions detailing the exact format of these supporting components, and a quick guide to writing NIH grants can be found through the NIH Examples of successful grants can often be found through your institution's office of research development. However, this chapter will focus on how to write a compelling scientific argument for grants, primarily for the NIH.

General definitions

A grant is an amount of money given by a funding agency (e.g., government body, professional society, private donor, etc.) that provides financial support for a proposed project. It can provide primarily salary support (common in training grants), money for supplies (small start-up grants), or both (e.g., NIH R01 grants). A contract is similar, but designed to obtain financial support for specifically defined tasks or deliverables such as developing a specified output or program. Cooperative agreements obtain financial support for work that will be developed and specified in collaboration with the funding agency. It is important to understand the different funding structures, as they have implications about what you can and cannot do within a specific project. When in doubt, ask! You can discuss it with the grant/contract contact person included on the RFA, the departmental contact in the office of sponsored programs at your institution, or your mentor.

Getting started

Once you have identified a research question and a potential funding agency or source, speak with the program officer for the RFA or RFP (request for proposals). This can help inform you whether there is interest in your topic and whether there are other potential funding mechanisms available. Additionally, interpersonal relationships are

Doing Research in Emergency and Acute Care: Making Order Out of Chaos, First Edition. Edited by Michael P. Wilson, Kama Z. Guluma, and Stephen R. Hayden.

© 2016 John Wiley & Sons, Ltd. Published 2016 by John Wiley & Sons, Ltd.

important: getting to know the program officer can be very helpful, as he or she can inform you of what is currently of importance and interest within their institute or organization.

Overall grant tone

Throughout the remainder of this chapter, you will notice a common theme cropping up – "This project can be done;" "We have the support;" "This is an important project;" For those who have ever made a successful sale's pitch, or obtained support from potential business investors, grant writing is much the same concept. In a formal and written fashion, you are trying to "sell" the reader on your idea and show them that you have every almost every resource lined up to complete the project, proving to them your project has a high chance of successful completion and that you are worth the additional investment.

As you write the grant, it may strike you "Why am I doing all of this work ahead of time? I can do much of this after I get funded." Firstly, if you feel the hypothesis is strong and important enough for you to go through the effort of writing the grant, you should consider doing the project regardless of whether you get funding from the current RFA or not. Secondly, all of the thought and effort you put into project development ahead of time makes everything later – the poster showing the results, the final journal publication – much, much easier. Thirdly, your project will have greater chances of successful completion after you have gone through the effort of multiple revisions of your research plan. Finally, as general advice, a small focused project has greater likelihood of being funded than a large diffuse project. Great success is built through a series of small steps.

The importance of grant application instructions

A key early step to a successful funding application is to obtain the grant application instructions and to go through them carefully and to follow them precisely. This may seem intuitive, but grants have been returned without review because the margins were not right or the font too small. Any deviation from the instructions – especially page lengths – is an easy way for the institutional officers or an overstretched grant reviewer to reject your proposal without reading it. A second and equally critical point is to know your deadlines! Most granting agencies, and particularly the federal government, have a specific date for grant submission and there is no flexibility for a late application. These deadlines are for the final submission – not for when you need to route it through your institution before submitting it to the funding source. Know your institutional guidelines for submission – does it have to be sent to them one week in advance or two weeks? Your institution needs to review and approve the proposal prior to its submission to the grant agency.

Often you will be able to obtain a copy of a previous similar grant that was successfully funded. Having a model for success can definitely enhance the quality of your grant, but be aware that the writing requirements or proposal structure may have changed, so always confirm that your formatting, style, and length are correct. Each funding agency will have its own grant format, but many follow the NIH model in general.

Writing the research plan

The Research Plan is the core of your project, in which you clearly and explicitly define your hypothesis and how you will conduct your research. In the current NIH format, it will contain four main components: Specific Aims, Significance, Innovation, and Approach.

Specific aims

The first section, Specific Aims, should quickly focus the reader to your research topic and your specific hypothesis. It should be one page, and is often the only page that unassigned reviewers will read. Items to be covered, albeit briefly, include: general long-term goals of the research; specific objectives of the proposal and the hypothesis to be tested; expected outcomes; and importance of the research project and its potential impact. Often, the first paragraph is scripted as follows: what is known in the specific research field; what is not known/current knowledge gaps in the field; how the current research project will fill the identified gaps; and why this is important knowledge. It commonly ends with the specific, testable primary hypothesis of the proposed research project.

> Injuries are the most common cause of death in persons aged 1–45 years of age. Pre-injury anticoagulant use has been shown to increase mortality in trauma. Emergency physicians and surgeons need to know what complications to expect when faced with a trauma patient on anticoagulants, but there are few data on bleeding rates in patients prescribed new anticoagulant medications like dabigatran. Our hypothesis is: Injured patients admitted to high volume, level 1 trauma centers on dabigatran are more likely to have bleeding complications, such as the need for transfusion, than injured patients not on anticoagulants when controlling for age, gender and comorbid conditions.

Significance

The Significance section will explain why your research topic and project are important. This section is usually 1–2 pages long (in a 12-page research plan). It may highlight critical barriers to progress in the field and how your research project will address them. You will also use this space to show how your project will improve the knowledge, technical capability, or clinical practice of the field. Within this section, you can give some thought as to how many people will be affected or how your project will change practice if the project is completed. A Significance section should answer the following questions: "Does this study address an important problem?" and "If our aims are achieved, what will be the result?" This section answers the "So what?" question – if you complete the research what difference would it make?

Innovation

The Innovation section tells how this project will challenge current practice or theories. This section is usually ½ –1 page in length. If your project uses a novel instrument, methodology, or approach, for example, "The ability of base deficit to predict mortality has never been examined in this population before," then use this section to describe how your project is unique. Note that there is a fine balance between innovative and impractical. You may have a new approach to a problem, but if it is not realistic or feasible within the bounds of the support provided by the grant, (e.g., "Evaluating chest pain in astronauts on the lunar surface"), it will be perceived as too risky and will not be funded. A common mistake of new grant writers is to promise too much for the scope of the grant. It is much better to do small projects well than to promise the world.

Approach

If the research plan is the heart of your grant application, then the Approach section is the heart of the research plan. This section is the critical component of the grant that will specifically describe what you plan to do and how you plan to do it. It is usually 9–10 pages in length and has a more in-depth discussion of the general points previously raised in the Specific Aims page. Here you will go into a more detailed discussion of the information conveyed in your introductory paragraphs, such as the history of the problem, the risks to public, and so on. Not every reviewer will read your Approach, but it is important for the assigned reviewer who will be evaluating your grant to understand the entire context of your project and what you plan to do.

Your Approach section will include a more expanded discussion of your hypotheses as well as your long term goals. This is the section where the grant writer displays their thought process and method of evaluating their stated hypothesis. This is your opportunity to show how all of your resources – patient population, institution, study methodology, and so on. – will fit to evaluate your hypothesis. You also need to state what steps (specific aims) you plan to do in order to successfully complete your project, in other words your overall experimental design with a concrete sequence of action and a specific work plan.

As part of the Approach, preliminary data are usually included. It is not an absolute requirement for all grants, but most funded grants, especially at the NIH level, will have some. It is an easy way to elevate the quality of your proposal. What exactly do we mean by preliminary data? Some sort of information related to your hypothesis – perhaps you did a pilot study looking at the question (often done in translational studies). Perhaps you have looked at your patient database and you already know you have at least 10,000 cases and 20,000 controls (clinical and epidemiological studies). In the former, you are showing "proof of concept" and the purpose of the grant is to fund you to fully investigate your idea. In the latter, you are building towards your power calculations. In both cases, preliminary data show feasibility. Often, preliminary data form the core of an upcoming publication. As described above, it gives evidence in favor of your hypothesis, it allows you to do some initial calculations on power, and it shows achievability. The point of the grant is to show the funding agency how important your question is and that you have a high-quality method of testing your hypothesis that is achievable with all of the resources you have available.

Within the Approach, you need to discuss the precise procedures and methods needed to be able to accomplish your experiment or answer your hypothesis and specific aims. With clinical research, this may be a discussion of how you will enroll subjects, test them, record the data and then analyze the results. You need to describe the overall study structure – are you going to conduct a retrospective case–control study, a multicenter prospective cohort study, or a double-blind, placebo controlled clinical trial? Additional components of discussing the experimental activities include how you will collect the data, how they will be managed and how they will be analyzed. A Gant chart is a good way to convey a complex schedule within page limits (Appendix 36.1).

If you are writing a training grant, this is also a good way to show when you will be in different stages of training and when you will graduate. Reviewers expect a high level of detail – they need to understand exactly what you are planning and how you will accomplish your research. If you are relatively new to research, this is where additional team support is critical. Get the input from an epidemiologist or biostatistician if you are carrying out clinical or public health research, or from a senior laboratory scientist if you are carrying out basic science research. The key is to be clear and understandable so the reviewer knows exactly what you will do, how you will do it and when you will do it.

Also, within the Approach section it is important to discuss potential problems as well as possible alternative strategies. No researcher, especially a junior researcher, knows exactly what will happen with their project. The reviewers want to see that you have carefully thought through the project, identified potential pitfalls, and have come up with ways to address problems or alternate strategies for success. This is where you prove to the reviewer you have a robust study design, and that, while you cannot foresee all contingencies, you can anticipate some solutions.

The budget and budget justification

The budget and budget justification are key components, for you, for your institution, and for the funding source. The budget will show how the money will be spent, while the budget justification will explain why it is being spent in this manner. These components should clearly support the research – if the expenditures are not consistent with the research plan and the approach, reviewers will raise questions. Do not forget – academic institutions take a percentage of grants as indirects (to support the administrative infrastructure). This varies depending on the type of grant, the rules of the funding source, and the location at which the research will occur. However, it can be upwards of 50% of your grant, depending on your institution.

Ethical considerations

When conducting research on humans or animals, you will need to obtain the appropriate institutional review and approval. This may be required prior to grant submission, but is frequently necessary prior to fund disbursement. If carrying out multisite or international work, this may require multiple approvals. Again, it is important that the reviewers and the funding agency have confidence that you will conduct your research ethically and within the appropriate federal regulations.

KEY POINTS

- Developing a successful proposal is a complex multistep task.
- Research is a collaborative effort. It is critical to develop a strong grant writing and research team.
- The grant should be structured based upon the funding agency's instructions.
- Key components of the proposal should include:
  - What is the gap in knowledge?
  - How will your work fill the identified gap?
  - Why is this important and innovative (the "so what" question)?
  - What have you (or your team) done in this area to show:
    - Expert knowledge
    - Prior experience
    - High likelihood of project success.
  - What are the environmental and personnel structures supporting the proposal?
- Have as many people as possible read your grant proposal prior to submission:
  - Include individuals from outside of your research area and even perhaps some lay readers. Their review can help make sure that it is readable, especially for a reviewer without knowledge in your specific research field.
- The NIH web site is a valuable source of further information (Appendix 36.2).

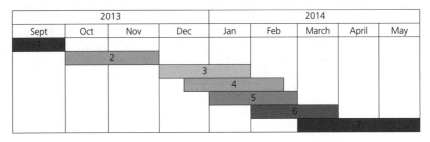

Figure A36.1.1 A representative Gantt chart.

Appendix 36.1 Gantt Chart

A Gantt chart is shown in Figure A36.1.1 describing the different stages of a research project: when each step is started, how long it takes, and when it should end. Note the key, and that the steps are listed chronologically, some steps occur concurrently. You should get information from your mentor on how long each of these steps is (e.g., IRB approval) or even run a small pilot to determine how long it will take you to enroll patients. You should also build into your timeline a factor of safety, to avoid delays.

Calendar/Mileposts
1 Study design and project proposal development: One month.
2 Institutional Review Board review and approval: Two months.
3 Project Implementation with inservices for support staff: 1–2 months.
4 Estimated data collection period: 1–2 months.
5 Estimated sample testing period: 1–2 months.
6 Data analysis: Two months.
7 Journal article writing and submission: Three months.
  Target Conference: ACEP, abstract submission date: Late April.

Appendix 36.2 Additional resources

- National Institutes of Health (2015) Grants & Funding. http://grants.nih.gov/grants/oer.htm (last accessed 16 May 2015).
- National Institutes of Health (2015) The K Kiosk – Information about NIH Career Development Awards. http://grants.nih.gov/training/careerdevelopmentawards.htm (last accessed 16 May 2015).
- The National Institute for Allergies and Infectious Diseases (2014) All About Grants: Tutorials and Samples. http://www.niaid.nih.gov/researchfunding/grant/Pages/aag.aspx (last accessed 16 May 2015).
- The National Institutes of Health Research Portfolio Online Reporting Tools: http://report.nih.gov/
- The National Science Foundation's (nd) Find Funding. http://www.nsf.gov/funding/ (last accessed 16 May 2015).
- Grants.gov (nd) Find Open Grant Opportunities. http://www.grants.gov (last accessed 16 May 2015).

CHAPTER 37

How to make an academic career: Developing a successful path in research

Deirdre Anglin and Michael Menchine

Department of Emergency Medicine, Keck School of Medicine of University of Southern California, Los Angeles, CA, USA

> *"I've just finished my Chief Resident year and am really excited and privileged to have been offered an academic position. I have an interest in disaster medicine and I would like to try my hand at research, although I haven't done much so far. This job is a great opportunity – I am going to be on the hospital disaster response team and want to figure out how to succeed."*
>
> Recent graduate/new faculty member

Congratulations! You are well on your way to an academic career for all the right reasons: you have decided that you want an academic career in a clinical setting, rather than a clinical career in an academic setting. You love the academic environment, the high level of education and teaching, innovation, and research that are involved with academics. Furthermore, you have already committed to pursuing research, one of the three pillars of academics (education, service, research). So, what else should you know before embarking on your research career in an acute care, clinical specialty?

Firstly, take a breath. Developing a research career takes a long time. Why, you ask? Because conducting meaningful, valid research is *really hard* and requires a knowledge base and skill set beyond what you have learned in residency. What is a good question? What study design should I use? How can I hire and manage staff? What data management services should I use? Who can help with the analytic plan? The writing? Funding? In our experience, many junior faculty members quickly become overwhelmed by these questions and begin focusing on non-research academic activities. We do not want this to happen to you. You have started off wisely by reading this book, which can help in answering these questions. But, perhaps more importantly, you should recognize that the training and experience you obtained in residency was predominantly clinical – and your patients will thank you for that. Whatever research training you received was probably unstructured and found in journal club or your periodic participation in projects with a faculty mentor. Becoming an independent researcher will require developing new skills that are distinct from the clinical expertise you have already gained, and this will take time. To put the time needed into perspective, a recent review from the National Institutes of Health (NIH) showed that, in 2011, the average age of an MD being funded for their **first** RO1 (the benchmark of independent research grants) was about 46 years. Now this may not be the time frame you or your new boss had in mind, but setting unrealistic expectations will put too much pressure on a bright but fledgling career. In order to conduct high quality studies you will need to have a robust research toolkit (Figure 37.1). And that takes patience to develop, something that many of us who practice in acute care settings do not have an overabundance of.

In our view, the academic toolkit is comprised of four categories: values, attributes, skills, and support. It is important to conduct an honest self-assessment and evaluation of your situation to determine what things are already in your toolkit and what deficiencies exist. While many young faculty already possess the necessary values and attributes to become successful researchers, fewer have the skills, and almost none have the time, mentoring, and financial support essential for success.

Doing Research in Emergency and Acute Care: Making Order Out of Chaos, First Edition. Edited by Michael P. Wilson, Kama Z. Guluma, and Stephen R. Hayden.

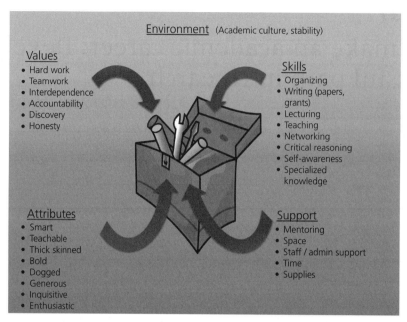

Figure 37.1 Components of an academic toolkit.

Here are key factors to take into consideration while developing the tools for a successful research career:
• Fellowship training
• Mentorship
• Choosing a research focus
• Profile of activities
• Challenges.

Fellowship training: Is it necessary?

Analytic, critical reasoning, writing, public speaking, networking, and organizational skills (among others) are crucial tools to add to your toolbox. You may gain these "on-the-job" by taking advantage of opportunities as they become available or pursing an advanced degree (i.e., MPH, MS, etc.) on your weekends and holidays. However, it is our opinion that undertaking a research fellowship is the best, or certainly the most efficient, way to gain these skills. Not only will you be able to obtain an advanced degree, but you will benefit from formal mentoring, specialized knowledge that you get from formal didactics, and the ability to apply for funding for the future. In addition, having a research fellowship to add to your credentials will make you more marketable and increase your potential for securing a job anywhere in the country.

It is important to be careful when selecting a research fellowship, in order to maximize the benefit you receive from the experience. Look for fellowships with the following characteristics:
• Reasonable clinical workloads (≤8 shifts per month so that you do not have to moonlight 4+ shifts a month).
• Adequate salaries.
• Presence of ACTIVE mentors.
• Track record of producing research scholars.
• Formal curricula.

Mentorship

Having mentorship is critical to building your successful research career [1]. Characteristics of great mentors include [2]:
• Taking a personal interest in you.
• Acting as a role model.
• Having knowledge, willingness and time to share their knowledge.

So, why is it so difficult to find a good mentor? Being a good mentor is extremely time consuming. A mentor must commit to spending time helping you develop well-thought-out research questions, research skills, critical thinking, writing skills, grant writing skills, and specialized knowledge [3]. Frustratingly, the time spent in mentoring relationships often feels "low yield" in the beginning. Projects are discussed, refined, critiqued, and frequently abandoned in favor of another possible study, seemingly setting you back to square one. An experienced mentor will recognize this as part of the research process and continue to promote an open forum for thoughtful discussion and, importantly, disagreement [4]. Unfortunately, if such a mentor exists around you, s/he may not have similar research interests. We believe that it is so essential to the development of your research career for you to have adequate mentorship that this should take priority over your own topical research interests.

The ideal mentor should have:
- Knowledge about the specific area or focus you intend to pursue as well as your career path.
- Availability to meet and hold open discussions on a highly regular basis (e.g., semi-monthly).
- A history of receiving extramural funding.
- Experience in publishing in high-quality journals.

It is probable that no one in your department meets all these criteria. As such, you should not feel limited to having a single mentor. In fact, since much of the research that is conducted in the acute care setting is multidisciplinary, it is often advantageous to have one or more mentors in other disciplines or institutions that can give you an "arms-length" assessment of the project and your progress [5], In addition to mentors, you may seek out advisors to provide you with specific information.

In the case where you are unable to find a single mentor, a few different approaches have been tried to fill in the gap. These include:
- Team mentoring: multiple individuals either in a group or separately provide mentoring in their areas of expertise. In this scenario, you must manage the mentoring relationship carefully and be clear about what you are attempting to gain from each member of your team.
- Peer mentoring: multiple individuals, often of similar academic rank, collectively provide advice and mentorship to each other. We advise that you take advantage of professional societies' (ACEP, SAEM, AAEM) interest groups, sections and task forces to identify like-minded individuals who can help in peer mentoring.

It is not a "niche": Choosing a research focus

> *"It is better to commit and change, than not to commit at all."*
>
> Mike Menchine

Now that you have decided to pursue the research "pillar" of academics you suddenly realize, "I'm interested in so many things, I'm not sure where to start!" This is why committing to an area early is so important. Without this commitment, young faculty are often paralyzed, not knowing what field to study, and as a result they do not study anything. Developing your area of focus will take time and most commonly require some course corrections. You cannot correct your course unless you have committed to going somewhere.

We use the term focus over the more popular term "niche" for a couple of reasons. Firstly, the very definition of a niche is something small and shallow. Your research should certainly not feel small (at least to you). You should feel passion about the topic and a genuine desire to answer questions related to it. Secondly, because niches are so small, it can be exceedingly difficult to pinpoint one when you are just beginning, particularly one that does not feel saturated by more experienced researchers. On the other hand, if you start with a general topic, such as prehospital medicine, you can continually focus in on more and more precise and meaningful questions. With a focus you will have a direction in which to move your career forward. As you move forward, you will be identifying mentors, refining skills, filling your CV with publications and other scholarly activities, and advancing your career. In the process, you should continue to keep your eyes open for new and innovative areas that are of interest to you. Changing your focus is not a bad thing, but rather part of a process of finding out what interests you most. Many seasoned researchers have had several foci during their careers.

When choosing a focus, there are several factors to take into consideration, including:
- Whether you have a mentor.
- The location/institution in which you practice.

- The patient population.
- The clinical pathology.
- Potential collaborators.

If you have a mentor, your research focus is your mentor's focus. This will enable you to learn the most and, hence, benefit the most from the mentoring relationship. Remember, be patient! Maintain your long-term vision, but also have short-term goals and plans. Independence will come later.

In addition, it is important to carefully look at healthcare delivery issues, unique characteristics of the patient population, and diseases that are prevalent among the patients presenting to the institution in which you practice. Think of your emergency department as your clinical laboratory. Much of your science will come from the observations and experiments you or your colleagues conduct there. It will be far easier to conduct research in a focused area if there are many potential study participants, rather than if you focus on something outside your common clinical practice. Importantly, you should view any change in the practice environment as an experiment, whether designed for research purposes or to solve a clinical or administrative function. Take advantage of these natural experiments (most often funded through the hospital or operations division of the department) to conduct evaluations, learn analytic strategies, and write up findings without having to spend years finding the funding to conduct your own controlled experiments. In many cases, existing national or local data sets may offer you less expensive ways of pursuing your focus and gaining research skills.

There are some fairly new types of research that are relevant to the acute care setting. These include:
- Translational research.
- Comparative-effectiveness research.
- Outcomes research.
- Multidisciplinary research.

Emergency medicine may be well positioned to be part of these newer research emphases.

Profile of activities

The profile of your academic activities will fall into the three pillars: education, research, and service. For promotion, you will be required to demonstrate excellence in at least one area and be good in the other two. Most often, faculty will be excellent in only one area (maybe two!); as the field of academic emergency medicine specializes and matures, it is increasingly rare to find faculty who are truly excellent in all three areas. As a researcher, you will need to show excellence in research, but still have activities in education and service. The ideal way to accomplish this is to leverage your activities so that they are synergistic and each activity counts for two. For example, if your Chair asks you to head up a committee (service) to decrease door-to-balloon times, you could simultaneously initiate a research project to study the outcome of the intervention you develop to get patients to the cath lab more quickly.

You should review your profile of activities annually prior to meeting with your Chair. You should also review your profile of activities when considering taking on an additional activity and ask yourself:
- How does this activity fit into my profile of activities?
- Does it fill a gap in my profile of activities?
- Does this activity overlap with my other activities, especially my research focus, or is it way out in left field?

You will be more successful if your profile of activities looks more like Figure 37.2a (Ideal profile of activities), rather than Figure 37.2b (Non-ideal profile of activities).

Service activities that align with a research career may include organizing journal club, being a member of your Institutional Review Board, becoming a journal reviewer, and organizing local and regional research conferences. Educational activities to consider in your profile of activities include developing and teaching research curricula for medical students or residents, mentoring students in their scholarly projects (importantly, mentored projects should have *your* focus), and lecturing at regional or national conferences.

Challenges

Navigating a research career is not for the faint of heart. Your colleagues who pursue academic careers centered on clinical education or even administration will likely have more initial success than you. They will receive teaching awards, be invited to head committees, and be appointed as associate clinical or educational directors while you are spending

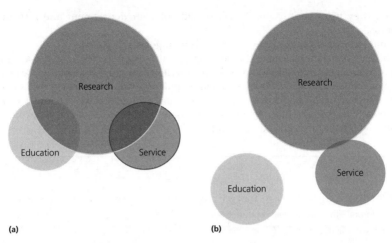

(a)   **(b)**

Figure 37.2 **(a)** Ideal profile of activities for a researcher; **(b)** non-ideal profile of activities for a researcher.

5–7 years developing a research agenda, finding mentors, and acquiring some key research skills. Research is expensive and funding is increasingly difficult to obtain. You will probably have to go through several rounds of grant writing and rejections before obtaining funding for your first project grant. You will have a similar experience when writing manuscripts. Rejections and revisions will seem like your whole life and frequently take a personal toll. During these times it is exceedingly important to maintain strong mentoring relationships, particularly with peer mentors who can help keep this in perspective and normalize the experience. You have got to keep your eye on the prize. The feedback you receive from rejected grants and papers are what will make you better in the future. If you accept the feedback and are talented and diligent, you will ultimately have the freedom to pursue answers to the pressing questions affecting our field.

Be selective in what you agree to take on and do not overpromise. It is important to learn to say "No" to the wrong opportunities. A classic example is being asked to handle the medical student clerkship. This often seems an attractive position to junior faculty, as it may come with some shift reduction and you will have the opportunity to interact with eager medical students keen to impress you. However, this task requires enormous amounts of time (orientations, individual meetings, writing letters) with little research yield and most likely will not fit within your focus. This should be an easy "no." However, it may be uncomfortable or impossible to say "no" to your boss or Chair! That is why it is crucial to communicate *early and often* with your Chair regarding your long-term research vision and shorter term goals, in order to gain their support and avoid them even asking you to do off-topic service activities.

To the greatest extent possible, service activities you engage in should be research-focused. As an example, many departments offer students research electives or operate student research associate programs that require faculty oversight. While the amount of work to organize and supervise many students is significant, doing so may fulfill an important service to your department and at the same time help develop an infrastructure that will directly benefit your personal data collection needs into the future. As with any service activity, be careful that the commitment is manageable in the context of your personal career development needs. You should also discuss the barriers you have encountered and needs that you believe you require to succeed as a researcher. Be careful not to come across as demanding or unreasonable when negotiating with your Chair over hours of clinical service. We suggest framing these discussions in terms of the skills you need to improve and strategies to gain them. For example, you may wish to take a course at the university for which you may need time/money or a preferential shift distribution. Rather than ask directly for these, demonstrate to the Chair the skills you need to develop and how these skills will increase chances of successful grant writing, manuscript preparation, or other department value. Ask for their support in helping you get these skills. Tell the Chair about the course. Perhaps the department can cover tuition costs or a temporary reduction in shifts, or perhaps the Chair can think of alternative resources to gain similar resources. Center the discussion around the skills that you need and how they will bring value to the department, rather than reducing this to an argument over four clinical hours a week.

Look for and create opportunities to get exposure for yourself and gain exposure to others in your field. This is important for your research career and also for future academic promotions. Attending professional meetings is a great way, especially if you plan ahead and arrange to meet with others who may be able to provide you with advice and insight. Do not be afraid to contact colleagues by telephone or e-mail to obtain their opinions. The next time you meet them, they will "know" you. Think outside of your department and institution when you are looking for collaborators.

Again, be patient and remember to take time to reflect on your goals and vision.

In summary, we believe that you will have the best opportunity to assemble the necessary tools for a successful research career by pursuing a research fellowship with an experienced mentor. In addition, selecting a research focus about which you are passionate and having a large patient population with the characteristics you wish to study will facilitate completion of the projects. Review your profile of activities on a regular basis to insure your academic progress is on track. Communicate with your Chair regarding your goals, your plans to accomplish them, and any barriers. Finally, be patient and keep your ultimate goal in mind!

KEY POINTS

- Strongly consider doing a research fellowship to assist you in gaining the necessary skills to be successful in research.
- Seek one or more mentors with different fields and strengths.
- Commit to a research focus and do not worry if you change your focus later.
- Learn how to say "no" to the wrong opportunities.
- Communicate your research agenda to your Chair.
- Keep in mind your overall profile of activities so that you say "yes" to the right opportunities and are prepared for promotion on schedule.
- Be patient!

References

1 Hollander, J.E. and Hsia, R.Y. (2012) Why do I need a mentor and how do I find one? In: V.S. Bebarta and C.B. Cairns (eds) *Emergency Care Research – A Primer*, American College of Emergency Physicians, pp. 11–17.
2 Cho, C.S., Ramanan, R.A., and Feldman, M.D. (2011) Defining the ideal qualities of mentorship: a qualitative analysis of the characteristics of outstanding mentors. *Am J Med*, **124**(5):453–458.
3 Carey, E.C. and Weissman, D.E. (2010) Understanding and finding mentorship: A review for junior faculty. *J Palliat Med*, **13**(11):1373–1379.
4 Detsky, A.S. and Baerlocher, M.O. (2007) Academic mentoring – How to give it and how to get it. *JAMA*, **297**(19):2134–2136.
5 Zerzan, J.T., Hess, R., Schur, E., *et al.* (2009) Making the most of mentors: a guide for mentees. *Acad Med*, **84**(1):140–144.

Glossary

Abstract   A summary of the contents of the scientific research paper. It contains a brief introduction of the study, the objective, the methods used, major findings, and a conclusion.

Academic Associate   Students who are able to participate in clinical research by helping the Principal Investigator collect data in the Emergency Department (ED) and learn from the staff in the ED – physicians, nurses, and so on. The students conduct research without interfering with the clinical operations of the department.

Academic Associate Program   A program that utilizes academic associates to collect data for research projects. It allows the research faculty to have enough coverage in the Emergency Department to continuously collect data without interfering with the clinical operations of the department.

Adverse Event   A harmful or undesirable medical occurrence in a human study participant. These include abnormal signs, symptoms, diseases, embarrassment, or loss of privacy that are temporally associated with the participants' involvement in the research study.

AHRQ (USA)   The Agency for Healthcare Quality and Research is experienced research groups who employ methodologically rigorous standards to predicting both scoping and large reviews.

Alternative Hypothesis (H_1)   The research hypothesis that suggests that a difference exists. It does not specify the size of different, it merely specifies that a difference is believed to exist. It states that there is a non-zero difference between the two groups studied with respect to variable(s) measured and it is inferred that the observed difference is due to effect(s) of the treatment.

Analysis Plan   Aids the researcher in choosing the most appropriate research methods, the tools required to measure data, and ensures that the data being collected are reliable.

Analysis of Variance (ANOVA)   Used for statistical inference to determine whether it is likely that at least two groups differ from each other, when parametric numeric data from three or more groups are compared.

Analytic Study   The observed group of subjects has a comparison or control group.

Animal Models   The study of animals that have characteristics similar to humans in their anatomy, physiology, or response to a pathogen in medical research in order to obtain results that can be used in human medicine.

Anonymity   The collecting of data that do not have any patient identifiers. Additionally, there is no link between response or information and a specific study participant.

Applicability   How well your results or findings apply to others. Ideally, your results would apply everywhere. However, your results may only apply to populations similar to that of your study participants.

Approach   This section of the grant proposal describes what you plan to do and how you plan to do it. It provides a more detailed description of the general points previously raised in the Specific Aims. It includes a more expanded discussion of your hypotheses as well as your long-term goals.

Attrition   Loss of study participants to follow-up, regardless of causation.

Authorship   Given to academics who make substantial contributions to the research project (i.e., concept, design, analysis, interpretation of data, etc.).

Autonomy   Having the freedom or independence to make your decisions. The individual has the capacity to understand and process information and the free will to volunteer without pressure. It ensures that researchers treat participants with courtesy and respect by allowing informed consent.

Baseline Variables   Descriptive patient information that should be collected for patients in both the control and experimental group of the study (i.e., age, educational status, etc.).

Basic Science   Any science that is fundamental to the study of medicine (i.e., anatomy, physiology, biochemistry, virology, etc.).

Bayesian Analysis   The means of assessing uncertainty. Using this analysis, clinicians can modify the pretest probability (the likelihood of being the true etiology) for each diagnosis based upon the presence or absence of individual diagnostic "tests", including history, physical examination, laboratory test results, and imaging.

Doing Research in Emergency and Acute Care: Making Order Out of Chaos, First Edition. Edited by Michael P. Wilson, Kama Z. Guluma, and Stephen R. Hayden.
© 2016 John Wiley & Sons, Ltd. Published 2016 by John Wiley & Sons, Ltd.

Belmont Principles   The three basic principles that provide the foundation for human subject research and the development of the IRB. These principles are autonomy (respect for persons), beneficence, and justice.

Benchmarking   A method used to establish a standard of excellence and comparing the functions or activities of the business with that standard.

Beneficence   Researchers must do no harm to research participants and ensure the research conducted is more beneficial than harmful.

Bias   A systematic error in a study, which can occur during participant selection, data collection, analysis, or reporting. Any factor that increases the likelihood of concluding one of the possible outcomes of the study for a reason other than being due to a treatment's inherent effect.

Biostatistics   Statistics that use data related to living organisms.

Blinded   The study participants, caregivers, and even researchers do not know which treatment is being administered.

Blinded Review   The reviewers do not know whom the author/s of the manuscript is/are.

Blocked Randomization   Ensures equal balance of patients in each group of the study (controlled and experimental), stratifying by time.

Budget   Shows how the money will be spent during the length of your study.

Budget Justification   Explains why the money is being spent in this manner.

Case–Control Study   An observational retrospective study that begins with an outcome then traces back to investigate exposures. It is a study in which two groups of subjects with the outcome of interest (cases) are matched to unaffected controls, and factors that may have contributed to their outcome differences are then assessed. When subjects are enrolled in their respective groups, the investigator already knows the outcome of each subject.

Case Report   A report of a single interesting clinical observation. This observational study cannot demonstrate any evidence of cause and effect, but it can suggest ideas for further research.

Case Series   A descriptive observational design with no control or comparison group. It is used to report the course and outcome of patients that have had a known similar exposure, disease, or treatment.

Causality   The relationship between cause and effect.

Center for Devices and Radiological Health (CDRH)   The U.S. FDA unit that serves the regulatory role for medical devices. The CDRH describes three stages for obtaining marketing clearance in the United States. First is to make sure that the product that you wish to market is actually a medical device as opposed to a drug. Second, you need to determine how the FDA might classify your device – which one of the three classes of perceived risk the device might fall into. The third stage of FDA clearance involves the development of data necessary to submit a marketing application to obtain FDA clearance to market.

Central Tendency   Three measures exist – mean, median, and mode. The mean is the arithmetic average of the data. The median is the mid-most observation, which has half of the data points lying below it and half lying above it. The mode is the most commonly observed data value.

Chi-Square   Used with nominal data to make statistical inference. There are two types – Chi-square test of independence and Chi-square goodness of fit test. The first compares data from two or more groups studied simultaneously, to determine whether they appear to differ statistically from each other. The second test compares a new sample's data against proportions observed from a previously studied comparison group. It determines if the new sample differs statistically from the comparison group.

Clinical Decision Instruments (CDIs)   Also known as clinical decision rules, are constellations of history or physical examination findings, and some laboratory test results, that can be used as valid and reliable probability estimates for disease or outcome. These tools aid healthcare providers to predict clinical outcomes with known sensitivity and specificity.

Clinical Queries   A PubMed feature that limits search results to "Clinical Study Categories". It allows the researcher to narrow the search results to make it more manageable to find articles/systematic reviews related to their research topic.

Clinical Research Organization (CRO)   A third party that acts on behalf of the research sponsor to verify subject welfare, adherence to study protocol, compliance with research regulations, and confirm database entries with source documents. It trains clinical investigators to assure that measurements are done uniformly across centers.

Clinical Trial Monitors   Outside groups employed by research sponsors to monitor study progression, events, and reporting.

Cochrane Database of Systematic Reviews   a leading resource for systematic reviews in health care.

Coercion   The practice of persuading a subject to participate by using force, threats, or even in the form of compensation. However, most review boards will allow a small amount of money for the participants' time and efforts.

Cohort Studies   The study subjects are grouped based upon whether or not they possess a purported risk factor for some specific disease. They are then followed across time to determine who develops disease, and who does not. Subjects in cohort studies cannot be randomly assigned to study groups. Most cohort studies are prospective studies; however, they are occasionally retrospective studies.

Collaboration   Allows individuals from a variety of backgrounds to apply their complementary skills to increase the effectiveness of the group. It can be as simple as members of the same department working together to something as complex as multiple universities working in conjunction with federal and industry interests.

Collaborators   Other scientists who you conduct research with. These individuals may provide you with valuable resources (i.e., knowledge or equipment) to that can help your joint projects. Working with collaborators allows you to participate in other studies as well as have them help you with your projects.

Community Consent   The agreement from local community leadership for the research project.

Compensation   Usually comes in the form of monetary support or the opportunity to coauthor scholarly works resulting from the study. It may also be in the form of resource materials derived from an industry study (i.e., laboratory equipment, reagents, etc.).

Compliance   In order for your research study to be carried out, the procedures imposed on your subinvestigators should not significantly impact work-flow, must not be technically unfamiliar to them, must not be unacceptable to a majority of them, and time windows for procedures and assessments should be ergonomic.

Conclusion   This section specifically and exclusively addresses the study objectives.

Confidence Interval   Shows the presence or absence of a statistically significant difference due to the treatment(s) in question; as well as gives information on the magnitude and precision of that effect.

Confidentiality   The information collected from patients has patient-identifying information or contains a link between response or information and a specific study participant.

Confounding   Study bias caused by confounding variables, which are associated with the independent and dependent variables of interest. A type of bias in which another variable, often unmeasured, causes changes in the dependent variable, but the independent variable of interest gets the credit or blame due to its association with the causative variable.

Contract   Designed to obtain financial support for specifically defined tasks or deliverables such as developing a specified output or program.

Cooperative Agreements   Used to obtain financial support for work that will be developed and specified in collaboration with the funding agency.

Cross-Sectional Study   A study used to describe the characteristics of a population at a specific point(s) in time or over a specific period of time. Such studies are used to assess the prevalence of acute or chronic disease, to measure the results of medical intervention, or to give census-like data. This type of study relies on data originally collected for other purposes and is typically used to develop hypotheses.

Database of Abstracts of Reviews of Effect (DARE)   A database that provides abstracts of systematic reviews that have been assessed for their quality. It evaluates the effects of the process and delivery of healthcare interventions in health care organizations.

Data Safety Monitoring Board (DSMB)   Is usually a panel of respected researchers not involved in the current trial but can provide their expertise and recommendations to study investigators. They periodically review and evaluate the collected data to ensure participant safety, conduct and progress, and the efficacy of the study. Additionally, the board makes recommendations on whether to continue, modify, or terminate the study.

Data Safety Monitoring Plan (DSMP)   Research plan that is submitted and provides adequate provisions for collecting data to ensure that participants are safe.

Descriptive Study   The observed study group has no comparison or control group.

Discussion Section   Revisits the introduction and explains how your study adds to the body of knowledge. It presents your interpretation of the main outcome measure or key results first.

Effectiveness   An all-encompassing term that measures a drugs ability to produce its indicated effect under usual or real world circumstances. It measures an overall treatment strategy more than a pure effect of treatment.

Efficacy   The measure used to determine a drug's ability to produce its indicated effect under ideal and controlled circumstances.

Equipoise   An equal distribution of study participants to different treatment arms of a clinical trial. Each participant enrolled has an equal chance to receive a treatment or a placebo and is enrolled before receiving the intervention.

Ethics   Pertains to or deals with morals and values.

Exclusion Criteria   Attributes that are present in a patient that disqualifies them from participating in a study.

Experimental Study   The researcher designs the intervention and measures a response to that intervention.

Expertise   Individuals who assist in carrying out the research study (i.e., volunteers, colleagues, subinvestigators).

External Validation   The quantification of the CDI in multiple settings and patient populations that differ from the one in which it was derived to ensure that the instrument works in disparate settings.

External Validity   The generalizability of your study results to other people and situations.

Falsifiability   The belief that for any hypothesis to have credibility, it must be inherently disprovable before it can become accepted as a scientific hypothesis or theory.

Feasibility Study   The assessment of the practicality of a proposed research study.

Fellowship   One of the most efficient ways to gain analytical, critical reasoning, writing, public speaking, networking, and organizational skills. It will give you the opportunity to benefit from formal mentoring, specialized knowledge, and the ability to apply for funding for the future.

Focus   The direction in which to move your career forward.

Food and Drug Administration (FDA)   The agency of the Department of Health and Human Services that requires manufacturers of drugs and medical devices to report any adverse events that they learn of themselves or which are reported to them. The FDA is responsible for investigating reports either before or after taking an action based on the report. They collect Adverse Event Reports from the Federal Adverse Event Reporting System and Vaccine Adverse Event Reporting System.

F-Ratio   Expressed as a point on a continuously distributed F-Ratio Curve. The curve has a specific shape and equations, dependent on the number of degrees of freedom of the numerator and the denominator used to calculate "F". It is translated to a statistical probability value by using the properties of the normal distribution.

Funding   Money provided by an organization or the government for a specific purpose.

Gantt Chart   A project schedule illustrating the start and finish dates of activities and the project itself.

Grant   An amount of money given by a funding agency that provides financial support for a proposed project.

Guidelines   General rules or pieces of advice for physicians and other health professionals, and/or healthcare providers, to follow in order to provide safe and quality care while conducting research.

The Hawthorne Effect   When an individual or group of individuals change(s) behavior due to being observed.

Hazard Ratio   Measures, over time, how often a specific event occurs in one group compared to how often it occurs in another group.

Health Insurance Portability Accountability Act (HIPAA)   Provides a set of national standards to protect and secure individuals' identifiable health information. It sets forth detailed regulations regarding the types of uses and disclosures of an individuals' personally-identifiable information.

Heterogeneity   The slight differences among studies in one or all of the domains associated with PICO-D.

Iatrogenic Events   Events caused by the physician.

Impact Analysis   Used to verify and quantify patient-centric or societal effectiveness and safety in real-world clinical practice.

Imputation   Inserting a value to replace missing data.

Inclusion Criteria   Attributes that are present in a patient that qualifies them to participate in a study.

Incorporation Bias   The test under observation is included in the criterion standard test.

Informatics   The study and management of electronic health records. For example, how and what information should be stored? How can patient privacy and maintenance of records be protected, yet easily available to healthcare providers?

"Information for Authors"   A page or website provided by journals that provide information and guidelines on how to submit a manuscript and what requirements need to be met.

Information Bias   The acquirement of biased information gathered from study participants. For example, recall bias relates to case–control studies: patients with disease are more likely to remember exposures they think relate to their disease than those without disease.

Informed Consent   The researcher(s) must provide relative information, answer any questions that improves the subject's understanding of the study, and obtain the voluntary agreement of the subject to participate in the study. The study participant is informed about all aspects of the research project so they can make an informed and educated decision regarding their participation.

Initial Review   An editor determines whether further peer review is warranted or not. At this stage, the editor may reject manuscripts if the subject matter is unlikely to interest the readers or if there are major flaws in the methodology, and so on.

Innovation   This section of the grant proposal tells how this project will challenge current practice or theories.

Institutional Animal Care and Use Committee (IACUC)   A committee that reviews and approves or disapproves grant protocols that use animal models.

Institutional Review Board (IRB)   Committees established to review and approve research studies that involve human subjects. The IRB ensures that all human subject research is conducted in accordance with federal, institutional, and ethical guidelines. The board reviews all research that involves human subjects while acting as an advocate for subjects' rights and welfare. It has the authority to modify research, conduct continuing reviews, observe/verify changes, suspend or terminate approval, and observe the consent process and research procedures.

Intellectual Property   Ideas or inventions that *you* created – designs, symbols, and so on.

Intention-to-Treat Analysis   All patients must be analyzed once they are randomized. It is a method used to analyze all patients, regardless of whether or not they completed or received the treatment being studied.

Internal Validation   The ability of the CDI to accurately distinguish patients with and without disease (or outcomes in prognostic situations).

International Research   Your coresearchers are from and in another country, gathering data in one or more countries, or your work is intended for readers outside of your own country. This research must take into account differences in culture, ethics, applicability, language, and presentation.

Introduction Section   Describes the historical background and significance of the topic, gives a brief review of previous and relevant literature to the current study, identifies gaps in current knowledge and states the rationale for the current study, and how the current study fills in these knowledge gaps. It states what is known about a subject, explains why further investigation is necessary, and concisely tells the reader what the authors have set out to do.

Justice   Ensures that the study procedures are administrated fairly to research participants.

Knowledge Translation   A process that attempts to bridge that gap between what is known and what is currently done in healthcare practice. Researchers assess and review bodies of scientific evidence in order to utilize research findings to improve healthcare practices and outcomes for the patients.

Limitations   The findings of the research study that cannot be generalized to the larger population. They are the major flaws of the study (i.e., small sample size, subjects lost to follow up, bias, lack of blinding, etc.).

Literature Search   The use of electronic textbooks, guidelines, systematic reviews, and article reviews of published literature to find quality references relevant to your research question. It allows the researcher(s) to become familiar with their research topic, its key concepts, terminology, and knowledge gaps in order to develop the focus of the project.

MAR   Missing at random – There is a relationship between the missing variable and some observed characteristic of the treatment population/other study related variables.

Material Safety Transfer Agreements   A legal contract that establishes the conditions and terms of transferring "tangible" research material between a provider, such as a principal investigator, and a recipient, such as a pharmaceutical company. It is used to protect the rights of both parties while documenting the transfer.

MCAR   Missing completely at random – There is no observed or unobserved relationship between the missing variable and any characteristic of treatment population or any other study related variables. The missing data are unsystematic.

Medical Devices   A large range of innovations from implantable devices to *in vitro* diagnostics. Anything that is not a pharmaceutical or a biologic is a "device" for regulatory purposes.

Mentor   A well-established investor who takes a personal interest in you and your career. A mentor provides guidance and advice to help you advance in your career.

Meta-Analysis   Data from multiple studies are combined, assessed for bias, homogeneity, and validity, and re-analyzed as a single, larger data set in the hopes of arriving at a consensus answer or more accurate estimate of effect.

Methods Section   This section of a paper explains what was done in the study and why. It describes what participants were selected for the study (inclusion and exclusion criteria), where the study took place, what type of study design was used (randomized control trial, observation, etc.). This section also provides information on how data were collected, recorded, and analyzed.

Minimal Risk   There is little to no harm or discomfort to the participating subject than that ordinarily encountered during daily life or during normal physical activity.

Misclassification Bias   Refers to the placement of participants in the wrong category, either of the dependent variable or independent variable.

MNAR   Missing not at random – There is a relationship between the missing variable and some unobserved variable or hypothetical outcome.

Multiple Linear Regression   An extension of a simple linear regression. This modeling tool permits an expression of how multiple independent variables influence a dependent variable.

National Institutes of Health (NIH)   Requires Data Safety Monitoring Plans for research it funds that involve human subjects

National Guideline Clearinghouse (NGC)   A resource available to the public that provides evidence-based clinical practice guidelines.

Negative Likelihood Ratio   The probability of a negative test result in patients with disease divided by the probability of a negative test result in patients without disease.

Negative Predictive Value   Relates to how likely a test will be negative when the disease is not present. "Of all the people who test negative, what proportion will not have the disease?"

NICE (UK)   The National Institute of Health and Care Excellence produces rigorous systematic reviews and health technology assessments.

Nominal Data   Rates, proportions, or frequencies of observations classed into named categories.

Non-Analytical Retrospective Study   Also known as a descriptive study. This type of study does not try to determine any quantitative relationship but tries to give us an idea of what is happening in a population.

Non-Parametric Test   Used when the data are not normally distributed.

Non-Significant Risk Devices   Devices that do not pose a significant risk to human subjects; for example, daily-wear contact lenses or contact lens solutions.

Normal Distribution   The mean, median, and mode are all very close to one another.

Null Hypothesis (H_0)   The hypothesis suggests that there is no difference between groups. It states that there is no difference between the two groups studied with the respect to the variable(s) measured.

Nuremberg Code   A set of ethical principles for research using human subjects created as a result of the Nuremberg Trials at the end of World War II.

Objectives   The results the research is looking for by the end of the study. The objectives summarize what should be achieved by the research project.

Observational Study   The researcher observes a study group and draws inferences about the effect of an exposure or intervention on subjects.

Odds Ratio   The ratio of odds of an event occurring in two different groups. For example, you might say that it is the odds of an event (or outcome) occurring in the intervention group compared to the odds of that event occurring in the control group.

One-Tailed Comparison   Looks for differences only in a specific direction when comparing groups with respect to characteristic

Operations Research   A method used for problem solving and decision making to provide meaningful and useful information for medical directors and the organization.

Ordinal Data   Numeric data collected using a rank-ordered scale (low to high or high to low).

Parametric Data   Interval or ratio data which can be expected to fit the Gaussian, or "normal" distribution. Ratio data have a minimum value of zero, while interval data can have a negative value.

Parametric Test   Deals with data that can be expected to be normally distributed and utilize the sample mean and sample variance for their calculation.

Peer Mentoring   Multiple individuals, often of a similar academic rank, collectively provide advice and mentorship to each other.

Peer Review   Reviewers read the entire manuscript in detail and note whether the authors have clearly defined their goals, explained their methods, thoroughly reported their findings, and justified their conclusions. Reviewers then decide if the manuscript should be accepted, revised, or rejected.

Personal Health Identifier (PHI)   Any information that identifies a patient; for example, demographics such as name, age, medical record number, gender, birth date, and so on.

Phase 1 Study   Generally a small study with few participants and a smaller budget with a shorter timeline that usually involve studying the pharmacokinetics and initial safety of the product.

Phase 2 Study   A study designed more for dose-finding. This type of study involves a group of participants who are affected by the illness or disorder targeted by the study and is given a range of doses to determine an efficacious dose range.

Phase 3 Study   These studies are typically prospective, multicentered, double-blinded studies which involve large numbers of patients. Power Analyses are important in setting up the needed number of subjects in each group to adequately compare efficacy and safety of the drug or device.

PICO-D   Focused details that all research questions should include – Population, Intervention (and Comparison treatment), Outcomes associated with the question and the Design to the question.

Pilot Test   A small-scale trial that is used to identify problems in your survey or intervention. A pilot survey may point out questions that are difficult to understand or even typing errors.

Placebo Effect   A phenomenon in which a fake treatment improves a patient's condition simply because the patient expects the treatment will help improve their health status.

Positive Likelihood Ratio   The probability of a positive test result in patients with disease divided by the probability of a positive test result in patients without disease.

Positive Predictive Value (PPV)   Relates to how likely a test will be positive when disease is truly present. "Of all the people who test positive, what proportion will actually have the disease?"

Postmarketing Surveillance   The ongoing monitoring of drug safety that occurs once a drug becomes commercially available.

Power   The probability that the study will reject the null hypothesis when the alternative hypothesis is true.

Preliminary Data   These give evidence in favor of your hypothesis, allow you to do some initial calculations on power, and show achievability.

Profile of Activities   Consists of three pillars – education, research, and service. You should be able to demonstrate excellence in at least one of these areas and be good in the other two. Depending on where you would like your career to go, you should take on activities that strengthen that particular skill.

Prospective Study   A study that follows a group of individuals who differ with respect to certain factors under study over time, to determine how these factors affect rates of a certain outcome.

Propositus   The reason for doing your study.

Publication Bias   Arises when a project with positive results is published compared to a similar project with negative results.

PubMed   A search engine available to the public that allows access to biomedical literature.

P-Value   An expression of how probable the numerical difference(s) observed within the study was/were obtained due to chance alone. A p-value of less than 0.05 is considered "statistically significant", leading the research to reject the null hypothesis.

Qualitative Study   A study designed to provide an in-depth understanding of an issue by investigating *why* and *how*. These studies typically consist of relatively small focused sample groups and less-defined questions with the resulting data categorized into patterns.

Quality Work   Doing a study with an interesting question, a strong design, and enough data so the results are believable with a relatively narrow confidence interval, a good analysis demonstrating where the results are applicable, and an interesting discussion.

Quantitative Study   Studies that are descriptive and causal. These studies are more common in clinical research and investigate the *what*, *where*, and *when* of the issue. They require large random samples with data that are numbers and anything measurable.

Random Allocation   All participants have a defined probability of assignment to a particular intervention. It is the best method of reducing bias during a research study.

Randomization   A way of minimizing confounding factors.

Randomized Control Trial (RCT)   The gold standard of clinical research. It is a method of research where the subjects being studied are randomly assigned to a controlled or experimental group.

Recruitability   Refers to three core concepts. 1. The incidence of your study condition-of-interest has to be high enough that you can complete the study in a reasonable time-frame. 2. Patients with the target-condition must be consentable. 3. A majority of patients with the target-condition have to want to consent to your study

Recursive Partitioning   Progressively subdivides the population into groups of patients with a particular outcome and can preferentially optimize sensitivity at the expense of specificity. It is a non-parametric modeling technique that is capable of assessing a large number of predictor variables with complex interactions.

Relative Risk   Estimates exposure to something that could affect the health of an individual/group. To calculate relative risk, you divide the proportion of patients in which the event occurred in the intervention group by the proportion of patients in which the event occurred in the control group. The result can be used to interpret both the directionality and magnitude of the relationship. For example, whether the risk of the event occurring in the intervention group is more or less likely to occur than in the control group, and to what extent.

Remote Consent   The agreement from the study participant through a phone call with a witness present.

Research Assistant   A researcher who assists in academic research.

Research Electronic Data Capture (REDCap)   A data collection system which is composed of close to one thousand institutional partners in 75 countries that has increased the productivity and streamlining of research studies. It is a secure web application that is designed to build and manage online surveys and databases that can be used for personal interviews, data collection from paper forms, and online surveys.

Research Plan   The core of your project, in which you clearly and explicitly define your hypotheses and how you will conduct your research.

Research Question   A question that is interesting to both you and the readers, can be answered ethically and within the time you have available, and can be translated into a hypothesis.

Results Section   Factual analysis of your data, framed entirely by the study objectives and based only on the statistical methodology you have specified.

Retrospective Study   Investigators look back at events that have occurred (i.e., looking back at a patient's medical history or their past lifestyle). This type of study is typically used to study rare diseases. This study requires less infrastructure and time to complete than prospective studies. It is relatively inexpensive, has readily accessible existing data, can generate hypotheses for prospective studies, and may only be the only ethical method for evaluating harmful treatments or bad outcomes.

Review Articles   The analysis and evaluation of research previously published by others.

"Revise and Accept"   The journal has decided to publish your manuscript as-is or after minor alterations are made.

"Revise and Reconsider"   You have been asked to make significant changes to your manuscript without the guarantee of publication.

Safety   Protection from danger, risk, or injury. Your study should "look" safe in order to be approved by the IRB, the study population, and the public. If the study is perceived as unsafe, the IRB may not approve the study and it will be difficult to convince patients to consent to the study.

Safety Study   A small, feasibility study in which a new intervention is tried out for the first time in a limited patient population and is carefully monitored to ensure it will not harm patients.

Sample Size   The size of a study group is chosen to maximize the chance of discovering a specific mean difference in the data collected.

Seed Funding   A small amount of money provided to begin a research project. The amount of money provided is relatively small because the project is still in a conceptual stage.

Selection Bias   Occurs during the process of selecting participants for the study intervention. It refers to an unrepresentative sample of a population due to improper randomization. The bias occurs due to a flaw during participant selection. For example, participants may be selected based on the proximity of the researcher, otherwise known as convenience sampling. Another example is non-response bias, where participants may not respond to surveys that have been sent out.

Sensitivity   The ability of a diagnostic test to reliably predict the presence of disease. "Of all the people who have disease, what proportion will test positive?"

Serious Adverse Event (SAE)   A harmful or undesirable medical occurrence in a human study participant. These include abnormal signs, symptoms, diseases, embarrassment, or loss of privacy that are temporally associated with the participants' involvement in the research study. An SAE is any adverse event that **causes hospitalization, is life threatening, disabling, or is teratogenic.**

Significance   A section of the grant proposal that explains why your research topic and project are important.

Significant Risk Devices   These devices present the potential for serious risk to health or safety of a subject. These include implants, devices that support or sustain human life, and devices that are substantially important in diagnosing, curing, mitigating, or treating disease.

Simple Linear Regression   A modeling tool that allows for the determination of the "line of best fit" between an independent variable and dependent variable, when the variation of the independent variable seems likely to cause variation of the value of the dependent variable. The slope of the regression line is an expression of covariance; how much the value of "Y" can be expected to vary for a given size of variation of the value "X" The coefficient "r^2" is used to convey the strength of the association between "X" and "Y".

Simple Randomization   Can be done by using a coin flip or random number table or generator. It is the easiest method to randomize patients at an equal ratio into each intervention group.

Specific Aims   This section of the grant proposal focuses the reader to your research topic and your hypothesis. This includes general long-term goals of the research, specific objectives of the proposal and the hypothesis to be tested, expected outcomes, and importance of the research project and its potential impact.

Specificity   The ability of a test to reliably predict the absence of disease. "Of all people who do not have disease, what proportion will test negative?"

Spectrum Bias   Relates to disease severity. Diseases are easier to diagnose when they are in their severe stages, and studies that include only severe cases will have an inflated estimate for sensitivity.

Standard Deviation   Explains the variability of parametric data and is used to quantify the variation in the data collected.

Standardized Difference   The difference between the means (the clinically important difference) divided by the population standard deviation.

Stratified Randomization   Allows organizing of participants by characteristics (age, sex), and then assigning treatment randomly to each strata.

Structured Critical Appraisal   A methodological process that is used to identify the strengths and weaknesses of research articles to assess their usefulness and validity. Critical appraisals evaluate the appropriateness of the study design for the research question.

Student T-Test   A method of statistical analysis that is used to compare two groups. It is a technique used to determine the probability that the two groups are the same or statistically different from one another.

Survey Methods   The sampling of subjects from a population and the relative survey data collection techniques (i.e., personal interviews, telephone interviews, mail surveys, etc.).

Sustainability   In order for the research study to be carried out, it must be financially feasible, have the appropriate support (expertise/industry partners), be adaptable to changes in the legislative or market landscape, and can be completed within a reasonable amount of time.

Systematic Review   An assessment and evaluation of existing evidence around a particular health topic. It is an organized method of locating, gathering, and evaluating literature on a health topic of interest. Systematic reviews provide measures of heterogeneity which informs our understanding of effects across studies.

Team Mentoring   Multiple individuals either in a group or separately providing mentoring in their areas of expertise.

Testable Hypothesis   A question that can be translated into an outcome and can be answered in a concrete way. For example, "Which drug is better?" could be translated to "Drug A is best for treating a particular (well-defined) condition as measured by mortality. "

Title   Headlines and answers the question posed by the research. It describes the design (if applicable) and grabs the attention of the reader.

Trip Database   A search engine available to the public that provides high-quality clinical research evidence.

Tuskegee Study   A study that involved 600 black men (399 with syphilis, 201 who did not) to record the natural history of syphilis. Researchers conducted the study without the patients' informed consent. They told the men that they were being treated for "bad blood", a term to describe multiple ailments including syphilis, anemia, and fatigue. However, the men did not receive any proper treatment needed to cure their illness. Men who participated in the study received free medical examinations, free meals, and burial insurance. The study was only supposed to be conducted for six months, but continued for 40 years.

Two-Tailed Comparison   Looks for whether two groups differ, but does not specify which direction.

Type I Error   Also known as a false positive, occurs when you incorrectly reject the null hypothesis (i.e., the null hypothesis is true, yet the inferential statistical tests applied to the study data led you to wrongly conclude that a statistically significant difference exists between study groups).

Type II Error   Also known as a false negative, occurs when you incorrectly accept the null hypothesis (i.e., the alternative hypothesis is true, yet your inferential statistical test found no statistically different difference between study groups).

Validity   the extent to which a concept or conclusion is logically sound.

Variance   The sum of squared deviations from the sample mean, divided by one less than the total number of observations. It measures how far a set of data points is spread out from the mean value.

Vulnerable Subjects   Pregnant women, prisoners, children, students and employees, minorities, economically and/or educationally disadvantaged or cognitively impaired persons, AIDS/HIV+ subjects, and terminally ill subjects.

Workup Bias   When patients with certain characteristics are referred for definitive testing.

Index

Doing Research in Emergency and Acute Care: Making Order Out of Chaos, First Edition. Edited by Michael P. Wilson, Kama Z. Guluma, and Stephen R. Hayden.
© 2016 John Wiley & Sons, Ltd. Published 2016 by John Wiley & Sons, Ltd.